Date Due

DEC 06 1999			
MAR 16 2001			
MAR 11 2002			
MAY 03 2002			
MAR 23 2005			
MAR 20 2006			
APR 07 2016			

Breast Ultrasound

Breast Ultrasound

A Systematic Approach to Technique and Image Interpretation

Christof Sohn, M.D.
University Gynecological Clinic
Frankfurt/M, Germany

Jens-U. Blohmer, M.D.
Department of Gynecological Oncology
University Gynecological Clinic
Charité Hospital
Berlin, Germany

Ulrike M. Hamper, M.D.
Department of Radiology
The Johns Hopkins Hospital
Baltimore, MD., USA

347 Illustrations
13 tables

Thieme
Stuttgart · New York 1999

Library of Congress Cataloging-in-Publication Data

Sohn, Christof.
[Mammasonographie, English]
Breast ultrasound: a systematic approach to technique and image interpretation / Christof Sohn, Jens-U. Blohmer, and Ulrike M. Hamper.
p. cm.
ISBN 3-13-111531-9, – ISBN 0-86577-722-5
1. Breast – Ultrasonic imaging. 2. Breast – Tumors – Ultrasonic imaging. 3. Breast – Diseases – Diagnosis. I. Blohmer, Jens-U. II. Hamper, Ulrike. III. Title.
[DNLM: 1. Breast Neoplasms – diagnosis. 2. Ultrasonography, Mammary – methods. 3. Diagnosis, Differential. WP 870S682m 1998a]
RG493.5.U47S6513 1998
616.99′24907543 – dc21
DNLM/DLC for Library of Congress 98-38151

This book is an authorized translation of the German edition published and copyrighted 1996 by Georg Thieme Verlag, Stuttgart, Germany. Title of the German edition: Mammasonographie. Ein systematisches Lehrbuch zur Technik und Befundinterpretation.
Some of the product names, patents and registered designs referred to in this book are in fact registered trademarks or proprietary names, even though specific reference to this fact is not always made in the text. Therefore, the appearance of a name without designation as proprietary is not to be construed as a representation by the publisher that it is in the public domain.

Rüdigerstraße 14, D-70469 Stuttgart
Thieme New York, 333 Seventh Avenue
New York, NY 10001 USA

Typesetting by Mitterweger, D-68723 Plankstadt
Printed in Germany
by Druckhaus Götz, Ludwigsburg

ISBN 3-13-111531-9 (GTV, Stuttgart)
ISBN 0-86577-722-5 (TNY, New York)

Contributors:

Cynthia I. Caskey, M.D.
Department of Radiology
University of Texas–Houston
LBJ General Hospital
Houston, TX., USA

Hans Junkermann, M.D.
University Gynecological Clinic
Heidelberg, Germany

Ulrich Siekmann, M.D.
Witten, Germany

Monika Schiesser, M.D.
University Gynecological Clinic
Heidelberg, Germany

Translated by Terry C. Telger

Important Note: Medicine is an ever-changing science. Research and clinical experience are continually expanding our knowledge, in particular our knowledge of proper treatment and drug therapy. Insofar as this book mentions any dosage or application, readers may rest assured that the authors, editors, and publishers have made every effort to ensure that such references are in accordance with **the state of knowledge at the time of production of the book.**

Nevertheless, this does not involve, imply, or express any guarantee or responsibility on the part of the publishers with respect to any dosage instructions and forms of application stated in the book. **Every user is requested to examine carefully** the manufacturer's leaflets accompanying each drug and to check, if necessary in consultation with a physician or specialist, whether the dosage schedules mentioned therein or the contraindications stated by the manufacturer differ from the statements made in the present book. Such examination is particularly important with drugs that are either rarely used or have been newly released on the market. Every dosage schedule or every form of application used is entirely at the user's risk and responsibility. The authors and publishers request every user to report to the publishers any discrepancies or inaccuracies noticed.

Any reference to or mention of manufacturers or specific brand names should not be interpreted as an endorsement or advertisement for any company or product.

Preface

Ultrasonography has gained an established place in the evaluation of breast masses. It complements radiographic mammography as a separate and equal modality effectively complementing modern breast radiology. Consequently, we felt there was a need for a textbook describing all the relevant aspects of breast ultrasound in a practice-oriented format.

The arrangement of chapters in the present book is intended as a systematic guide to performing breast ultrasound examinations. Particular attention is given to differentiation between benign and malignant lesions. This is appropriate, in view of the rising incidence of breast cancer and the growing clinical importance of ultrasound, which has particular advantages over mammography in the differential diagnosis of breast masses in young women. In addition, meticulous sonographic imaging can identify with confidence a subgroup of women who have lesions in which the likelihood of malignancy is low enough for biopsy to be avoided. This, in turn, may result in improved patient care, reducing patient discomfort, morbidity, and mortality and ultimately decreasing the overall cost of health care.

New techniques in breast ultrasound, such as three-dimensional sonography, blood flow imaging, and ultrasound contrast agents, are also described here. However, it should be noted that blood flow imaging is still primarily a research application. At present, it does not offer very much assistance in differentiating between benign and malignant lesions in ordinary clinical settings.

Frankfurt/Berlin/Baltimore
Fall 1998

Christof Sohn
Jens-U. Blohmer
Ulrike M. Hamper

Contents

1 Introduction

Ultrasonography has become an indispensable imaging modality in the evaluation of breast disorders. To avoid misunderstandings, it should be stressed initially that breast ultrasound is not in competition with other diagnostic modalities, notably radiographic mammography. Breast ultrasound complements mammography, rather than replacing it, and both modalities should form a diagnostic unit in the evaluation of breast diseases.

It should also be noted that neither ultrasound nor mammography can provide histological evaluation of the breast parenchyma or a focal abnormality. The sonographic appearance of a focal lesion correlates with the histological findings in many, but not all, cases.

The physical examination, mammography, and cytology are the three traditional mainstays of breast diagnosis. Through these methods, it has been possible to reduce breast cancer mortality by approximately one-third in postmenopausal women (Kaiser et al. 1993, Shapiro et al. 1971). During the past 20 years, however, epidemiological studies in Western industrialized nations have shown a rising incidence of breast cancer that is most significant in premenopausal women (Andersson et al. 1988, Brenner et al. 1990). There are valid concerns about the use of mammography in these women, many of whom are of childbearing age. Another problem is the limited usefulness of mammography in the radiographically dense breasts of young women (Bassett et al. 1991).

With the development of high-resolution ultrasound scanners in the 1980s, breast ultrasound gained a role in the early diagnosis of breast cancer. An experienced examiner using this dynamic sectional imaging technique can detect small focal abnormalities within the dense breast parenchyma of young women. Since there is no ionizing radiation, even pregnant patients can be examined without risk.

As a result, ultrasound has become an integral part of the diagnostic management of focal breast lesions during the past 10 years.

Differentiating between normal tissue variants and pathological changes can be a difficult task. Not all neoplastic lesions can be demonstrated by ultrasound, or even by mammography. Moreover, breast ultrasound is a relatively subjective procedure that depends critically on the experience and thoroughness of the examiner and the quality of the equipment.

The female breast is a complex organ consisting of parenchymal tissue (glands and ducts), subcutaneous and retromammary fat, and a suspensory framework of connective tissue. The relative proportion of these tissues is both age-dependent and highly variable from one individual to another. This accounts for the extreme diversity of the sonographic findings in the breasts of different women. The breast is also a dynamic organ that shows changes during the course of the menstrual cycle. Sonographic breast patterns can even vary from side to side in the same individual.

The onset of puberty is marked by growth of the lactiferous ducts, increased hydration of the breast stroma, and proliferation of the connective tissue that forms along the breast parenchyma. Mature breast tissue contains 15 to 20 main lactiferous ducts that extend back from the nipple to the individual lobular units. The breast parenchyma exhibits marked cyclic variations during the menstrual cycle. Increased hydration in the postovulatory phase can lead to edema, with dilation of the ducts and proliferation of the terminal lobules. There may be associated fluid discharge from the nipple. When menstruation occurs, the glandular tissue returns to a "resting" state.

Pregnancy is associated with marked enlargement of the lobules as glandular tissue replaces much of the intralobular and interlobular connective tissues.

Some involutional changes begin as early as the fourth decade of life. These early changes bear no relationship to the further involution that occurs at menopause. Both mammography and sonography show a decrease of tissue density in the involuted breast.

Menopausal involution is characterized by a regression of the glands and lactiferous ducts and their replacement by fat and connective tissue. The breast parenchyma loses its typical lobar architecture.

Thus, the presence or absence of proliferative stimuli at various phases of the menstrual cycle and in various stages of life influence the radiological appearance of the breast. Usually, these changes are as clinically silent as breast masses, but an anxious or knowledgeable woman may notice breast changes and seek diagnostic evaluation.

The present chapter concludes with a brief historical review of breast ultrasound. Subsequent chapters explore the current indications for breast ultrasound and its role as a diagnostic tool. Guidelines are offered on selecting equipment and on the technique for performing a breast ultrasound examination. Since normal ultrasound findings depend on the age of the patient, attention is given to the changes in sonographic breast anatomy that occur normally with aging. A knowledge of these physiological changes is essential so that abnormalities can be recognized. The benign or malignant nature of breast lesions is assessed on the basis of standard sonographic views. The typical ultrasound features of specific breast lesions are illustrated, and criteria are presented for differentiating benign from malignant masses. The book also reviews sonography of the axilla and explores the role of ultrasound in the follow-up of breast cancer and in the augmented breast. A special chapter deals with Doppler sonography in the differential diagnosis of focal sonographic lesions, presenting guidelines for practical application and the interpretation of findings. Fine-needle aspiration and automated core biopsy of breast masses under sonographic guidance offer key advantages over mammographically guided needle procedures. The book concludes with a look at new trends in breast ultrasound, such as three-dimensional imaging and the effect of drugs on the results of Doppler investigations, as well as a short chapter on the current status of contrast agents and their application to breast ultrasound.

This book is intended to provide the examiner with a systematic framework for the practical performance of breast ultrasound examinations. Explanations in the text are therefore supported by numerous illustrations covering the sonographic features of the normal breast and of typical benign and malignant breast disorders.

Historical Development of Breast Ultrasound

It took 50 years for diagnostic ultrasound to evolve from "hyperphonography" and A-mode displays to modern, high-resolution real-time imaging and color Doppler sonography using high-frequency electronic transducers and digital image storage and processing. A few of the historical milestones involved are reviewed here.

Pohlmann and his colleagues first reported in 1939 on the frequency-dependent absorption of ultrasound in human tissue. In 1942, Dussik published an article "On the Possibility of Using High-Frequency Mechanical Vibrations as a Diagnostic Aid," and termed the technique "hyperphonography."

During the 1950s, Wild and Reid in the United States were the first researchers to use A-mode technology for ultrasound examinations of the female breast.

In the 1960s, comparative studies on ultrasound breast imaging were carried out using water immersion, breast compression, and contact transducers. These ultrasound scanners operated at frequencies of 2.0–2.5 MHz.

As early as 1969, Kratchowil and Kaiser, using compound B-mode scanners and contact transducers operating at 1.5–6.0 MHz, analyzed acoustic shadows as a means of differentiating between benign and malignant breast masses. Important technical innovations came from Japan, where focusing transducers in the 5–10 MHz range were used. The gray-scale technique, introduced into breast ultrasound in the late 1960s, offered a large dynamic range that improved discrimination between intramammary structures (Kelly-Frey 1985).

In the 1970s, the experience of Jellins and colleagues with the Octoson unit (3-MHz water-immersion scanner) led them to recommend sonography as the imaging procedure of choice for every woman under 30 years of age (Jellins et al. 1975).

Color imaging systems were tested during the 1970s, and real-time B-mode scanners were in use for breast imaging by the end of the decade.

Starting in the early 1980s, technical advances focused on the development of high-frequency transducers (5 to 13 MHz) that could provide enhanced resolution with an adequate imaging depth over a focal range from 0.5 to 5 cm.

In Germany, the groups of B. J. Hackelöer (1986), W. Leucht (1992), and J. Teubner (1983, 1985a, b) were among the pioneers of breast ultrasound. Hackelöer et al. (1986) and Leucht (1992) tested the accuracy of various sonographic criteria in the differential diagnosis of breast masses. Teubner et al. (1983, 1985a, b) carried out tests to determine the way in which various technical factors (sound frequency, ultrasound unit, offsets) affected the resolution and appearance of normal anatomical structures in the female breast. In the United States, significant pioneering work in breast ultrasound was performed by Fornage (1993) and his group (1989, 1992), Jackson (1990, 1995) and her group (1986, 1996), Mendelson (1994), Parker et al. (1991, 1994, 1995a, b, 1996), Stavros and Dennis (1993), and Stavros et al. (1995).

Results achieved in the 1980s cannot compare with the results of breast examinations performed with the modern ultrasound instruments of the 1990s. Current research and development in breast ultrasound are focusing on new techniques of blood flow imaging, three-dimensional sonography, and the use of ultrasound contrast agents.

2 Basic Technical Principles of Breast Ultrasound

Breast ultrasound is a highly specialized discipline in the field of ultrasonography. It is usually performed by an experienced examiner who is assumed to have a detailed knowledge of the basic physics of diagnostic ultrasound. For this reason, we can limit the discussion of ultrasound physics here to key concepts that have particular relevance in breast imaging. It is also important to review potential artifacts, given the importance of recognizing these phenomena in breast images and using them as sources of diagnostic information (e.g., acoustic shadows). Equipment settings are also discussed and illustrated, owing to their critical influence on breast sonograms.

Physics

The principle of ultrasonography is straightforward: ultrasound pulses of a particular frequency are transmitted into the tissues, and the returning echoes are received and processed to generate an image of the underlying tissue. Because different tissues interact with ultrasound in different ways, different levels of acoustic energy are reflected back to the transducer.

Ultrasound energy is subject to two basic processes as it travels through tissues: *attenuation* (absorption) and *scattering* (reflection). These two processes, plus the variations of sound velocities in different media, are responsible for the specific ultrasound characteristics of tissues.

An important phenomenon in diagnostic ultrasound is *acoustic impedance* (Fig. 2.**1**). It is defined as the relationship of the acoustic pressure ("driving force") to the molecular motion that is induced within the medium. Even a low acoustic pressure will cause the molecules in a medium of high density and low compressibility to vibrate. But the molecules in highly compressible media such as gases must be deflected to a greater degree before they will vibrate. The interface between two adjacent media of different compressibility produces an *impedance mismatch*, i.e., an acoustic boundary that can reflect sound waves. Because the acoustic impedances of differ-

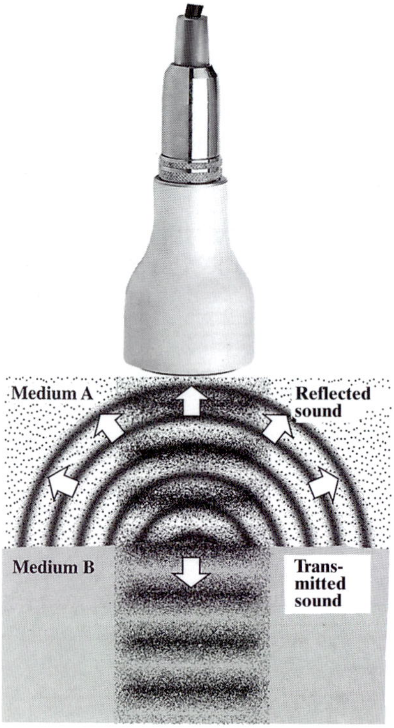

Fig. 2.**1** The passage of sound waves from one medium into another medium with a different acoustic impedance.

ent human tissues are very similar, only a very small part of the ultrasound energy is reflected at the interface between acoustically dissimilar tissues, while most of the energy (more than 99 % on average) is transmitted through. Since the impedance mismatch between air and tissue is extremely large, very little energy passes through an air-tissue interface, and virtually all of the incident ultrasound is reflected. Boundaries between soft tissue and bone also reflect a large portion of the ultrasound energy (about 50 %). Most of the transmitted energy is then lost to attenuation, leaving very little energy that can return to the transducer as echoes from structures located within or past the bone.

Another phenomenon, well known in optics, is *diffraction*. When ultrasound passes through a small orifice or travels along the boundary of a structure whose sound speed is much different from that of the adjacent tissue and the beam strikes an interface at an angle, the sound energy may be diverted from its original path. Since image generation is based on the assumption of a straight path of sound travel, diffraction can result in minor spatial distortions – mainly refraction.

The frequency dependence of *attenuation* is of central importance in ultrasound imaging. Ultrasound transmitted at lower frequencies will travel farther through tissues than higher frequencies. For example, an ultrasound wave at 3 MHz will lose one-half of its intensity after traversing about 3 cm of soft tissue, whereas a wave at 7 MHz will undergo the same attenuation after only 1 cm.

The transmission and reception of ultrasound waves by a transducer are based on the *piezoelectric effect*, discovered by the Curie brothers in 1880. This effect describes the ability of crystal structures to induce an electrical potential when mechanically deformed, and conversely to undergo mechanical deformation when exposed to an electrical potential. Transducers that transmit and receive ultrasound waves operate by this principle. When an alternating voltage is applied to a piezoelectric crystal, the crystal will expand and contract at a similar frequency, emitting a sound wave that has the same frequency as the applied voltage. The returning sound waves then produce a rhythmic mechanical deformation of the transducer face, generating an electrical voltage.

The piezoelectric crystals used in ultrasound transducers typically have a moderately wide *bandwidth*. This means that a crystal vibrates optimally at its *resonant frequency* and is capable of emitting sound waves at a bandwidth of 60–80 % of the frequency. The resonant frequency depends on the material and thickness of the crystal, and determines the operating characteristics of the transducer.

Sonographic Terms and Techniques

Among the various modes of information display that are used in diagnostic ultrasound, the *B-mode image* (brightness modulation, B-scan, two-dimensional imaging) is by far the most common. Two other basic display modes are *A-mode* (amplitude modulation, A-scan) and *M-mode* (time-motion display). Only B-mode imaging is used in examinations of the breast.

Two-Dimensional B-Mode Imaging

Real-time scanners have completely replaced manual compound scanners in modern diagnostic ultrasound. B-mode imaging derives its name from “brightness modulation,” meaning that echoes are displayed on the monitor as illuminated spots whose brightness is proportional to the amplitude of the echoes received. The ultrasound is transmitted by electronically switched crystal arrays, or by moving crystals (see below). The array emits numerous ultrasound beams that enter the tissue in a linear or fan-shaped pattern, and it receives the reflected ultrasound energy in the same position. Based on an assumed sound velocity of 1540 m/s in tissue, the returning echoes are processed according to their arrival time (i.e., their distance from the transducer), and are processed and displayed line by line, generating a two-dimensional cross-sectional image of the scanned tissue plane.

Particularly with B-mode technique, the ultrasound energy emitted by a crystal has the shape of a conical beam several tenths of a millimeter in diameter. As a result, the individual lines that are assembled to make up a complete image have a certain spatial extent that determines the *resolution* of the beam. Resolution is defined as the ability to discriminate two closely adjacent objects as being separate structures. Two types of resolution are distinguished: lateral resolution and axial resolution. Lateral resolution characterizes the ability to discriminate adjacent objects in a line perpendicular to the axis of the beam. Lateral resolution is inversely proportional to the width of the beam, and it also depends on the number and density of the adjacent transmitted and received sound beams. Because a high-frequency transducer emits a narrower beam than a low-frequency transducer, higher-frequency arrays offer superior resolution (in the range of 0.1–1.0 mm).

Since a narrow sound beam provides better resolution, modern transducers use electronic focusing to shape the beam. This is accomplished by pulsing the individual crystals with slight time delays, in a manner that deflects the crystal emissions and creates *focal points* along the axis of the beam. These focal zones can be varied both in number and in their distance from the transducer (Fig. 2.**2**).

Axial resolution is the ability to distinguish two objects that are on a line parallel to the sound path. Axial resolution is degraded by the fact that the ultrasound crystal "rings down" in its vibration, adding a degree of spatial length to the emitted pulse. Modern scanners have an axial resolution of 0.1–1.0 mm.

There are various ways in which the transmitting and receiving crystals can be assembled in a transducer. Designs range from a single-crystal transducer to linear and curved arrays consisting of many transducer crystals that are electronically interconnected.

Linear array (Fig. 2.**3a**). A linear-array transducer consists of a large number of small crystals (usually 128) arranged in groups that function alternately as transmitters and receivers. Ultrasound is emitted from the transducer in parallel scan lines. The linear array provides uniform resolution over the full depth of the image field.

Convex array (Fig. 2.**3b**). A convex or curvilinear array consists of numerous separate crystals that are arranged in groups along a curved scanning surface. The radius of curvature is greater than 25°, producing a beam divergence of 60–90°. The main advantage of a curved array is its superior imaging capabilities in the near and far field. It also provides broad near-field coverage, avoiding the narrow apex of the sector format.

Sector transducer (Fig. 2.**3c**). A sector transducer has a more convex face than the curved array, with less than a 25° radius of curvature. This produces a very wide-angle beam in the far field (> 90°), but gives very narrow coverage at close range. One advantage of sector probes is their small contact area, which permits scanning through small acoustic windows (e.g., the intercostal spaces, endovaginal or endorectal scanning, etc.). Concerns about geometric distortion by sector probes are unfounded, but the reduced density of the scan lines, particularly in the far field, results in poorer lateral resolution. Sector transducers may be of the mechanical or electronic type.

In a *mechanical* transducer, a single crystal may be oscillated or "wobbled" through a certain arc as it alternately transmits and received sound, or several crystals (usually 3–5) can be rotated on a circular path and alternately transmit and receive. Because of their mechanical action, these transducers are subject to wear, and require maintenance. Also, the quality of the transducer

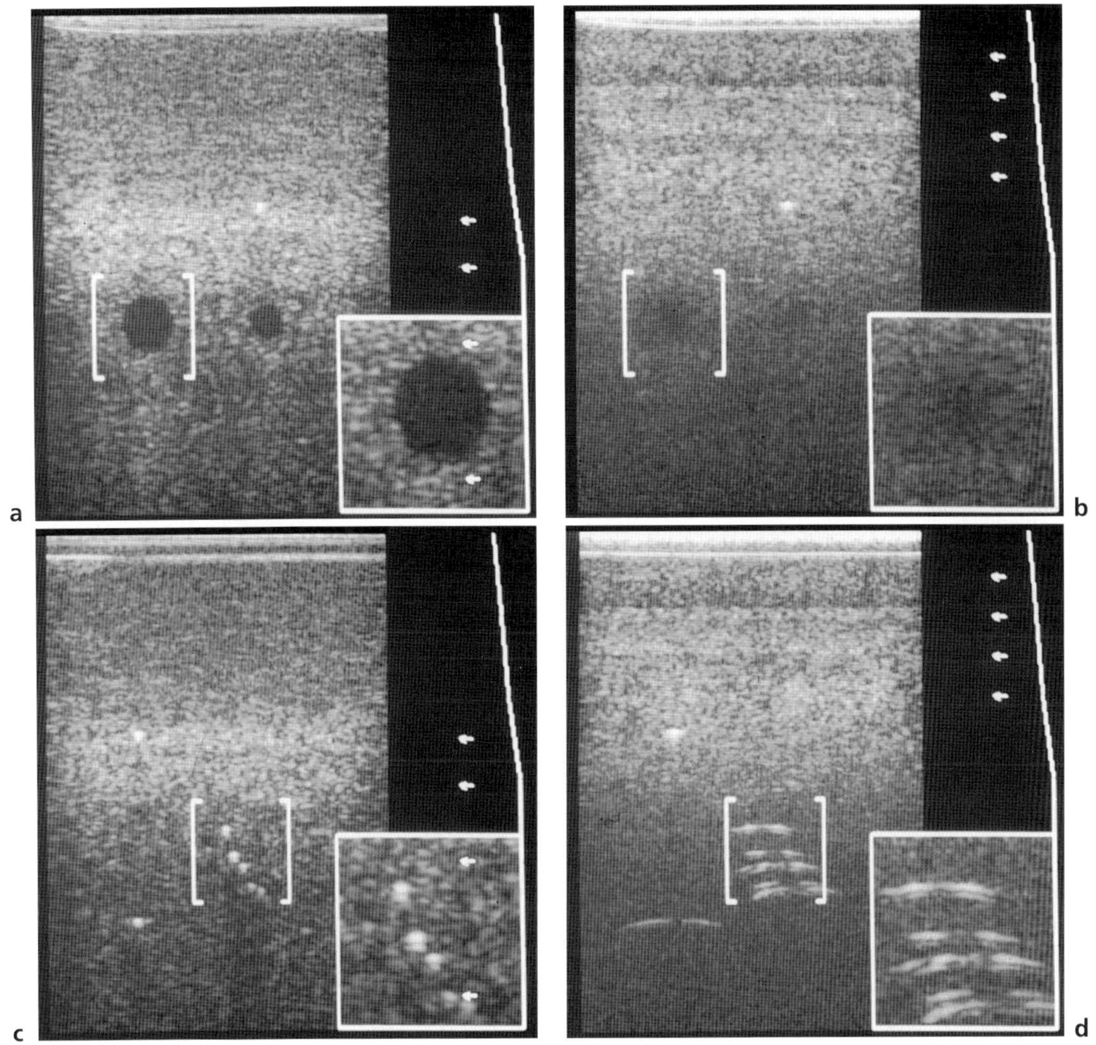

Fig. 2.2 **a–d** Effect of focal zone placement on the appearance of different structures. **a** The tubes are visible in cross-section because they are located within the focal zones. **b** When the focal zones are moved upwards, the tubes are not defined. **c, d** A similar effect occurs with thread targets imaged in cross-section: the threads are well defined in **c,** and poorly defined in **d.**

relies on extremely precise fabrication and adjustment by the manufacturer.

The *electronic* variant of the sector probe is the *phased-array sector transducer*, consisting of a convex assembly of separate crystals comparable to a very short linear-array system. But unlike the linear array, all the crystals in the assembly contribute information to every scan line in the image. The crystals can be pulsed in a particular sequence to shape and steer the beam. Controlling a phased-array transducer requires sophisticated electronics, so this type of system is very costly.

The *annular-array sector transducer* uses a combination of mechanical and electronic technology (Fig. 2.**4**). The transducer consists of several annular crystals arranged in concentric rings, and a wobbler mechanism sweeps the beam through the tissues. Cur-

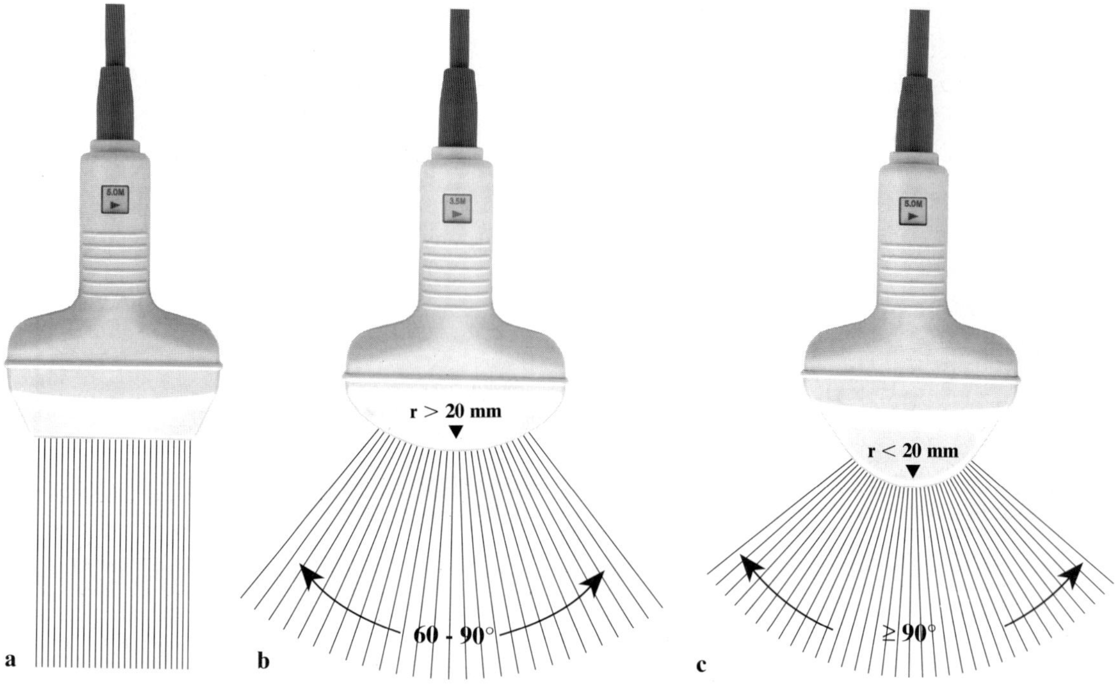

Fig. 2.**3a** Linear array, **b** convex array, **c** sector scanner.

rently, this is the only technology that provides rotationally symmetrical focusing, which minimizes section-thickness artifacts.

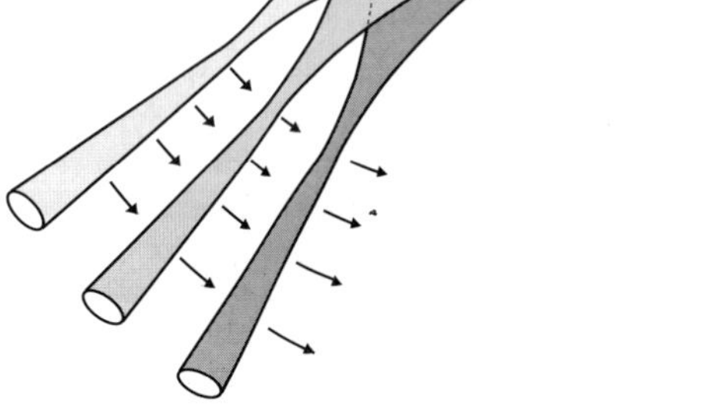

Fig. 2.**4** Annular-array sector scanner.

Time Gain Compensation (TGC) (Fig. 2.**5**)

Because ultrasound waves lose energy as they travel through tissues, the echoes returned from deeper structures are weaker than those from more superficial structures. Thus, the echoes from greater depths must be amplified more than echoes from the near field, in order to ensure that all echoes are displayed at their true intensity. Time gain compensation (TGC) accomplishes this by amplifying signals in proportion to the attenuation caused by the depth of the reflector. At the same time, TGC must allow for individual and interindividual variations in the absorption and reflection characteristics of the examined tissues, and ultrasound units are therefore equipped with slide switches for manually adjusting the TGC slope.

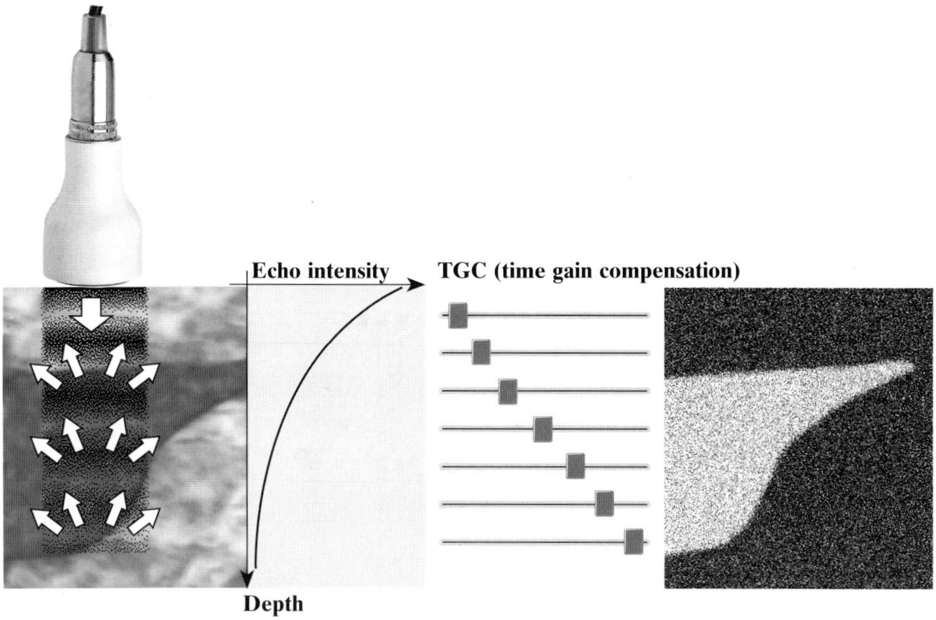

Fig. 2.5 Time gain compensation (TGC) corrects for attenuation caused by the transit time of the ultrasound beam.

Ultrasound Artifacts

Artifacts are a central problem in diagnostic ultrasound; they must be properly recognized and interpreted so that an accurate diagnosis can be made. The most common imaging artifacts and their causes are reviewed below.

Side-lobe artifact (Fig. 2.**6**). All piezoelectric crystals emit secondary, off-axis lobes around the primary beam. When a side lobe encounters a strong reflector, the echoes are interpreted as occurring at varying distances from the emitting crystal along the transducer axis. Side-lobe artifacts may appear as geometric figures on the monitor. Modern ultrasound units can suppress this artifact by using transit-time calculations to filter out laterally incident pulses.

Section-thickness artifacts (Fig. 2.**7**). Because the scan plane has finite thickness, echoes originating from the edges of the beam may be projected into the image plane.

Noise (Fig. 2.**8**). Every electronic device produces unwanted intrinsic signals – short, low-level pulses that create a uniform, stippled pattern of spurious signals. Since TGC amplifies the echoes from deep objects more than superficial ones, it also increases the noise level. As a result, the noise signals may be more intense than the echo signals and obscure tissue details. The onset of this phenomenon defines the *maximum imaging depth* of an ultrasound unit.

Acoustic enhancement (Fig. 2.**9**). Distal or posterior enhancement occurs when the ultrasound beam passes through a fluid-filled cavity. Because the ultrasound traverses the fluid medium without absorption or reflection, the echo signals proximal and distal to the fluid have the same intensity. As a result, tissues lying behind the fluid appear more echogenic than tissues of equal quality and depth lying adjacent to the fluid-filled cavity. This phenomenon is useful for recognizing fluid-filled breast masses at ultrasound (cysts, hemangiomas, etc.).

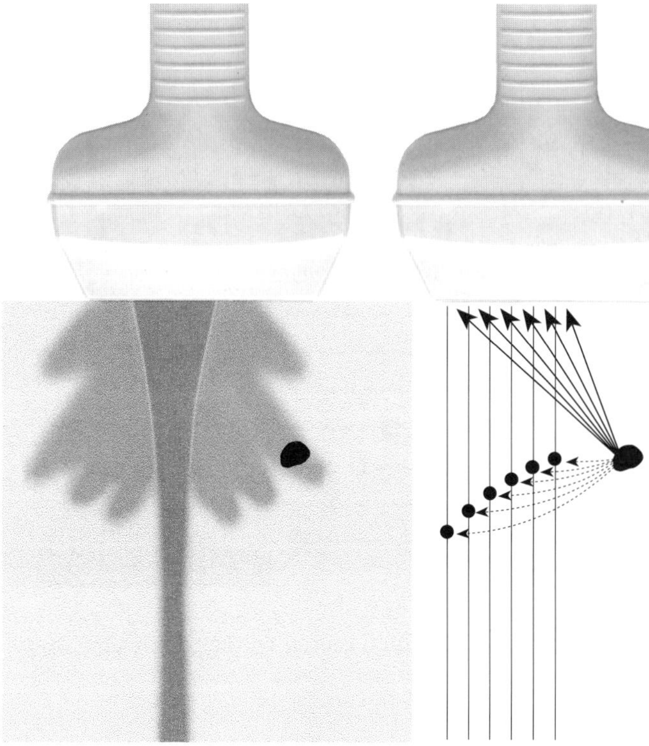

Fig. 2.**6** The origin of side-lobe artifacts.

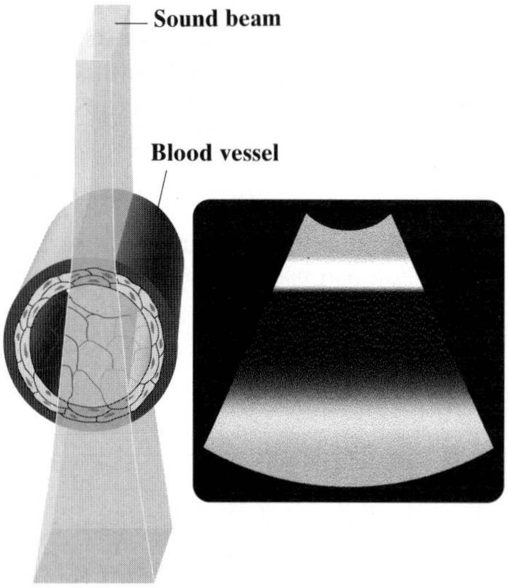

Fig. 2.**7** The origin of section-thickness artifacts.

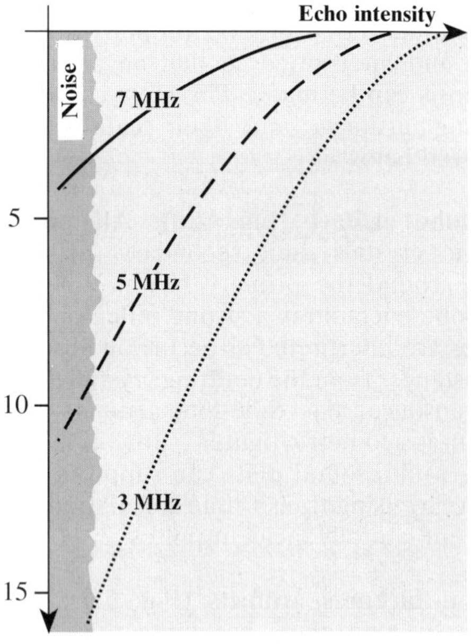

Fig. 2.**8** Electronic noise as a limiting factor for ultrasound imaging depth.

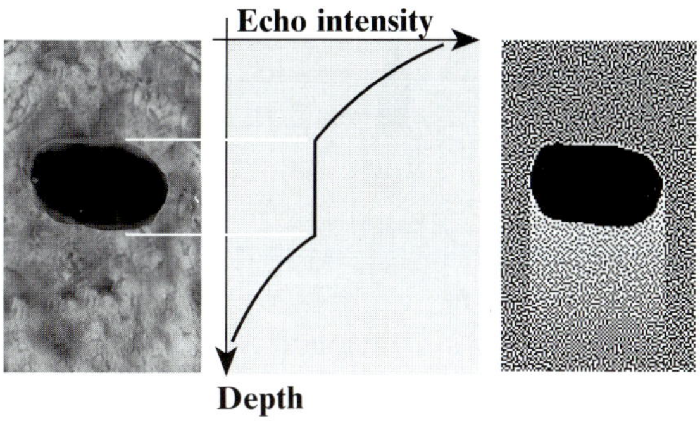

Fig. 2.9 Posterior acoustic enhancement.

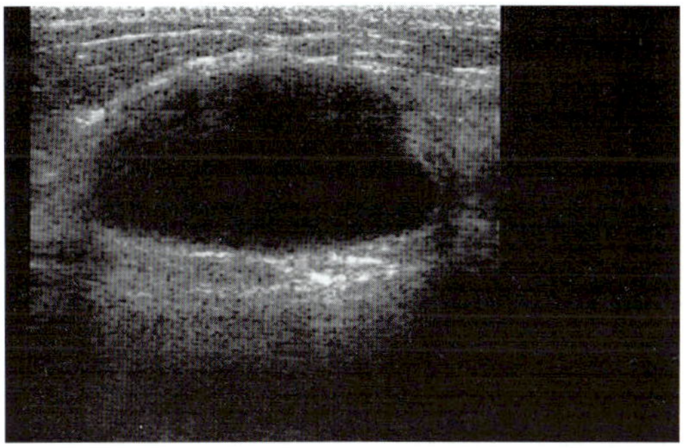

Fig. 2.10 A breast cyst, showing bilateral edge shadows and central posterior enhancement.

Edge shadows (Fig. 2.10). Edge shadows are band-like shadows that project distally from the lateral edges of a rounded structure. Several explanations have been offered for this phenomenon, the most likely being that a high reflectivity at the tangential sites combined with high attenuation and diffraction in those areas reduce the amplitude of echoes from reflectors behind the edges of the mass in comparison with adjacent areas.

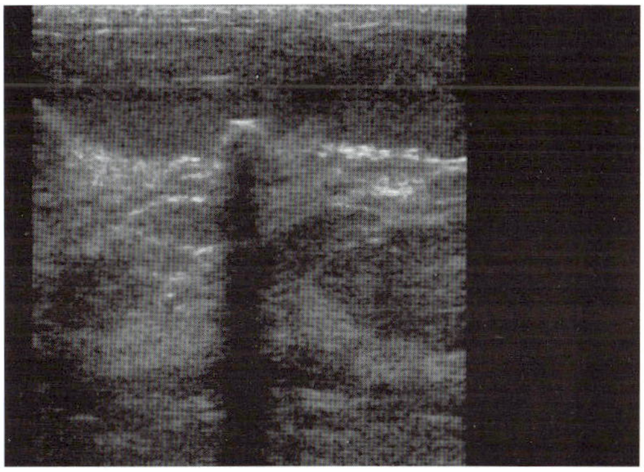

Fig. 2.11 An acoustic shadow cast by a macrocalcification in the breast.

Shadowing distal to bone and air (Fig. 2.11). Because bone and gas-filled cavities are strongly attenuating and create a large impedance mismatch, they pose a barrier to ultrasound penetration. Little or no ultrasound energy is available behind these structures to produce echoes that can be imaged; consequently, the region "shaded" by these barriers appears devoid of echoes and is called an acoustic shadow.

Reverberations (Fig. 2.12). Multiple reflections may be generated when an ultrasound pulse encounters a strong reflector with a large surface area. A large percentage of the ultrasound energy is reflected back and, on reaching the transducer, is not only received but reflected back into the patient from the transducer face, making several round trips between the transducer and the original reflector. As a result, the tissue structure generates multiple echoes that are displayed at equidistant intervals. This phenomenon occurs when the strong reflector is located very close to the transducer, or when the medium between the transducer and reflector is highly conductive to sound. Reverberations are commonly seen in examinations of the bladder, for example.

Geometric distortion. Ideally, it is assumed that ultrasound follows a straight path through the tissues, traveling at a constant

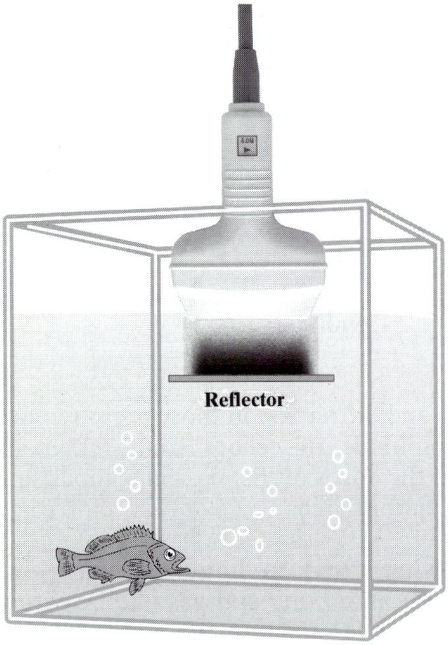

a

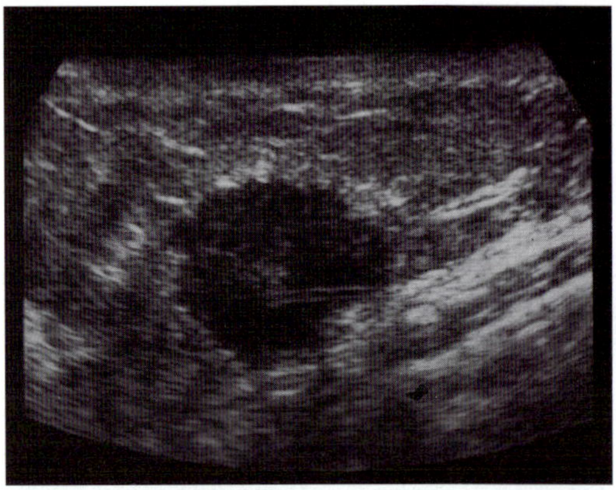

b

Fig. 2.12 Reverberations. **a** Principle. **b** Reverberations in a breast mass, caused by the built-in offset of an annular array transducer.

velocity of 1540 m/s. But in reality, the sound alters its path as a result of diffraction and refraction, and it has different velocities in different media. Because these changes are not factored into the image generating process, small geometric image distortions can result. Despite the very small deviation, this artifact can cause difficulties in ultrasound-guided needle procedures.

Mirror-image artifact. This artifact occurs when the ultrasound pulses encounter a strong oblique reflector at a 40–50° angle. If a pulse reflects off the strong interface before encountering a real structure, it will register the structure as occurring on the other side of the interface, creating a spurious mirror image of the real structure.

From the above discussion, it is clear that the highest possible frequencies should be used in diagnostic ultrasound to ensure optimum resolution. A 5-MHz transducer is commonly used in obstetric ultrasound, as this frequency allows for deep imaging and modern technology is available for analyzing the returned signals. A 7.5-MHz probe is a good general-purpose transducer for breast imaging and generally can be used even in large breasts. Small breasts and superficial structures can be examined with newer, high-frequency transducers at 7.5–13.0 MHz, offering superb image quality.

Imagers and Transducers

Ultrasound equipment manufacturers offer imagers and transducers for breast ultrasound that operate in the frequency range of 5–15 MHz. A 5-MHz or 7.5-MHz transducer is recommended for routine use. If the operating frequency (resolution) is too high, even normal breast tissue may show a nonhomogeneous profusion of details that can mask pathological changes. In Germany, official standards adopted in 1993 specify the minimum quality criteria for breast ultrasound imaging equipment used by physicians enrolled in health care funds:

- In terms of safety, the equipment must conform to IEC standard 1157.
- The examination must be performed with a B-mode imager.
- Scanning mode: linear or curved array with a built-in offset, or sector scanner with a built-in offset.
- Nominal frequency: 5.0–7.5 MHz.
- Working range: 0.5–4.0 cm. With a linear or curved array, the transmission focus should be adjustable to depths of 0.5–1.7 cm, 1.5–3.5 cm, and 3.0–5.0 cm. Linear arrays with a nonconforming focal depth must be provided with a variable offset. Curved arrays and sector scanners must have a built-in offset with a linear coupling surface. For sector scanners with a fixed focus, the focal point must be located at a depth of 1.0–2.0 cm.
- Zoom display: the monitor display must have a temporal and axial resolution of 0.02 ms and 0.15 mm.
- Width of image field: at least 5 cm at a depth of 1.5 cm and no more than 8 cm at or below the skin surface; a maximum scanning angle of ± 20° is permitted for curved arrays and sector scanners.
- Depth of image field: at least 5 cm.
- Frame rate: at least 15 images per second with a single focus.

In the United States, all ultrasound systems used for breast imaging or any other application must be approved by the Food and Drug Administration (FDA).

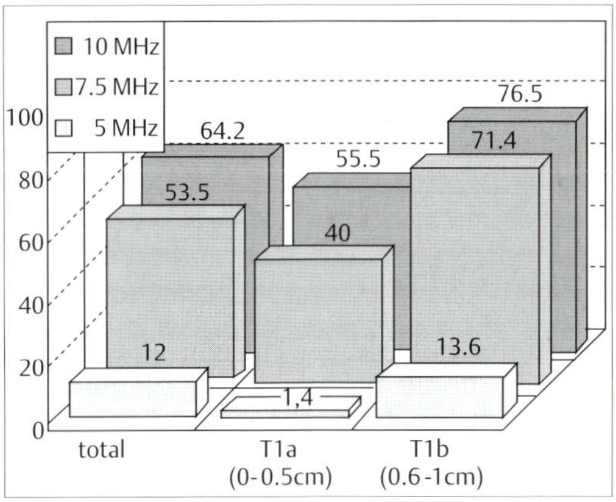

Fig. 2.**13** Sensitivity of various ultrasound frequencies in the detection of nonpalpable breast masses (in percentages, after Catarzi 1992).

Table 2.**1** Values for maximum axial resolution, compared with frequency.

Frequency (MHz)	Resolution (mm)
3.5	0.440
5.0	0.308
7.5	0.205
10.0	0.154
13.0	0.118

The operator selecting an ultrasound system should make sure that the system conforms to established standards. It should also be determined whether the transducer conforms to the nominal specifications stated by the manufacturer. For example, many instruments do not focus precisely in the region indicated on the monitor, but shift the zone of maximum sharpness up or down. Every examiner should become familiar with these characteristics before performing an examination.

It is a basic rule in diagnostic ultrasound that as the operating frequency increases, resolution improves while imaging depth decreases. The 7.5-MHz transducer provides a good trade-off between imaging depth and resolution. High-frequency probes also provide better sensitivity for blood flow measurements. Comparative studies have shown, moreover, that higher transducer frequencies are more sensitive than lower frequencies in the detection of nonpalpable breast masses (Table 2.**1**, Fig. 2.**13**).

Technical Recommendations

The following recommendations are offered for ultrasound units and transducers used in breast examinations.

Linear Transducer

Advantages. With electronic linear transducers, the focal depth can be freely selected (dynamic focusing) (Kremkau 1993), and multiple focal points can be selected to increase lateral resolution over the full depth of the image. The near focal region often starts at a depth of only 0.5 cm, providing a clear, detailed image of breast tissues just beneath the skin. These transducers do not require an offset that would make the probe heavier and perhaps more difficult to handle. Instruments with a deeper focus can be used with an offset to move the focal region closer to the skin. Electronic transducers are light and do not vibrate like some mechanical transducers. Also, they are more resistant to being bumped or dropped than mechanical transducers with their sensitive internal components. The large number of piezoelectric elements in the transducer ensure good resolution throughout the field of view. A sector transducer is useful for evaluating suspicious palpable and mammographically visible breast lesions, but is not suitable for locating clinically and mammographically occult lesions because of its limited sector format (Madjar et al. 1993).

Frequency Range 5–13 MHz

Advantages. Lateral resolution defines the ability to discriminate two objects in a line perpendicular to the beam axis; axial resolution defines the ability to distinguish two objects on a line parallel to the beam axis. Lateral resolution improves as the wavelength of the ultrasound decreases and thus as its frequency increases. Modern instruments with frequencies of 7.5 MHz or higher have a resolution of approximately 0.2 mm, meaning that they can define structures as small as 0.2 mm in diameter, depending on the location of the lesion in the breast and on the surrounding tissues (Mendelson 1993). Axial resolution can be improved by using a broad-bandwidth transducer-i.e., one containing special nonpiezoelectric damping materials that generate waves of low frequency in addition to the higher-frequency waves from the piezoelectric crystals. This "broad-band technology" produces focal regions at various levels in the scan plane, and provides almost uniform resolution over the full depth of the image. As the imaging depth increases, the proportion of low frequencies in the transmitted sound automatically increases.

There are no precise definitions of what constitutes a "high" axial or lateral resolution.

A very high operating frequency (13 MHz) provides excellent lateral resolution in the near field, but gives relatively poor axial resolution at greater depths (Hardy et al. 1990, Madjar et al. 1993).

Contrast Resolution

The more bits of information that can be stored in the ultrasound scan converter (i.e., the more gray-scale levels that can be assigned to a pixel), the better the contrast resolution of the system. Contrast resolution increases with the number of bits per pixel. Current ultrasound systems image at 6 to 8 bits per pixel.

Monitor

Modern ultrasound units can provide a resolution of 512 × 512 pixels, with 8-bit encoding of gray levels for each pixel stored by the scan converter. This requires a screen capacity of 250,000 pixels with 256 gray levels. The resolution of the monitor should at least be equivalent to that of the ultrasound unit.

Ergonomics

The transducer should be light and easy to hold. It should be possible to operate display controls with one hand. Equipment for photographic documentation should be within easy reach.

Useful Options and Features

- A zoom feature (1 : 1 to 8 : 1) provides a close-up view of the internal structures of cysts, mammary ducts, and solid masses.
- Postprocessing. Image data stored in memory can be manipulated by altering the brightness levels, for example, to improve the discrimination of intramammary structures. A classic example of postprocessing is taking a "soft" parenchymal image and converting it to a "hard' image for evaluating the heart or blood vessels (e.g., in prenatal ultrasound).
- Color B-mode. The technique of color-coding the gray levels in a B-mode image has been known for some 30 years (Kelly-Frey 1985), but has become clinically practical only since the advent of fully digitized data acquisition and storage in modern ultrasound systems. By adding more levels of appreciable contrast to the image, the color display permits the examiner to discern finer differences within the tissue texture (Fig. 2.**14**).
- Displaying the TGC slope and focal zone carets at the edge of the screen is helpful in checking for optimal adjustment of the technical parameters.
- It is helpful to have organ and directional annotations displayed on the monitor. Best is a pictogram of the breast in which the position of the transducer can be entered with a trackball.
- Digital imaging processing and storage increase the accuracy of the sonographic information, in part by minimizing transmission errors and losses. This can improve the ability to distinguish between tissue structures.
- Color Doppler sonography (CDS) is a technique that may assist in the differential diagnosis of indeterminate breast masses.
- It may be helpful to have an extra 5-MHz probe for patients with very large breasts, where the 7.5-MHz probe may provide

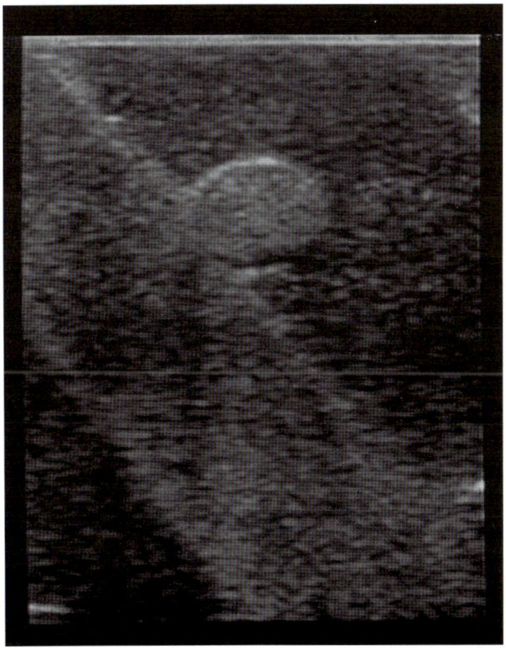

a

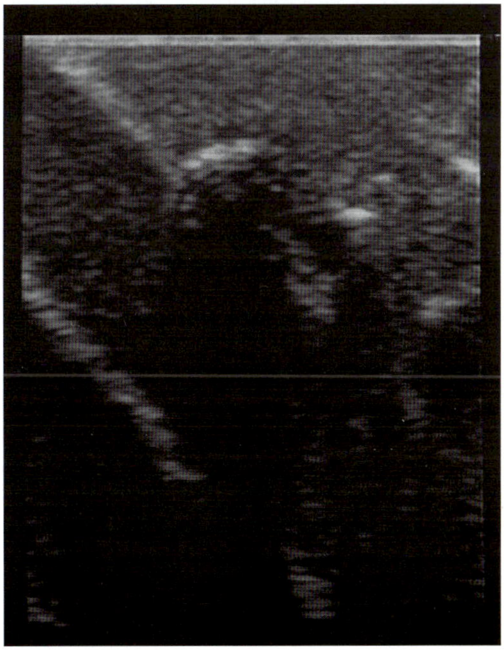

b

Fig. 2.**14 a, b** Each pair of panels shows an anechoic structure and a hypoechoic structure imaged by breast ultrasound transducers produced by various manufacturers. The variation in the quality of the various images is easily seen.

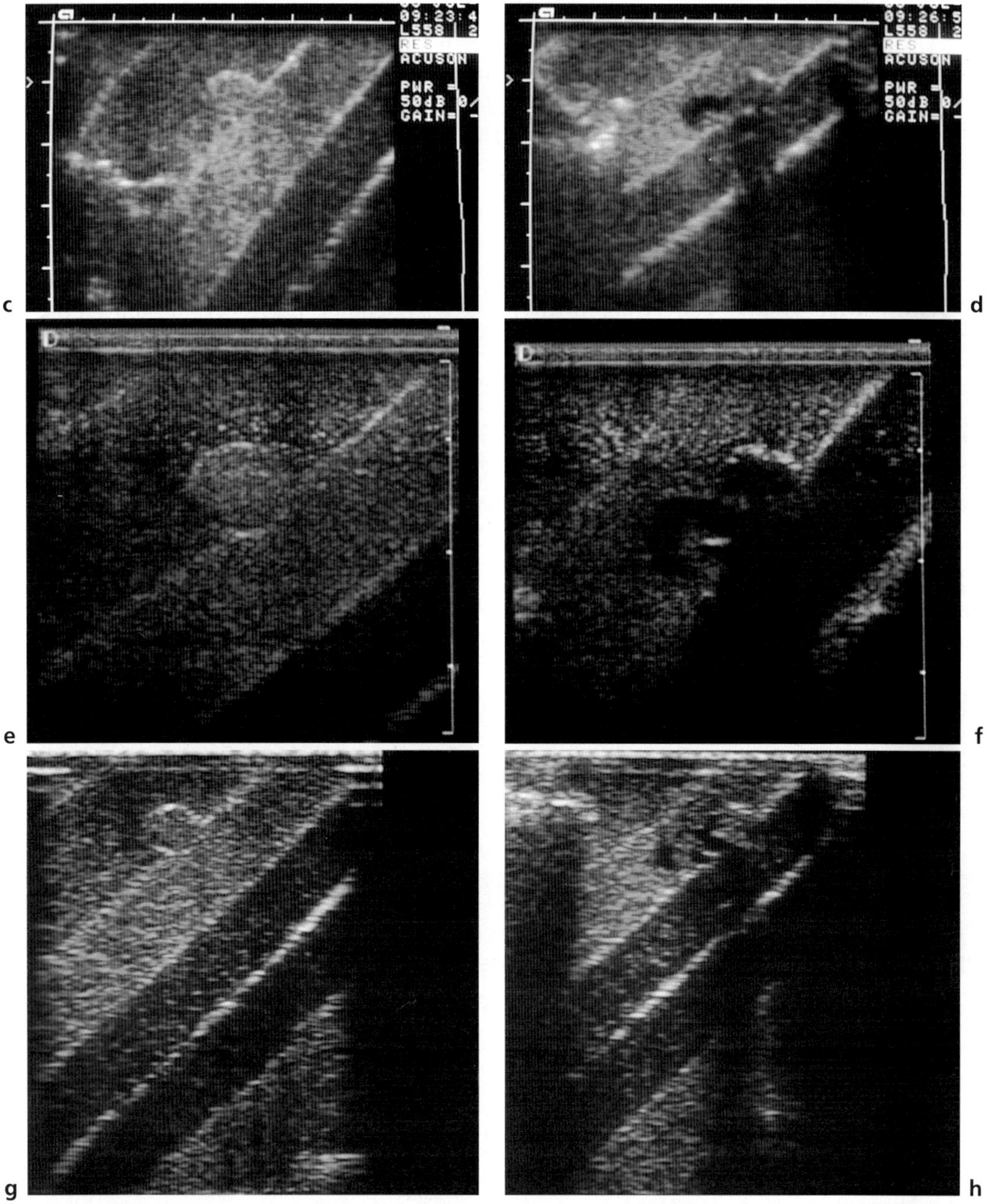
09:23:4
L558
RES
ACUSON
PWR =
50dB
GAIN=
09:26:5
L558
RES
ACUSON
PWR =
50dB
GAIN=

Fig. 2.**14 c–h.**

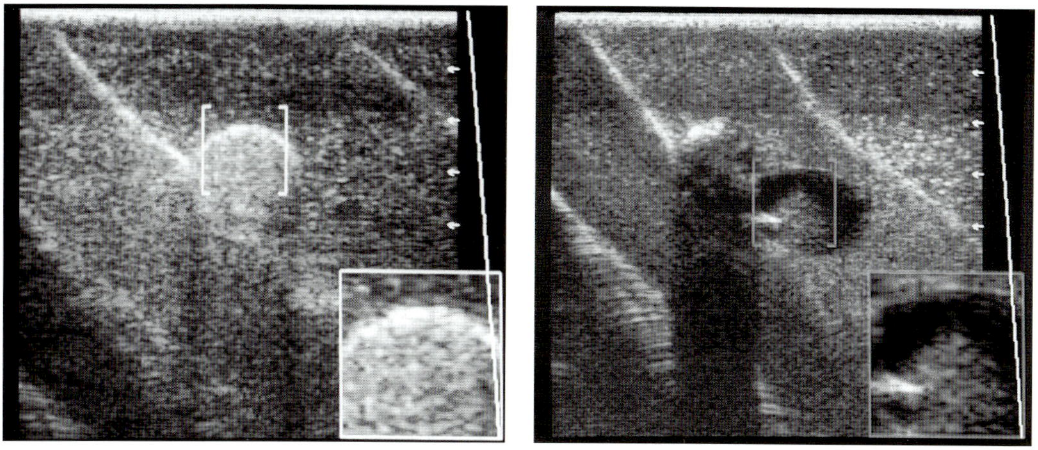

Fig. 2.**14** i–j.

insufficient depth range even at the highest power setting. The lower the frequency, the greater the penetration. Broad-band transducers automatically decrease their transmission frequency with increasing depth.
- Another useful option is a videotape unit for recording dynamic phases of the examination (e.g., the compressibility of a breast mass).
- Electronic storage media (optical disks, SyQuest, Streamer, etc.) provide an economical means of storing ultrasound images without data loss or degradation. Images stored in this way can be integrated into the examination report.

Selecting a Breast Ultrasound Unit

The best way to select an ultrasound unit is not to study its technical parameters but to "field test" the unit by performing a breast examination in a patient. An acceptable unit for breast ultrasound must define all aspects of the normal sonographic anatomy of the female breast and allow equal visualization of superficial and deep structures.

Offsets

An offset or standoff is generally unnecessary for linear transducers that are designed for breast ultrasound, as these instruments provide very good resolution at close range (0.5 cm). An offset may be needed, however, to differentiate intracutaneous structures (atheromas, lipomas).

With a convex array or sector scanner, near-field resolution was improved in the past by using an offset to raise the transducer above skin level and move the focal zone into the superficial region of interest. The "waterbag technique" should not be used, as it is very difficult to obtain full breast coverage through a waterbag that has to be constantly moved about during the examination. One disadvantage of a built-in offset is that it can cause troublesome reverberations (Fig. 2.**12**). Modern high-frequency transducers currently available for breast imaging allow superb near field resolution obviating the need for standoff techniques.

Equipment Settings

There are no "universal" equipment settings that can be recommended, but some general guidelines can be offered. One is to switch on the ultrasound unit several minutes before use; some monitors need warm-up time in order to give an optimum picture. Also, the monitor adjustments should be checked frequently, since they critically affect the ultrasound image, regardless of other settings. The brightness and contrast controls are adjusted by the gray-level scale on the monitor until the maximum gray level appears completely black and the first gray level is a brilliant white.

In other respects, the equipment settings should be tailored to the specific examination. An example in obstetric ultrasound is fetal echo cardiography. While fine, "soft" instrument settings are best when screening for fetal anomalies, coarser, "hard" settings should be used for fetal cardiac imaging to bring out the details of interest.

Every modern ultrasound unit can be preset to any of several basic setting configurations that can be accessed for specific applications and require only minor tailoring adjustments. These preset modes are a great convenience, and their use is strongly recommended.

Initial Settings

No settings are optimal for every system, but we can offer recommendations based on personal experience (Table 2.**2**).

The operator should seek the help of a sonographer or manufacturer's representative in choosing the settings that will define all the anatomical details described on p. 25. These settings may be permanently entered and activated when the breast ultrasound transducer is connected to the unit, or the operator may select the settings at the start of the examination (regardless of the basic unit).

Table 2.2 Recommended initial settings for ultrasound scanners for real-time breast ultrasound.

Parameter	Selection
Dynamic range	High (50–70 dB)
Overall amplification	Low
Contrast	Medium setting
Line density	High
Frame rate	High

The TCG slope, including the near and far gain components, should be tailored to each individual breast by adjusting a series of slide switches. Superficial structures should not appear "washed out" (swamped with echoes), and deeper structures should not appear too dark.

Resolution Tests for Different Scanners

Several transducers from different manufacturers tested on the same ultrasound phantom under identical conditions show how markedly the image quality can vary among different instruments. It should be noted that while this test is informative, it is by no means comprehensive and is based on an arbitrary selection of instruments (Fig. 2.**14a–j**).

3 Current Role of Ultrasound in the Evaluation of Breast Masses

Mammography traces its origins to the year 1913, when Salomon of the Berlin Charitè Hospital used roentgen rays to examine breast masses (Salomon 1913). The method developed rapidly, and by the 1960s mammographic screening programs had been instituted whose efficacy is documented by the decline in breast cancer mortality in postmenopausal women who have been screened (Frischbier 1994, Fournier 1993). Breast ultrasound has lagged behind mammography in its development, due in part to a perceived lack of need for diagnostic methods other than mammography (Kelly-Fry 1985). It has been shown, however, that breast ultrasound is superior to mammography in its ability to detect focal abnormalities in the radiographically dense breasts of adolescent women (Fornage et al. 1987, Madjar et al. 1994). Thus, breast ultrasound is still a relatively young modality.

Some researchers claim that ultrasound is approximately 90 % sensitive in the detection of breast carcinoma (Harper et al. 1993). Others claim that ultrasound is not useful for differentiating between benign and malignant tissue (Kindermann and Willgeroth 1993, Mendelson 1993) and is not capable of establishing whether a mammographically suspicious focal lesion is malignant or benign (Finlay et al. 1994). Breast ultrasound using current technology cannot detect preinvasive lesions or intraductal disease (Mosny and Nitz 1994). A recent study by Stavros et al. (1995) demonstrated that although there is a significant overlap in sonographic characteristics between benign and malignant lesions, ultrasound imaging can identify a subgroup of nodules in which the certainty of malignancy is low enough to avoid biopsy. Therefore, applying excellent sonographic technique and strict adherence to sonographic criteria for benign and malignant lesions, breast sonography improves the specificity for the majority of both benign and malignant breast nodules.

It is also clear that ultrasound is not a substitute for mammography. Madjar et al. (1991), for example, missed some breast cancers in a selected patient population (women hospitalized with a focal breast lesion), particularly in fatty breasts. Without physical examination and radiographic mammography, these carcinomas would have been missed with ultrasound alone. It would be a mistake, however, not to check the initial mammographic diagnosis or equivocal radiographic findings by means of breast ultrasound (Mosny and Nitz 1994).

> Breast ultrasound is an adjunct to primary mammography. There is no statistical evidence that ultrasound can reduce breast cancer mortality when used as an *exclusive* screening modality. Consequently, breast ultrasound is not a substitute for mammography.

Current Indications for Breast Ultrasound

Diagnosis and differential diagnosis:

- Every palpable mass in the breast and axilla, particularly in women under 30 years of age and in pregnant and lactating women (Madjar et al. 1994, Mendelson 1993).

- Radiographically dense breast that is difficult to evaluate by mammography (Madjar et al. 1994, Mendelson 1993).
- Prior to planned tumor excision for staging, and to exclude multicentric disease (Kindermann and Genz 1993).
- For the investigation of a suspicious focal lesion detected by mammography or magnetic resonance imaging (MRI) and for the preoperative localization of a nonpalpable mass (Mendelson 1993).
- A mammographically detected mass that is suspicious for carcinoma, or is not unequivocally benign (Finlay et al. 1994, Mendelson 1993).
- Surveillance of masses that are benign by physical examination, mammography, and sonography.
- A mammographically detected mass that may be a cyst or fibroadenoma. Sonography can determine whether the mass is cystic or solid (Kindermann and Willgeroth 1993, Mendelson 1993).

Postoperative and post-therapeutic follow-up:

- Screening for tumor recurrence after mastectomy or the insertion of a breast implant; see Chapter 17 (Mendelson 1993).
- Checking the integrity of breast implants and diagnosing fibrous capsular contracture; see Chapter 17 (Audretsch 1975, Baldt et al. 1994).
- Postoperative evaluation of hematomas, seromas, and inflammatory processes (Blohmer et al. 1994, Caccialanza et al. 1994).
- Evaluating the response of puerperal or nonpuerperal mastitis to treatment (Blohmer et al. 1994).

Other indications:

- Surveillance of breast cancers that have been "downstaged" by chemotherapy or irradiation (Forouhi et al. 1994, Kedar et al. 1994).
- Mastodynia.
- Carcinophobia.
- Ultrasound-guided booster irradiation of the tumor bed after breast-conserving surgery (Leonard et al. 1993).
- Ultrasound-guided abscess drainage (Karstrup et al. 1993).
- Ultrasound-guided biopsy of suspicious breast lesions (Fornage et al. 1992, Parker et al. 1991, 1994, 1995a, 1995b, Parker and Burbank 1996).

A controversial indication for breast ultrasound is in women who refuse mammography because of radiation exposure or apprehension about pain.

Breast ultrasound is *the* modality for gaining an initial impression in patients who present with breast symptoms in the office setting, and for investigating findings that are equivocal with other imaging procedures.

Even the "classic" indication for breast ultrasound – differentiating between cystic and solid masses – can significantly reduce the number of biopsies that are performed on benign breast cysts (Mendelson 1993).

Principles of the Examination

An examiner carrying out breast ultrasound should note the following principles:

- The most important examination for the early detection of breast cancer is breast self-examination by the patient. Even today, it is the method by which most breast cancers are detected (Kaiser et al. 1993, Kindermann and Willgeroth 1993).
- The patient's personal and family history should be taken before an imaging study is performed. This information should include:
  - Any "lumps" felt by the patient herself.
  - Presenting complaints (mastodynia, premenstrual discomfort).
  - Any familial occurrence of breast cancer.
  - Number of previous pregnancies and childbirths.
  - Previous surgical and therapeutic procedures on the breasts.
  - Use of hormones (hormone replacement, oral contraceptives).
  - Previous breast examinations (mammograms) during the past year.

- The examiner should inspect and palpate both breasts before the ultrasound examination and, if necessary, during the course of the examination.
- A unilateral nipple discharge, especially when bloody, should be investigated by cytological examination and ductography.
- Every suspicious palpable mass and every focal lesion that is not definitely benign in the imaging analysis should be biopsied or excised and histologically evaluated, if necessary using immunohistochemical techniques (Blohmer et al. 1994).
- The ultrasound unit should be suitable for breast imaging. Small masses may be missed by an instrument not designed for breast ultrasound (e.g., a vaginal probe).
- The examination should not be rushed, and images should be closely scrutinized during the examination and properly documented.
- A true sonographic focal lesion warrants appropriate further investigation (Fig. 3.**1a**) if it is seen in at least two planes (with the transducer rotated 90°) and is reproducible.
- Every structure that appears abnormal to the examiner is permanently documented in at least two planes (laser printer, videotape, electronic storage media), and the location of the lesion is indicated.

Algorithm for Evaluating Breast Masses

Ultrasound occupies a key position in the evaluation of breast masses, regardless of whether the mass is initially detected by palpation or mammography. Every diagnostic workup of breast lesions should include physical examination, mammography, and sonography.

Experience in recent years has confirmed the value of magnetic resonance imaging (MRI) for the exclusion of additional lesions prior to breast-conserving surgery and in the follow-up of breast cancer to differentiate scar tissue from recurrent carcinoma (Heywang et al. 1989, Kaiser et al. 1993).

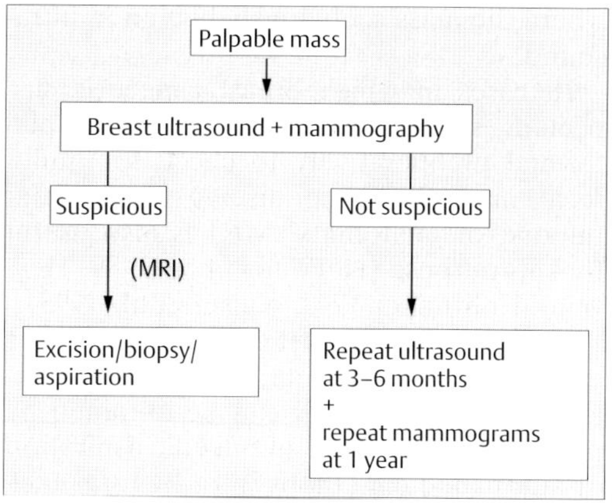

a

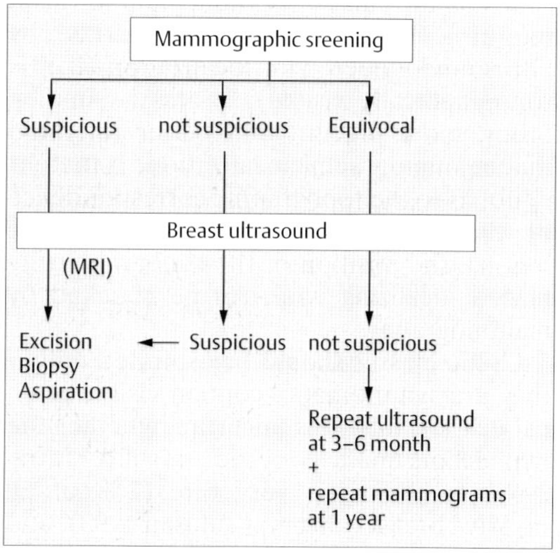

b

Fig. 3.**1 a, b** Algorithms for the differential diagnosis of breast masses. **a** The palpable mass is primary, and imaging studies follow. **b** Mass detected by mammographic screening.

The role of ultrasound in breast cancer follow-up is described in Chapter 12.

The flowcharts in Fig. 3.**1** show the standard algorithms that are followed in the evaluation of breast masses.

In patients with a palpable breast mass (Fig. 3.**1a**), immediate sonography is advised to obtain initial information that is useful for benign/malignant differentiation. An individual diagnostic workup and schedule can then be formulated. This sequencing avoids delays in cases in which there is sonographic suspicion of breast cancer, and it offers immediate reassurance in cases where the mass is obviously benign at ultrasound.

In cases in which breast cancer is suspected, sonography should also be performed preoperatively to check for multifocal or multicentric disease, intraductal tumors, or bilaterality. MRI is also useful for this purpose (Heywang et al. 1989, Heywang-Köbrunner 1992, Kaiser et al. 1993).

If any of the diagnostic procedures raises a suspicion of carcinoma, histological evaluation is required. This can be obtained by percutaneous biopsy (fine-needle aspiration or automated core biopsy), or by total excision of the mass. A nonpalpable mass requiring excision should be marked by ultrasound-guided wire localization (if it is sonographically visible), as this is simpler, faster, more precise, and better tolerated than mammographic localization. If there is doubt as to the topographic correspondence of the mammographic and sonographic lesions, the position of the sonographically placed localizing wire can be checked by mammography.

Cystic masses should be aspirated only if they are symptomatic, contain visible internal echoes, or if it is uncertain whether the hypoechoic mass is cystic or solid. Intracystic carcinoma is very rare (2% of all invasive breast cancers) (Tulusan 1993), and there is no guarantee that cytological examination of the cyst aspirate will disclose the cancer. At the same time, however, the availability of cytological findings (e.g., cells showing atypical proliferation or intracystic malignancy or an acellular aspirate) may be helpful in planning further treatment. Another rationale for cyst aspiration is to relieve painful breast tension that appears to be caused by breast cysts. Of course, the aspirate in such cases should be cytologically examined.

If any of the diagnostic procedures raises even a low index of suspicion, further sonographic follow-up is essential and should be supplemented by follow-up mammograms taken at the recommended intervals.

If a nonpalpable breast mass has been detected by either mammography or sonography, the other of the two modalities should be performed to supplement the initial study (Fig. 3.**1b**). Thereafter, the workup follows the algorithm for evaluating palpable breast masses.

If an ultrasound follow-up examination is selected, it should be performed three to six months after the initial breast ultrasound to ensure that in case the first examination was false-negative (e.g., a small, indeterminate lesion), necessary surgical treatment can still be provided without dire consequences for the patient. Short-interval sonographic follow-ups theoretically increase the diagnostic accuracy and pose no radiation hazard to the patient. As in mammography, the intervals between examinations may be increased after the initial follow-ups.

The mutually complementary diagnostic procedures reviewed in Fig. 3.**2** can establish the benign or malignant nature of a breast mass with a high degree of confidence and, in cases of malignancy, can stage the lesion prior to surgery. Various biopsy methods are available that can further increase diagnostic accuracy (Parker 1994). This approach allows the physician to discuss plans for operative and medical management with the patient in an expeditious fashion and formulate an optimum plan for the operation (including the surgical

- Palpation: detection, localization, benign/malignant differentiation
- Mammography: detection, localization, benign/malignant differentiation, intraductal component, multifocality, preoperative localization, biopsy/aspiration
- Ultrasound: detection, localization, benign/malignant differentiation, multifocality, axillary involvement, preoperative localization, route of approach, biopsy/aspiration
- MRI: detection, localization, benign/malignant differentation, multifocality, relation to surroundung tissues (pectoral fascia), axillary involvement

Fig. 3.**2** Preoperative management, including all diagnostic measures for selecting a stage-appropriate treatment method.

approach, incision, and extent of the resection) that is appropriate for both oncological and reconstructive requirements (Audretsch et al. 1995). This applies to segmental resections (negative margins, isolated intramammary focus) as well as mastectomy.

The goal of all breast cancer therapy is local tumor eradication combined with appropriate measures for curative and palliative systemic control.

Some examples of the complementary roles of the various diagnostic procedures are shown in Figs. 8.**30**, 8.**36**, and 8.**48**.

Microcalcifications in Breast Ultrasound

One disadvantage of ultrasound is that most currently available units cannot clearly demonstrate clusters of microcalcifications in the breast. There is still controversy as to whether newly emerging technologies in modern high-resolution scanners can accomplish this. Figure 3.**3** illustrates the possible sonographic correlation of mammographically visible calcifications in the glandular breast tissue.

The question of whether there is really a need to demonstrate breast microcalcifications with ultrasound has not yet been answered. This modality has its own specific criteria that are applied in the differential diagnosis of breast masses (Chapter 6). The availability of these criteria may indicate that, in contrast to mammography, there is no strict need to evaluate microcalcification patterns.

The diagnosis of breast carcinoma in situ is a different matter. This lesion is not detected by ultrasound because, since there is no invasive disease, there is no change in tissue echogenicity. In the study by Potterton et al. (1994), ultrasound detected a focal lesion in only one of 26 cases in which mammography had demonstrated microcalcifications with no definable mass. Micropapillary intracystic carcinoma in situ may produce internal echoes in cysts (Tulusan 1993), but a benign/malignant differentiation cannot be made on the basis of sonographic findings. Only mammography can demonstrate the typical calcification associated with carcinoma in situ. Presently, mammography is the only modality suitable for the early detection of breast cancer, comparable in importance to the cytological screening of preinvasive cervical carcinoma.

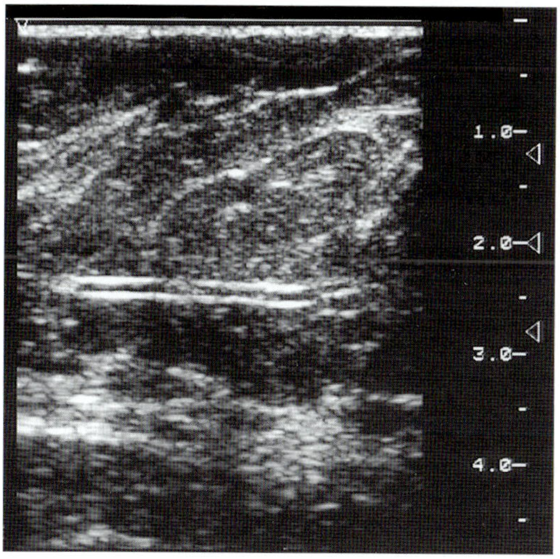

a

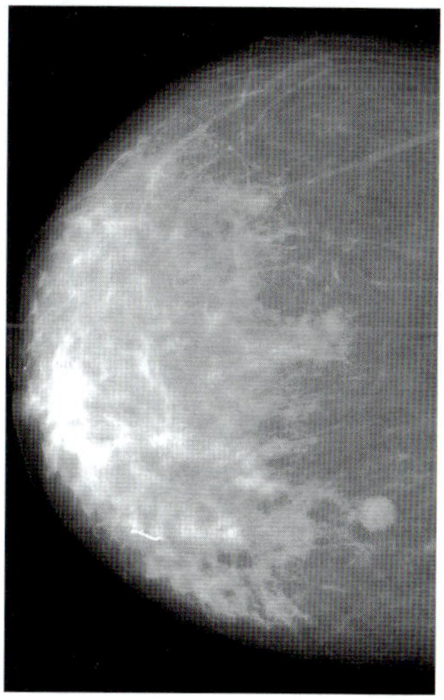

b

Fig. 3.**3 a, b** Calcifications.**a**Sonographic appearance of a calcified vein wall. **b** Corresponding mammogram of the calcific structures, which are seen most clearly in the upper quadrants. A lower-quadrant cyst is also visible.

4 Practical Guidelines for Performing Breast Ultrasound

Procedure

The initial equipment settings are selected (Chapter 2), the patient's history is taken, and the breasts are palpated in a warm and well-lit examination room. With the head of the couch tilted slightly upward, the patient lies supine with her arms folded behind her head. This position flattens the breasts against the chest wall and shortens the acoustic path length, thus increasing the amount of energy returned from the tissues and improving the image quality. In this position, the female breast has the approximate shape of a symmetrical cone, making it easier to conduct a systematic examination.

To improve sound transmission into the patient, acoustic gel is applied to the skin of the breast to be examined. This eliminates any air pockets between the transducer and skin that could reflect the sound waves back and keep them from reaching deeper tissues. A generous amount should be used so that the examination will not have to be interrupted to apply more gel. Figure 4.**1** shows the effect of poor acoustic coupling caused by insufficient gel between the skin and transducer. The room should be darkened to eliminate troublesome screen reflections and create optimal conditions for perceiving image details.

The transducer is held perpendicular to the skin (Fig. 4.**2**). This shortens the sound

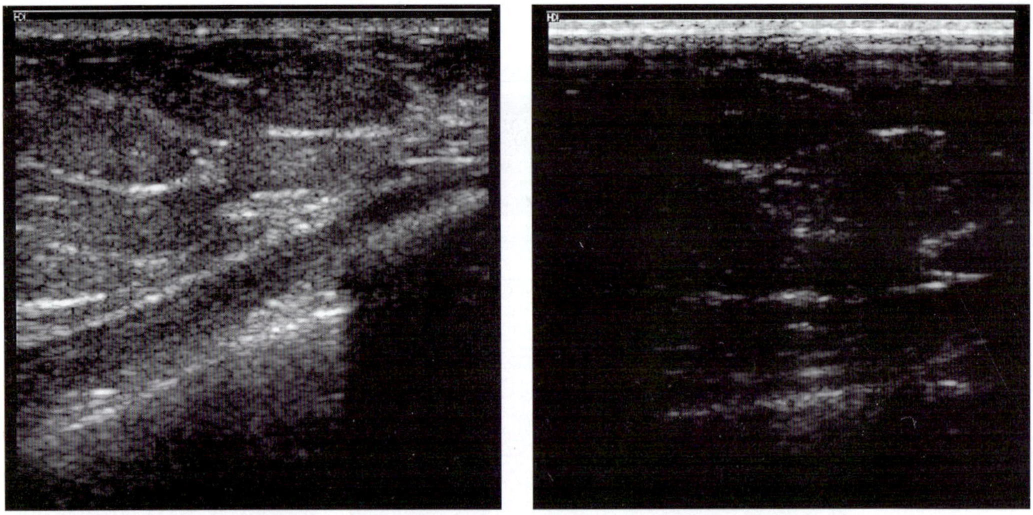

a b

Fig. 4.**1 a, b** Effect of acoustic gel on ultrasound image quality.**a** An adequate amount of gel provides good acoustic coupling and good definition of deep echoes, as it allows the sound waves to reach deeper tissues with sufficient energy. **b** With the transducer in the same position but coupled with insufficient gel, most of the sound is immediately reflected by an air pocket on the skin, so that little energy is able to penetrate to deeper levels.

Fig. 4.2 Transducer positioned at the correct 90° angle relative to the skin surface.

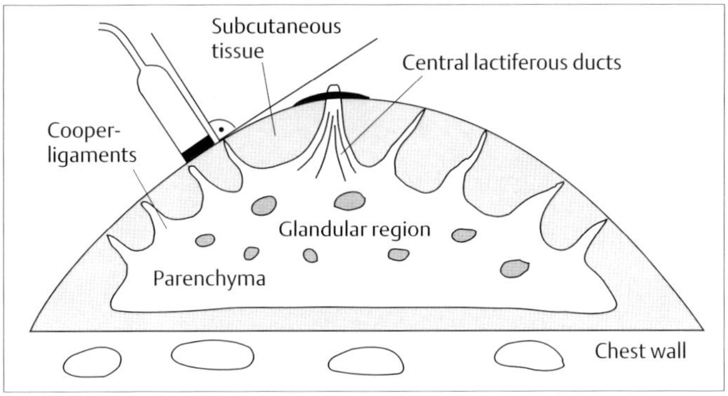

path through the tissues and reduces sound absorption, again resulting in a better image. Figure 4.**3** illustrates the effect of transducer angle on image quality.

The focal zones are adjusted to produce a sharp image encompassing the full thickness of the glandular tissue. If the glandular tissue is so thick that areas near the chest wall are poorly imaged even at the highest power setting, the focal zone can be restricted to a single focal point placed at the deep border of the breast parenchyma (Fig. 4.**4**). The number of focal zones should also be reduced if image generation becomes too slow (reduced frame rate).

The recommendations given on p. 8 should be followed in adjusting the time gain compensation (TGC). By keeping the left hand on the TGC controls at all times during imaging, the operator can respond at once to changes in slice thickness and echogenicity.

The selected image size should be sufficient to permit all breast structures from the skin to the chest wall to be evaluated (Fig. 4.**5**). Otherwise, lesions that are small or located near the chest wall may be missed.

In our laboratory at the University of Heidelberg, the examination is started by placing the transducer below the inframammary crease and scanning in a lateral-to-medial direction. The transducer is then moved upward by half its own width, and the breast is scanned from medially to later-

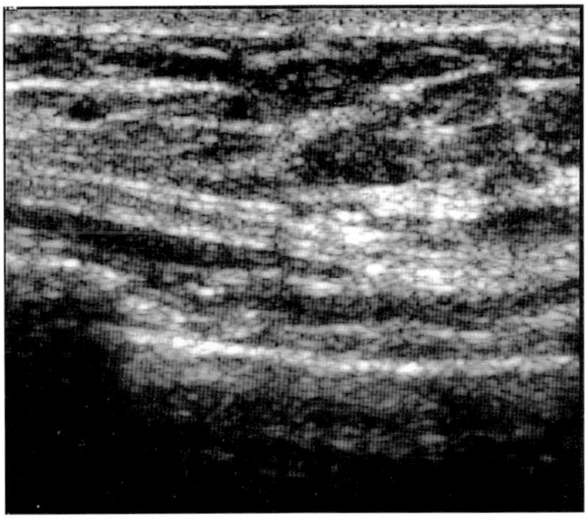
a

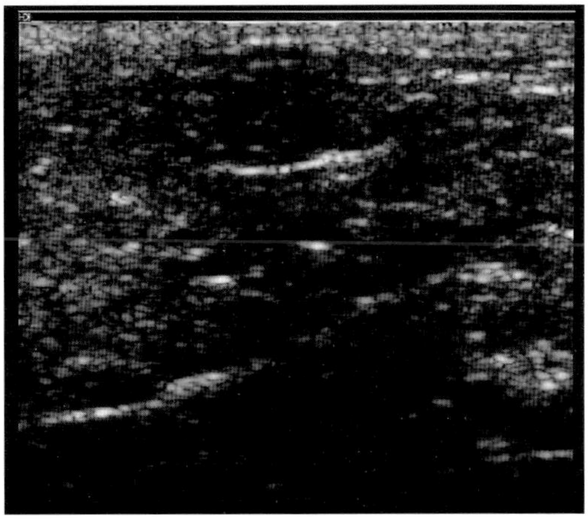
b

Fig. 4.**3 a, b** Effect of transducer orientation on image quality. **a** With the transducer oriented at the correct 90° angle, the sound waves traverse the glandular tissue on the shortest path. Sound absorption is minimal. **b** When the transducer is held at an oblique angle at the same site, image quality is poor.

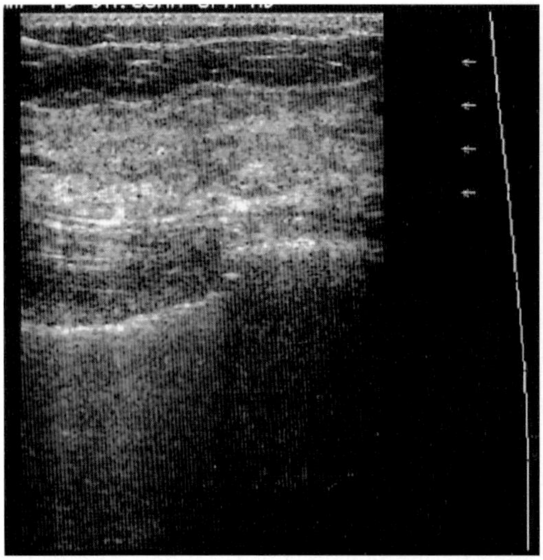
a

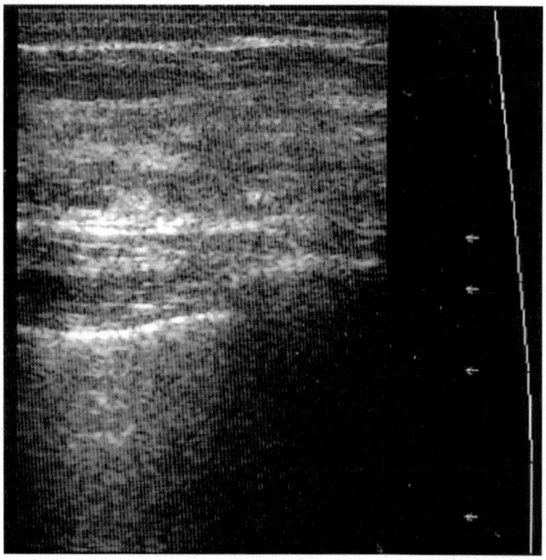
b

Fig. 4.4 a, b Effect of focal zone placement on image quality. a The focal zones have been placed within the region of interest, providing good general definition of anatomical detail. b With the transducer in the same position, the focal point has been moved deeper, causing the anatomical detail to appear less sharp.

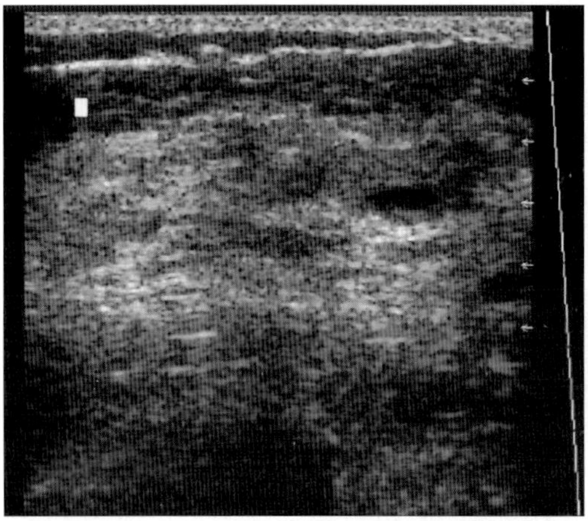
a

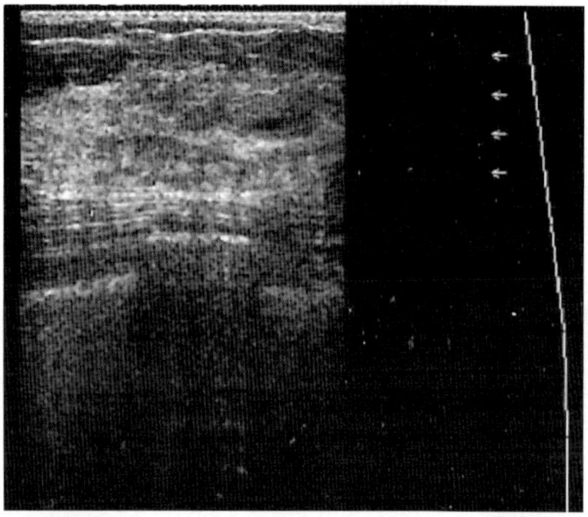
b

Fig. 4.5 a, b Effect of selected image size on the depiction of anatomical structures. a With optimum selection of the image size, all structural details of the subcutaneous, mammary, and retromammary tissue layers can be satisfactorily evaluated. b A smaller image size has been selected without moving the transducer. The air-filled chest occupies half the image, and the mammary layer appears too small. It is difficult to evaluate anatomic detail.

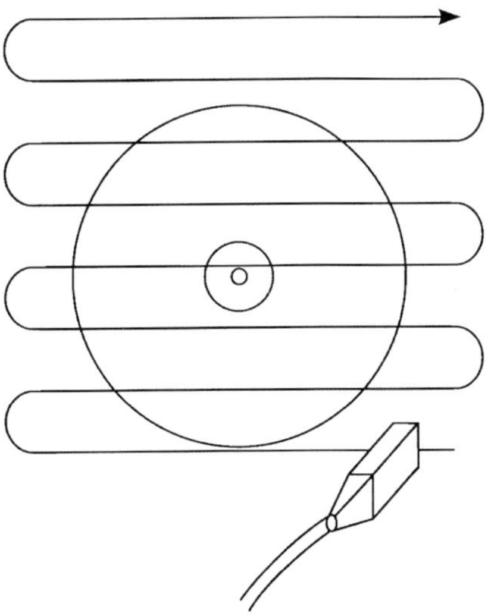

Fig. 4.6 A meandering transducer pattern provides complete ultrasound coverage of the breast.

ally. This overlapping scan pattern is continued up to the level of the clavicle (Fig. 4.**6**).

Next, the subareolar region is examined by angling the transducer (Figs. 4.**7**, 4.**8**) or by pushing the nipple slightly to one side. This part of the examination is important, since in 31 % of cases a second retroareolar cancer will accompany a carcinoma that is detected in one of the other breast quadrants (Tulusan 1993). If the transducer is held perpendicularly, almost all of the sub-

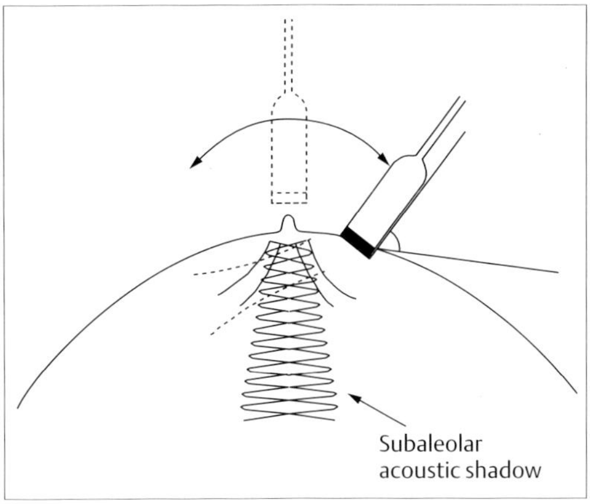

Fig. 4.7 Diagram of the subareolar shadow and the transducer angle used for scanning the subareolar region.

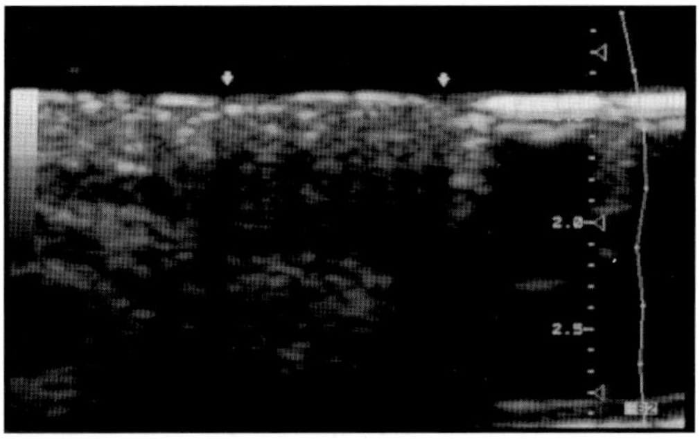

Fig. 4.**8** Sonographic appearance of the nipple. An offset is used to define the surface of this structure more clearly. The edges of the nipple are marked with arrows.

areolar region is obscured by shadows (Fig. 4.**9**). It has been theorized that this shadowing is caused by strong scattering of the sound waves by central ducts that are oriented parallel to the beam and by surrounding fibrous and fatty tissues. As the sound waves impinge on these acoustically mismatched structures at an acute angle, a highly reflective interface is created that keeps the energy from penetrating to deeper levels (Teubner et al. 1983).

Next, the transducer is moved in a circular path around the areola to image the central ducts in longitudinal section (Fig. 4.**10**). This aids in the detection of intraductal echoes.

Transducer pressure can be applied to the breast tissue both to improve image quality and to evaluate the compressibility of breast masses (Fig. 4.**11**). Compression can improve resolution at deeper levels by shortening the sound path and thus reducing energy losses (Teubner et al. 1985a, b).

Gentle transducer pressure is also helpful for checking the integrity of the Cooper ligaments. Ligaments not involved by tumor will show a springy recoil when local pressure is applied and then released.

Frequently, the Cooper ligaments cast acoustic shadows (Fig. 4.**12a**) that disappear when the breast tissue is compressed (Fig. 4.**12b**). The shadows from uncompressed ligaments result from the total reflection (Snellius' law) of sound that impinges on the ligaments at a shallow angle (Teub-

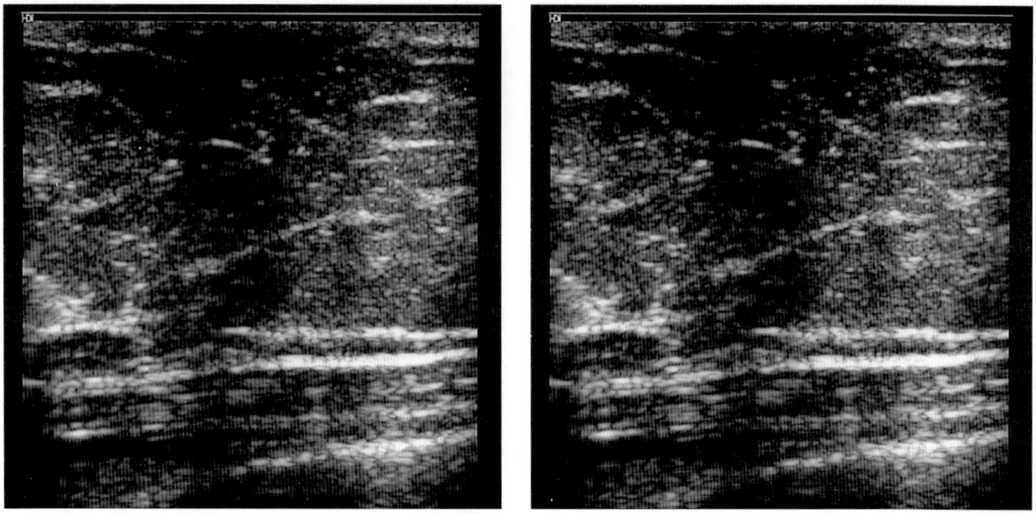

a b

Fig. 4.**9 a, b** Sonographic appearance of the subareolar shadow. **a** This scan plane does not permit evaluation of the subareolar region. **b** The subareolar image is improved by angling the transducer and increasing the gain setting.

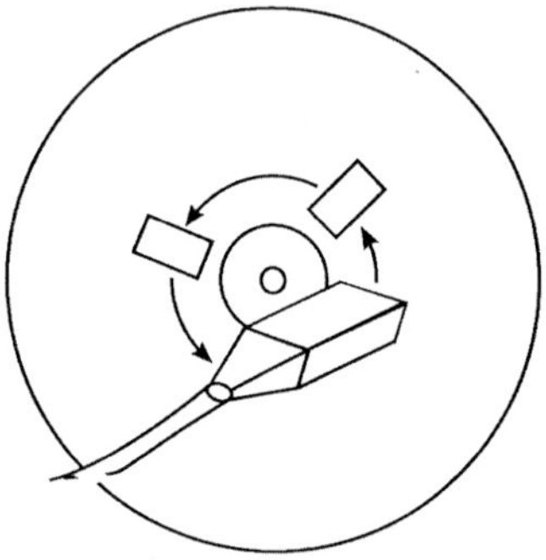

Fig. 4.**10** Scanning in a radial pattern around the areola provides a long-axis view of all the central lactiferous ducts, and may define intraductal structures.

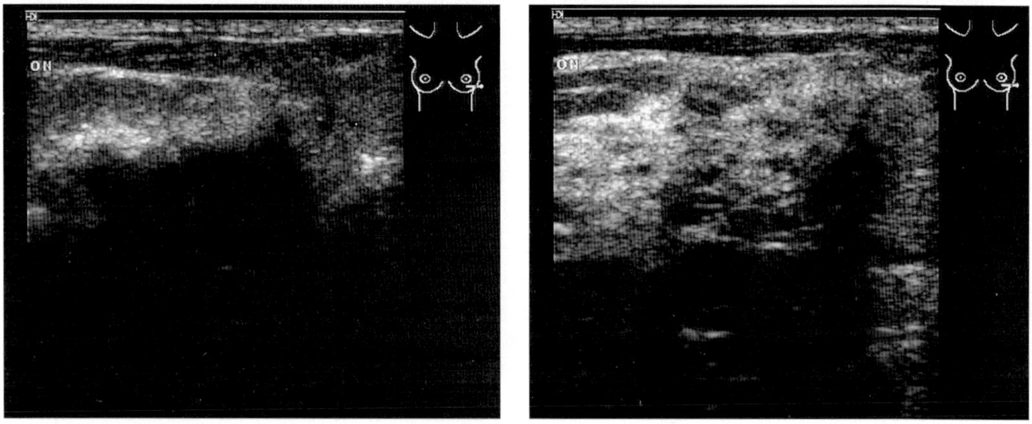

a b

Fig. 4.**11 a, b** Effect of transducer pressure on image quality. **a** When pressure is not applied, the breast tissue is difficult to evaluate. Acoustic shadows obscure much of the glandular region. **b** When pressure is applied to the transducer, the breast tissue can be evaluated.

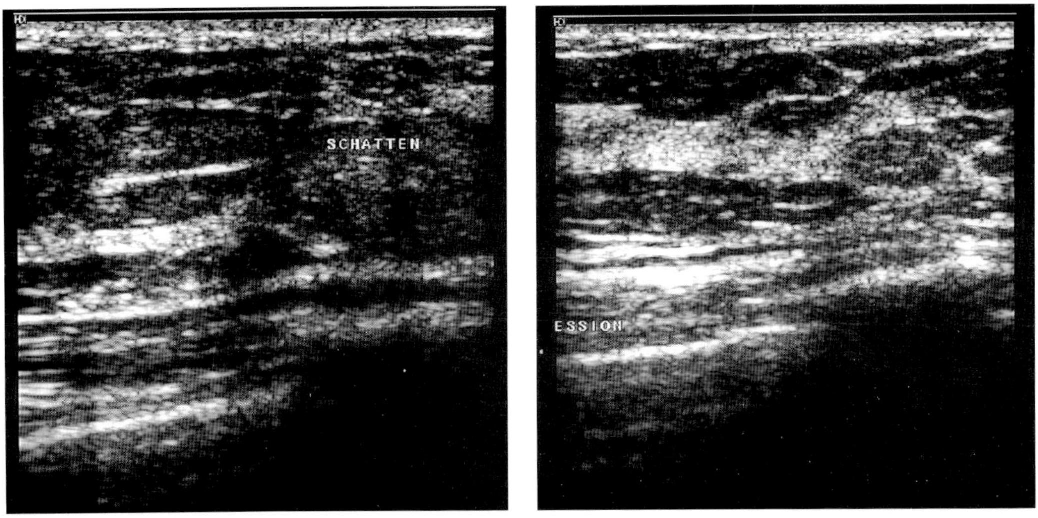

a b

Fig. 4.12 a, b Posterior shadowing from the Cooper ligaments. **a** Acoustic shadows appear behind several subcutaneous Cooper ligaments. They are caused by the total reflection of ultrasound that encounters these structures at a certain angle. **b** Applying transducer pressure alters the angle of the Cooper ligaments relative to the beam, and the shadows disappear (although slight attenuation is still seen).

ner et al. 1983). Compression alters the beam-ligament angle, so the shadows disappear.

Any circumscribed mass that is detected by the meandering or other scanning protocol should be examined in multiple planes by angling and repositioning the transducer as needed. This will provide the examiner with a three-dimensional mental picture of the breast mass. Typical sonographic criteria for benign/malignant differentiation may be visible only in certain planes, or a

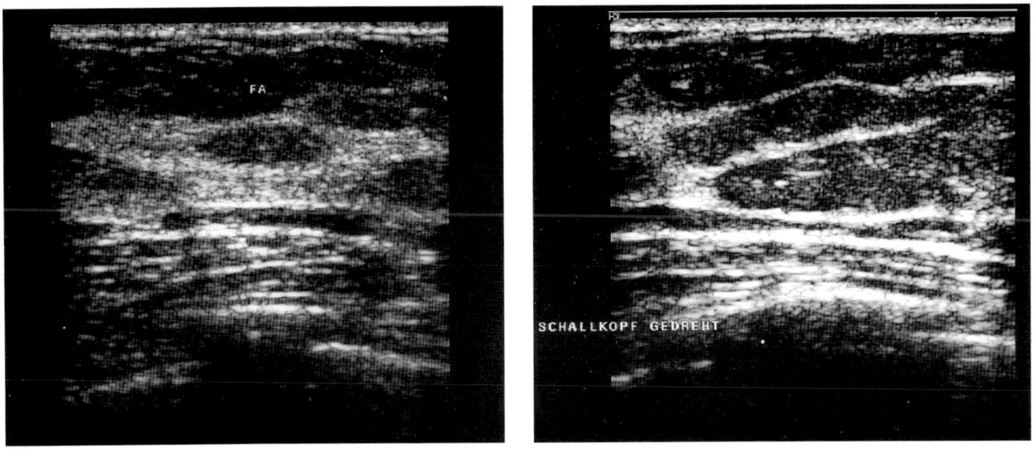

a b

Fig. 4.13 a, b Sonographic appearance of a fat lobule in a partially involuted breast. **a** This structure could be mistaken for a fibroadenoma on this image plane. **b** When the transducer is rotated 90°, the continuity of the structure with the rest of the fatty tissue becomes apparent. This technique is useful for excluding a fibroadenoma or other circumscribed lesion.

presumed focal lesion may be identified as a mammary lobe or fat lobule when imaged in cross section (Fig. 4.**13**).

For completeness, the examination should then proceed to the axilla (Chapter 11).

The examiner may elect to repeat the meandering scan pattern, this time starting at the top of the breast and working downward and scanning at right angles to the initial planes.

A complete bilateral breast ultrasound examination should always include both breasts and both axillae.

Our protocol, which is based on patterns of disease seen in cytological preparations, is not the only option. Madjar et al. (1991), for example, recommend diagonal scanning patterns. Stavros et al. (1995) recommend systematic evaluation of the breast using radial and antiradial scanning techniques in a clockwise fashion. Whatever technique is used, it is essential to ensure that any particular scanning pattern provides complete coverage of the intramammary and axillary tissues.

5 Sonographic Anatomy of the Female Breast and Changes with Aging

Since pathological changes alter normal breast anatomy, it is essential for the examiner to be familiar with and able to recognize normal anatomy (Fig. 5.**1**).

Normal Anatomy

The glandular tissue of the breast (the breast parenchyma or glandular region) is a cone-shaped region situated around the nipple, with a superolateral extension to the axilla (the axillary tail). As a result, most of the glandular tissue is located in the upper outer quadrant of the breast. The relative proportions of glandular and fatty tissue in the breast change with age (see below). The breast parenchyma consists of 15–20 mammary lobes, each of which is connected to the nipple by a lactiferous duct. The lobes are separated from one another by interlobar connective tissue. Just before entering the nipple, each of the 15–20 main ducts expands into a dilated segment called the lactiferous sinus. Each lobe consists of 30–80 lobules, which contain the milk-producing elements of the breast. The lobules in turn are composed of 20–40 terminal units or acini, which are surrounded by hormonally responsive intralobular connective tissue.

Between the skin and glandular tissue of the breast is a layer of subcutaneous fat of variable thickness. The fat is permeated and supported by connective tissue septa. A thin fascia forms the boundary between the fat and glandular tissue. The Cooper ligaments are strands of connective tissue that traverse the breast parenchyma from the pectoral fascia to the skin, forming a mechanical connection between these structures and the glandular tissue. Lesions of the breast parenchyma can cause dimpling of the skin through traction on the Cooper ligaments or through carcinomatous or inflammatory infiltration of the ligaments. Interposed between the glandular tissue and the pectoral muscle fascia is a thin layer of retromammary fat that allows the breast parenchyma to move relative to the chest wall. Infiltration of this layer causes deep carcinomas to become fixed to the pectoral fascia.

At about 20–30 years of age, initial involutional changes occur as the parenchyma of the breast is replaced by fatty and connective tissue. Changes occur in the shape and consistency of the breast. Starting at about age 30, the connective tissue of the breast becomes relatively less abundant, while the proportion of fatty tissue increases. The fat content of the breast decreases after menopause. These processes occur at different rates in different individuals. Hyalinization of the residual connective tissue (regression) combined with an increased proliferation of hormonally responsive epithelial and mesenchymal components of the glandular tissue lead to the various forms of "fibrocystic change" (Chapter 7). These changes are attributable to a progesterone deficit caused by the more frequent occurrence of anovulatory cycles after age 35, leading to a state of estrogen dominance (Feldmann and Schindler 1995).

Normal Sonographic Anatomy

A good ultrasound unit will depict and clearly differentiate all the *layers of the breast* (Fig. 5.**1**) (Venta et al. 1994). These features are listed below in the order of

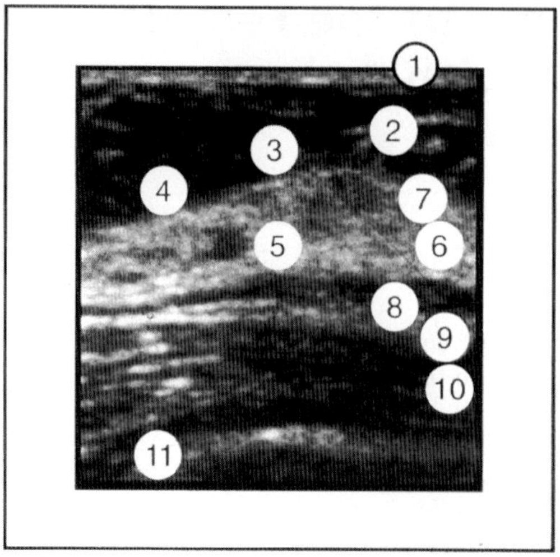

a

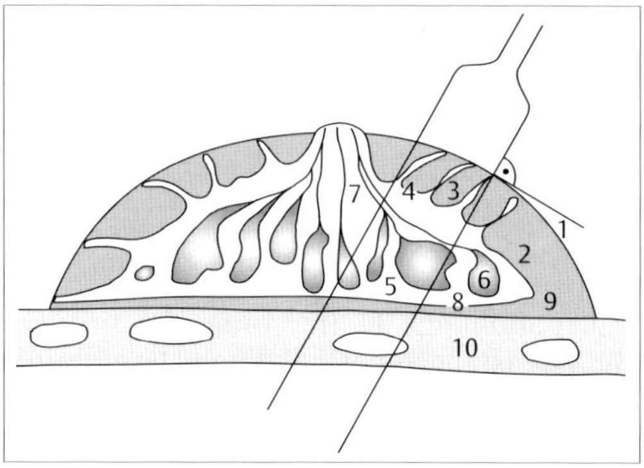

b

Fig. 5.**1 a, b** Normal sonographic anatomy. The numbers on the sonogram correspond to the numbered anatomical structures in the drawing. 1 Skin, 2 Subcutaneous fat, 3 Cooper ligaments, 4 Superficial fascia, 5 Glandular tissue, 6 Lobule, 7 Lactiferous ducts, 8 Deep fascia, 9 Retromammary fat, 10 Muscle and fascia, 11 Rib

their occurrence from the transducer to the chest wall:

1. The skin appears as an echogenic (bright) band immediately below the transducer.
2. The subcutaneous fat, traversed by:
3. The Cooper ligaments, which appear as a hypoechoic (dark) layer criss-crossed by bright lines that extend to the skin.
4. The superficial fascia covering the breast parenchyma forms a hyperechoic band separating the subcutaneous tissue from the mammary gland.
5. The structure of the breast parenchyma is reminiscent of a sponge with large pores.
6. The hypoechoic "pores" are the lobules, which must be clearly distinguishable from the surrounding breast tissue. The interlobar connective tissue has an echogenicity between that of the fascial layers and the fat.
7. The lactiferous ducts and particularly the subareolar lactiferous sinuses appear as narrow, hypoechoic channels traversing the "sponge" of the breast parenchyma.
8. The deep fascia appears as a thin echogenic band separating the glandular region from the chest wall.
9. The retromammary fat determines the mobility of the breast parenchyma on the pectoral fascia. It appears as a narrow, hypoechoic (dark) seam interposed between the breast parenchyma and the muscle fascia.
10. The pectoralis fascia is very echogenic. The pectoralis major muscle appears as a hypoechoic layer with an internal pattern of parallel linear echoes.
11. The rib surface appears as a broad, convex, echogenic stripe with posterior acoustic shadowing. If the breast parenchyma is thin, the rib may be visible as an elliptical structure with smooth margins. The ribs of older women have an echogenic center caused by internal calcification. The intercostal muscles appear as hypoechoic areas between the ribs.

The ribs should not be mistaken for breast masses if their relation to the muscle fascia is noted. Also, moving the transducer cephalad or caudad will demonstrate an adjacent "mass" of identical appearance.

Since the structure of the female breast changes with age, its sonographic appearance also changes during the life cycle.

Childhood

During childhood, the breast undergoes longitudinal growth like the rest of the body. Two to three years prior to menarche, the mammary gland visibly enlarges. The lobules gradually differentiate, and the ductal structures form an arborizing network. The breast parenchyma appears sonographically as a small island of retroareolar tissue. In cases of precocious puberty with concomitant thelarche, this parenchymal island is enlarged. The lobules are not yet fully formed and are not sonographically visible (Fig. 5.2). Ultrasound shows a homogeneous tissue of moderate echogenicity.

Adolescence

Development of the mammary lobules commences after menarche and continues until about 20 years of age. When menarche occurs, the lactiferous ducts enlarge within the surrounding connective tissue and replace most of the fatty tissue. The adolescent breast consists almost entirely of glandular tissue with very little fat. The lobules are not fully developed until the first ovulation occurs. At this stage the breast consists of 15–20 lobes surrounded and supported by interlobar connective tissue. Each lobe contains 30–80 lobules, which are separated by hormonally sensitive intralobar connective tissue.

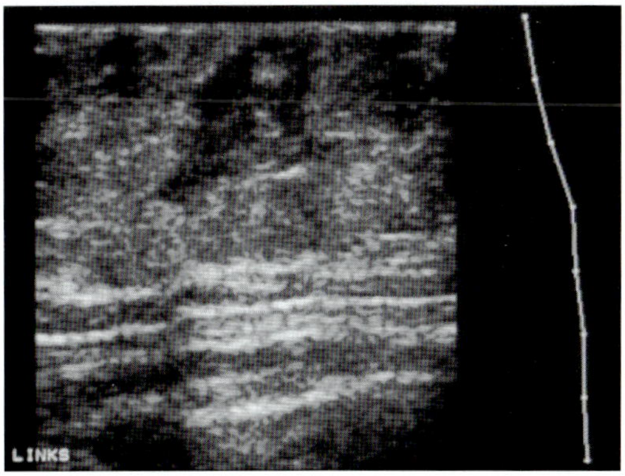

Fig. 5.2 Sonographic appearance of a juvenile breast at thelarche.

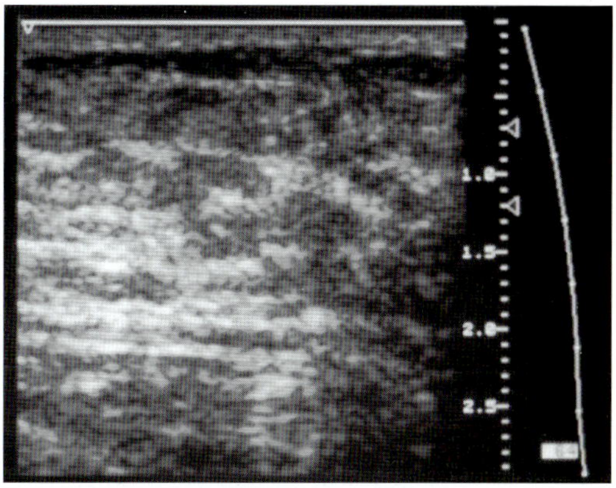

Fig. 5.3 Sonographic appearance of an adolescent breast at age 14.

Cysts may develop at an early age due to incomplete development of the terminal ductules. The excessive proliferation of intralobular connective tissue can lead to the development of fibroadenomas, which may regress spontaneously if less than 1 cm in size (Barth and Prechtel 1990).

Sonography shows a relatively echogenic, homogeneous glandular region in which the parenchyma and connective tissue are virtually indistinguishable. The subcutaneous and retromammary fat layers appear thin and hypoechoic. The supramammary fascia is strongly echogenic (Fig. 5.3). The prominence of this sonographic pattern varies from one individual to the next, however (e.g., in the width of the subcutaneous fat layer).

The adolescent breast is difficult to evaluate radiographically because of its high stromal content, so ultrasound is the preferred modality for investigating palpable breast masses in this age group (Barth and Prechtel 1990).

Sexual Maturity

Starting in the third decade of life, the interlobar connective tissue gradually regresses and is replaced by fat. The breast at sexual maturity is approximately 30 % fat, more than 50 % connective tissue, and 10 % to 35 % parenchyma (Barth and Prechtel 1990).

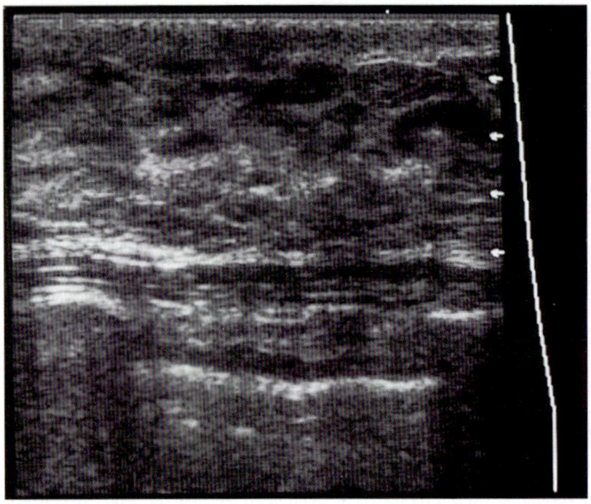

Fig. 5.**4** Sonographic appearance of the breast at sexual maturity.

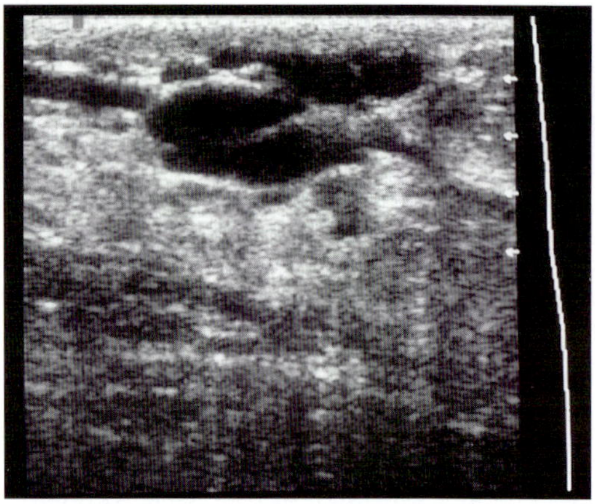

Fig. 5.**5** Lactiferous ducts showing central dilation and containing small, suspicious internal echoes (warranting further investigation or follow-up).

This change in the relative amounts of the various breast tissues can be demonstrated with ultrasound. Breast sonography in multiparous women commonly shows ectasia of the central lactiferous ducts (Figs. 5.**4,** 5.**5**).

Pregnancy

During pregnancy, the glandular parenchyma prepares for lactation. Almost all the connective tissue of the breast is replaced by glandular tissue. As gestation proceeds, the subcutaneous fat layer becomes thinner, while the ducts enlarge. These changes can be seen on breast sonograms in pregnancy (Fig. 5.**6**). Sonographic assessment of the breast tissues is difficult at this stage, however, due to the high fluid content of the breast, the heterogeneity of the tissues, and the generally thickened and enlarged glandular region.

Lactation

The ductal structures, notably the central ducts, are dilated during lactation. The fat content of the breast decreases in favor of lactating glandular tissue, so the subcutaneous fat layer is thinned. Just prior to nursing, the secretion-distended lobules are visible sonographically as cystlike hypoechoic structures. The lactating breast, like the breast in pregnancy, is difficult to evaluate with ultrasound. It may be helpful to reexamine the breast shortly after nursing, when the mammary layer is thinner and the structures traversed by the sound waves are less heterogeneous (less scattering, less juxtaposition of enhanced and attenuated areas; Fig. 5.**7**).

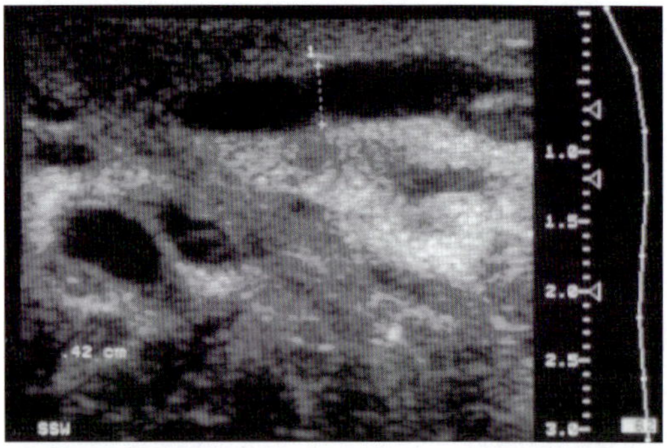

Fig. 5.**6** Sonographic appearance of the breast parenchyma in the 34th week of pregnancy. The ducts are dilated (to more than 4 mm in diameter), and glandular tissue has replaced much of the subcutaneous fat.

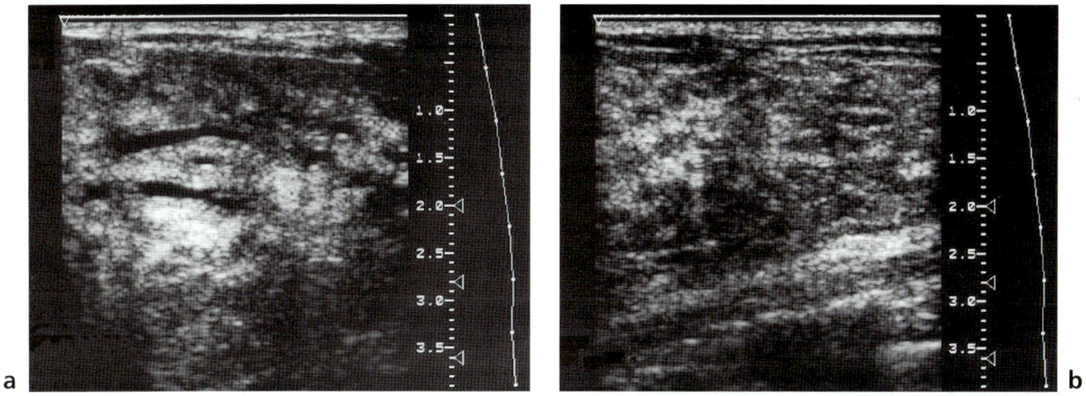

Fig. 5.**7** **a, b** Sonographic appearance of a lactating breast. **a** Note the thin subcutaneous fat layer and dilated lactiferous ducts. Enhancement behind these ducts alternates with areas of attenuation, making the sonogram difficult to interpret. **b** The breast tissue is easier to evaluate immediately after nursing. The normal sonographic anatomy of the glandular tissue is seen (see Fig. 5.**1**).

Perimenopause and Postmenopause

Since the majority of breast cancers are diagnosed in this age group, a knowledge of normal, age-appropriate sonographic changes is important so that asymptomatic cancers and other abnormalities can be recognized.

Starting at about *40 years of age*, the lobules and lobes atrophy and undergo fibrofatty replacement. The timing, rate, and extent of these changes vary in different individuals. The breast at age 40 is approximately 20 % fat, 60 % connective tissue, and 10 % to 35 % parenchyma (Barth and Prechtel 1990). At ultrasound, islands of residual parenchyma are clearly visible as small, hypoechoic "pores" within the dense (fibrotic), hyperechoic connective tissue. The Cooper ligaments are thickened. Interspersed among the parenchymal islands are connective tissue septa that still trace the outer boundaries of the former mammary lobes. A honeycomb-like pattern is produced (Fig. 5.**8**). The physiological hormonal alterations that occur at this age (persistent follicles) create an imbalance between regression and proliferation, leading to the development of small retention-type cysts. The cysts appear sonographically as round, smooth-bordered, hypoechoic to anechoic structures 5 to 10 mm in diameter within the hyperechoic connective tissue. Often they are too small to show posterior acoustic enhancement. Central dilations of the main ducts (up to 10 mm) are commonly seen, and are a normal age-related feature (Fig. 5.**9**) (Barth and Prechtel 1990). These changes are observed in all women, and are difficult to distinguish from fibrocystic change (Chapter 7).

By *50 years of age*, fat already makes up 40 % of the breast tissue, connective tissue up to 55 %, and parenchyma only 5 % to 20 %. There are still about 35 % of women in this age group who show an overall breast pattern comparable to that in women of reproductive age (Barth and Prechtel 1990).

Starting at about *60 years of age*, involution of the mammary lobules progresses rapidly. Fat and connective tissue each make up about 50 % of the breast tissue, which is less than 10 % parenchyma. Ductal cysts and papillomas reportedly occur in 50 % of women in this age group (Barth and Prechtel 1990) (Fig. 5.**10**).

By *80 years of age*, the breast parenchyma has disappeared completely in 71 % of women (Barth and Prechtel 1990), having been replaced by fat.

Involution may be classified as lipofibromatous (predominantly fat, Fig. 5.**11**) or fibrolipomatous (predominantly connective tissue, Fig. 5.**8**).

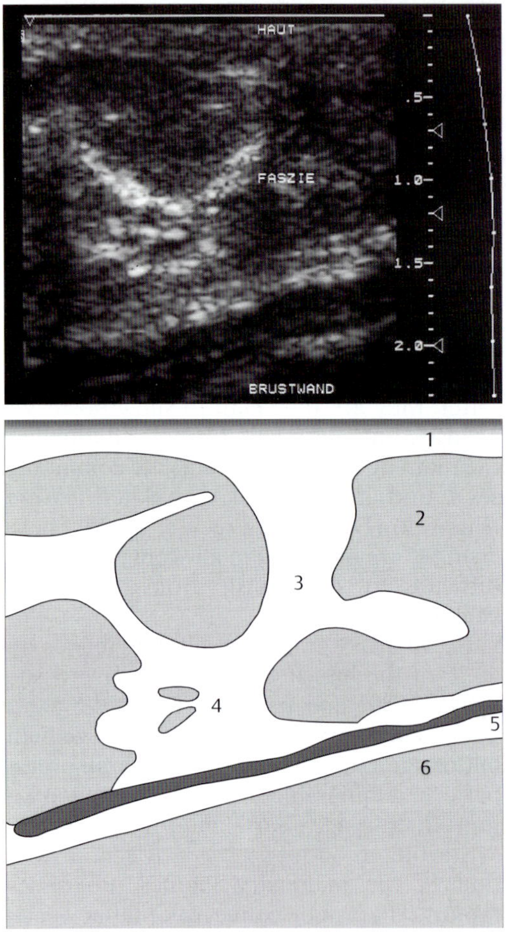

a

b

Fig. 5.**8 a, b** Markedly increased fat content is seen in this partially involuted breast. The superficial fascia and Cooper ligaments are broadened and hyperechoic as a result of hyalinization. **a** Sonographic appearance. **b** Schematic drawing. 1 Skin, 2 Subcutaneous fat, 3 Broadened, hyperechoic Cooper ligaments and fasciae, 4 Residual glandular tissue, 5 Thin fatty layer between the residual glandular tissue and pectoral fascia, 6 Chest wall

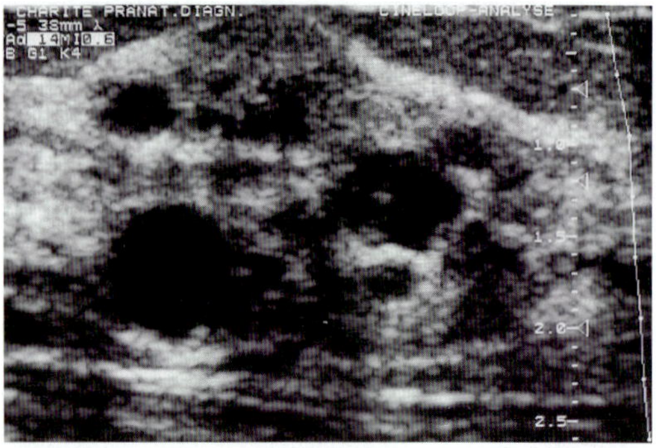

Fig. 5.**9** Dilated central ducts with terminal cysts. The cysts show anechoic centers, narrow borders, and posterior enhancement.

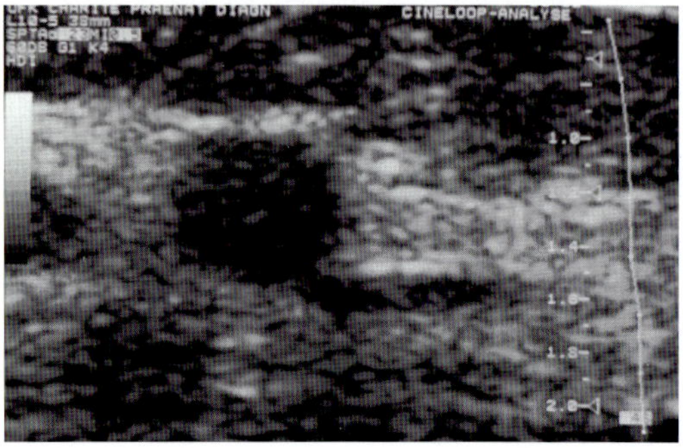

Fig. 5.**10** A cyst located at the end of a lactiferous duct.

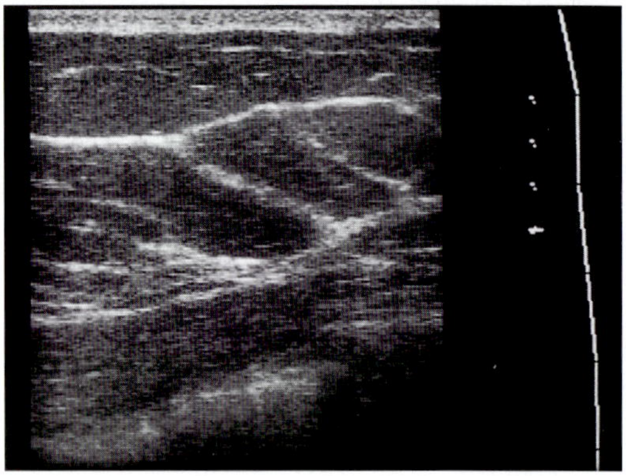

Fig. 5.**11** Lipomatous pattern of breast involution. The predominant tissue is fat (hypoechoic). A few connective tissue septa (hyperechoic) permeate the fatty tissue.

Effect of Drugs, Chromosome Abnormalities, and Morphological Defects on Sonographic Breast Anatomy

Hormone replacement delays involutional changes in the breast (Fig. 5.**12**). Serial mammograms in women on estrogen therapy may also show an increase in breast parenchyma (Barth and Prechtel 1990). About 35 % of perimenopausal women who benefit from hormone therapy have a high content of breast parenchyma, and the rest have about a 20 % content of parenchymal tissue (Barth and Prechtel 1990) – still sufficient to be responsive to hormonal stimulation.

Many women who start hormone replacement therapy complain of bilateral mastodynia. This is attributed to tension exerted on the proliferating lobules by the surrounding connective tissue, which has undergone age-related fibrosis. Ultrasound can exclude a focal lesion as a possible cause of the mastodynia. Local or systemic progestin therapy will improve complaints in many of these women.

Accessory breast tissue in an axillary location exhibits the same structure as ordinary breast tissue (Fig. 5.**13**). It first becomes noticeable as a result of enlargement during pregnancy. A history of axillary discomfort during lactation may direct attention to the anatomical cause of the sonographic finding.

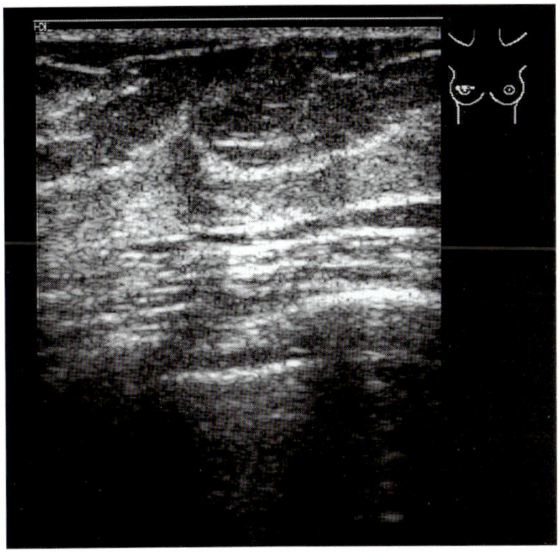

Fig. 5.**12** Sonographic appearance of a previously involuted breast, one year after the onset of hormone replacement therapy.

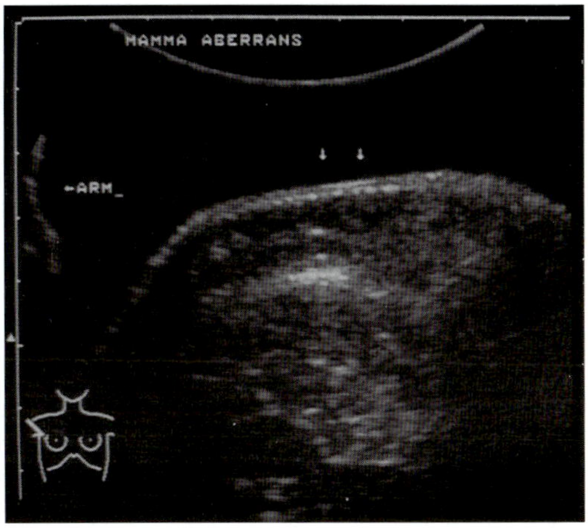

Fig. 5.**13** Accessory breast tissue in the axilla during lactation (5-MHz sector transducer with a fluid offset).

Patients on long-term immunosuppressant *corticoid therapy* show complete lipomatous breast involution after taking the medication for several years.

Patients with *Turner's syndrome* who have received hormone replacement therapy show an alteration in breast architecture (Fig. 5.**14**). Ultrasound does not show the typical lobar structure with surrounding fibrofatty tissues. Apparently the mammary lobes form only when a complete chromosome set is present (the type of sex chromosome is immaterial, as demonstrated by the normal architecture of the breast parenchyma in gynecomastia). The glandular tissue occupies a layer between the subcutaneous fat and pectoral fascia.

Gynecomastia

The glandular tissue in one or both male breasts may enlarge to several centimeters, or can reach the size of a fully developed female breast (Chapter 7). The enlarged

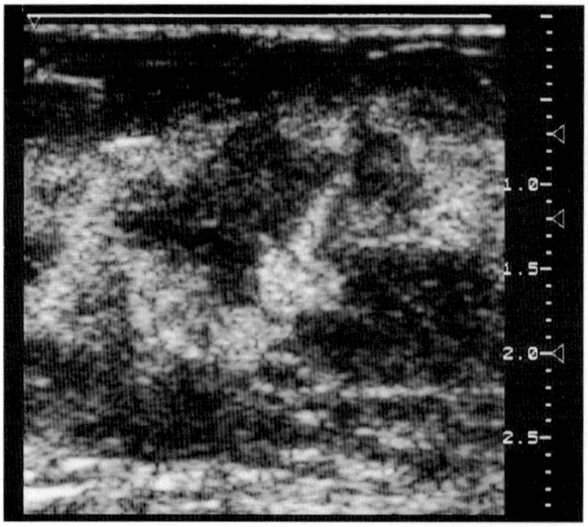

Fig. 5.**14** Breast sonogram in a woman with Turner's syndrome who had received hormone replacement therapy. The arrangement of the tissue layers-skin, fat, glandular tissue, thin fat layer, chest wall – is the same as in women with a complete chromosome set, but the sonographic appearance of the structures within the glandular layer is abnormal.

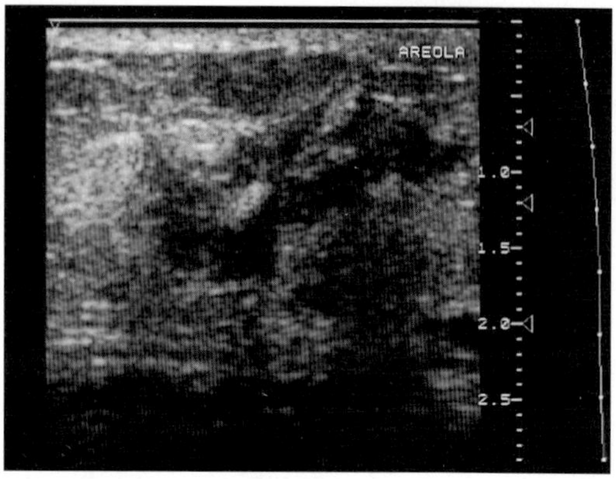

Fig. 5.**15** Gynecomastia. Subareolar ultrasound scan in a man who had taken tamoxifen for prostate cancer (without breast irradiation). The sonographic appearance of the breast is indistinguishable from that of a hormonally responsive female breast.

male breast is subject to all the diseases of the female breast, except those relating to pregnancy.

The sonographic appearance of gynecomastia is indistinguishable from that of a normal female breast. The breast ultrasound of young males usually demonstrates the sonographic features of juvenile mammary tissue (Fig. 5.**15**; cf. Fig. 5.**2**).

6 Sonographic Criteria for the Differential Diagnosis of Breast Masses

Ultrasound imaging of the breast has been improved in recent years by the advent of high-resolution scanners that provide a lateral resolution of 0.5 mm and up to 256 shades of gray (Anton et al. 1993, Konishi 1992, Madjar et al. 1991, Mendelson 1993).

Studies evaluating the sonographic differentiation of benign and malignant breast masses have either focused on establishing criteria for differentiation suggesting a benign or malignant nature (Hackelöer et al. 1986; Teubner et al. 1983, 1985) or, more recently, have started with a particular histological type of lesion and described its sonographic features (Teubner et al. 1993; Stavros et al. 1995). In practice, the radiologist interpreting breast images rarely works from known histological types, and usually has to rely on primary and secondary sonographic criteria in differentiating benign and malignant lesions (Hackelöer et al. 1986; Stavros et al. 1995). From a practical standpoint, it is best to start by evaluating each of these phenomena in the differentiation of focal sonographic lesions before considering how the various degrees and combinations of these criteria are manifested in association with specific histological entities.

Ultimately, the radiologist has to determine whether percutaneous biopsy or excision of a breast lesion is warranted on the basis of the sonographic findings. Thus, a knowledge of the ultrasound criteria that suggest malignancy, along with a knowledge of normal sonographic anatomy, is one of the most important examiner-dependent factors in breast ultrasound.

This chapter describes each of the acoustic phenomena that are associated with breast masses, and considers their predictive value for benign/malignant differentiation. They are the sonographic criteria for the differential diagnosis of breast masses. We address the key question of which criteria in high-resolution ultrasound are useful for evaluating the benign or malignant nature of breast masses, and which are not.

To answer this question, a study was conducted at the Department of Obstetrics and Gynecology of the Charité Hospital in Berlin, in which the preoperative ultrasound findings in 310 women were analyzed and compared with the postoperative histological findings (Blohmer et al. 1995b).

All ultrasound findings were evaluated prospectively on the basis of sonographic criteria known from the literature: central echogenicity of the breast mass, posterior acoustic phenomena, internal echoes, edge shadows, borders, axial orientation, compressibility, mobility, and architectural disruption.

The postoperative histological evaluation was then used to classify the focal lesions of the 310 patients into two groups (malignant and benign), whose characteristics are shown in Table 6.**1.** Ninety-seven of the 310 lesions were carcinomas (prevalence 31.3 %), 22 of which were larger than 2 cm.

The frequency of occurrence of each ultrasound parameter was determined retrospectively for each patient group. The odds ratio (OR) between the two groups is useful as a measure of diagnostic accuracy. The OR expresses the relative risk that a breast carcinoma is present when a certain ultrasound finding is observed.

Table 6.**2** shows the frequency of positive ultrasound findings in both patient groups and the calculated odds ratios. All the para-

Table 6.1 Postoperative histological and cytological diagnosis.

Focal lesion	Number of cases
Invasive ductal and lobular carcinoma	94
Mucinous or medullary carcinoma	3
Benign lesions	213
Fibrocystic change	148
Cysts	110
Fibrosis	38
Fibroadenomas	65
Total	310

meters except for internal echoes show statistically significant differences in the frequency of positive ultrasound findings between the benign and malignant groups.

Central Echogenicity

Definition

Focal lesions in breast ultrasound may be anechoic (black, Fig. 5.**9**), hypoechoic (gray, Fig. 6.**1**), or hyperechoic (white, Fig. 6.**2**). The lesions are detectable when their echogenicity contrasts with that of surrounding tissues, such as an anechoic cyst (Fig. 5.**9**) or hypoechoic carcinoma (Fig. 6.**1**) contrasting with the brighter echoes of the breast parenchyma, or a hyperechoic area of fibrosis (Fig. 6.**2**) contrasting with the lower-level echoes of surrounding fat. Hyperechoic lesions are sometimes described as hyperdense, and hypoechoic lesions as hypodense.

The echogenicity of the largest area of a focal lesion determines whether its center is described as anechoic, hypoechoic, or hyperechoic. For example, if hyperechoic regions are predominant over less echo-

Table 6.2 Frequency of the sonographic criteria for benign and malignant breast lesions and the calculated odds ratios.*

Parameter	Benign lesion	Breast carcinoma	Odds ratio (95 % confidence interval)
Hypoechoic	193/213 (90.6 %)	79/97 (81.4 %)	$p < 0.05$
Internal echoes	81/213 (38.0 %)	29/97 (29.9 %)	n.s.
Axial orientation (vertical or round)	100/213 (47.0 %)	77/97 (79.4 %)	$p < 0.001$
Borders	7/213 (3.3 %)	90/92 (92.8 %)	$p < 0.001$
No edge shadows	83/213 (39.9 %)	94/97 (96.6 %)	$p < 0.001$
Posterior attenuation	50/213 (23.5 %)	74/97 (76.3 %)	$p < 0.001$
Noncompressibility	63/213 (29.6 %)	90/97 (92.8 %)	$p < 0.001$
Architectural disruption	7/213 (3.3 %)	86/97 (88.7 %)	$p < 0.001$

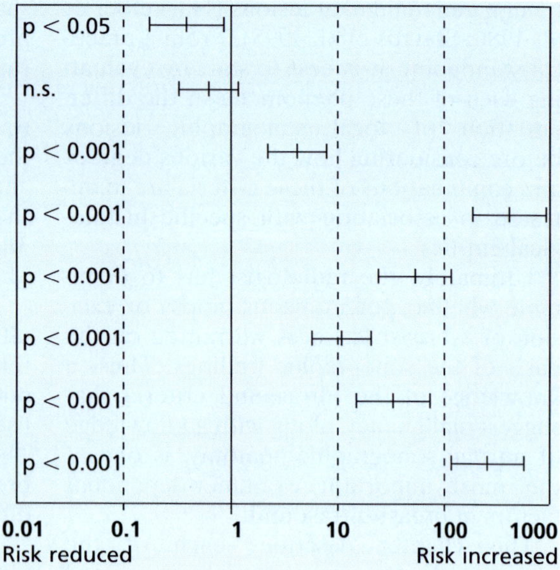

* Measure of the risk that a carcinoma is present when that sonographic criterion is observed.

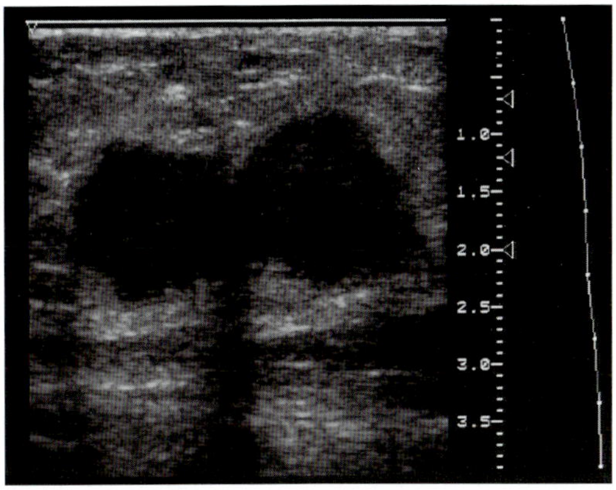

Fig. 6.**1** Sonographic appearance of a bifocal, cellular, invasive lobular breast carcinoma. Both foci are hypoechoic and have narrow but irregular borders. They show posterior enhancement and thin, bilateral edge shadows. In contrast to cysts, the lesions are not compressible and have a vertical orientation (see Fig. 8.**46**).

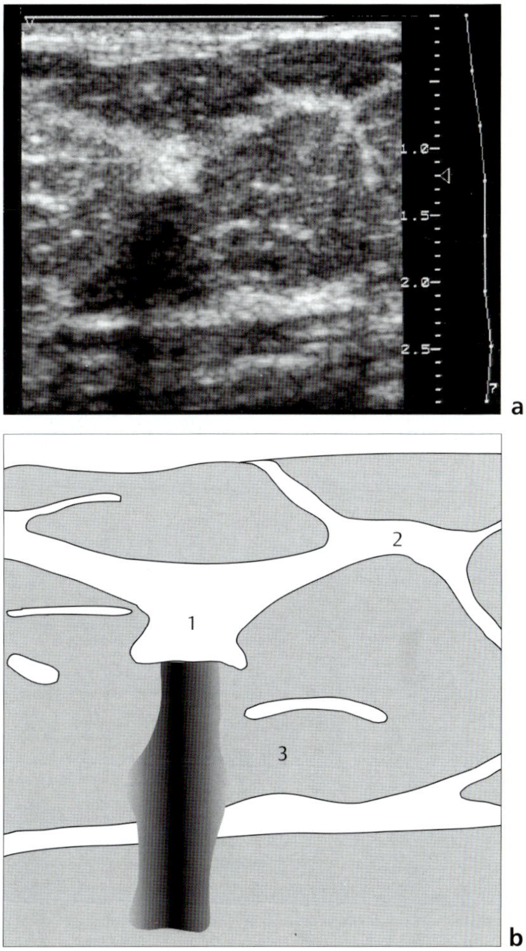

Fig. 6.**2a** Sonographic appearance of circumscribed fibrosis involving the connective tissue septa of a partially involuted breast. The architecture of the breast is unchanged. The fibrotic area is hyperechoic and shows posterior attenuation. **b** Corresponding diagram.
1 Fibrosis, 2 connective tissue septa, 3 posterior attenuation.

genic ones (Fig. 6.**3**), the lesion is classified as hyperechoic.

Usefulness in Differential Diagnosis

A mass that is hypoechoic relative to the breast parenchyma has an odds ratio (OR) of approximately 0.45 (Table 6.**2**), meaning that the risk of breast cancer as the cause of this finding is reduced by about 50 % when a hypoechoic lesion is found. Thus, low echogenicity is not a useful parameter for benign/malignant differentiation, and echogenicity in general is of little or no help in evaluating a breast mass. Most carcinomas, cysts, and fibroadenomas are hypoechoic or anechoic; circumscribed fibrosis and certain carcinomas are hyperechoic.

If the focal lesion is located at a depth of more than 3 cm in the (hyperechoic) glandular tissue, it is difficult to classify the lesion as definitely anechoic or hypoechoic.

The central echogenicity of a breast mass is helpful for locating the mass, however, since by definition the echogenicity of a non-isoechoic mass contrasts with that of the surrounding tissues.

Internal Echoes

Definition

Internal echoes are structures whose echogenicity contrasts with (and usually exceeds) that of the predominant echogenicity of the surrounding mass. Internal echoes may be coarse-textured or fine-a

b

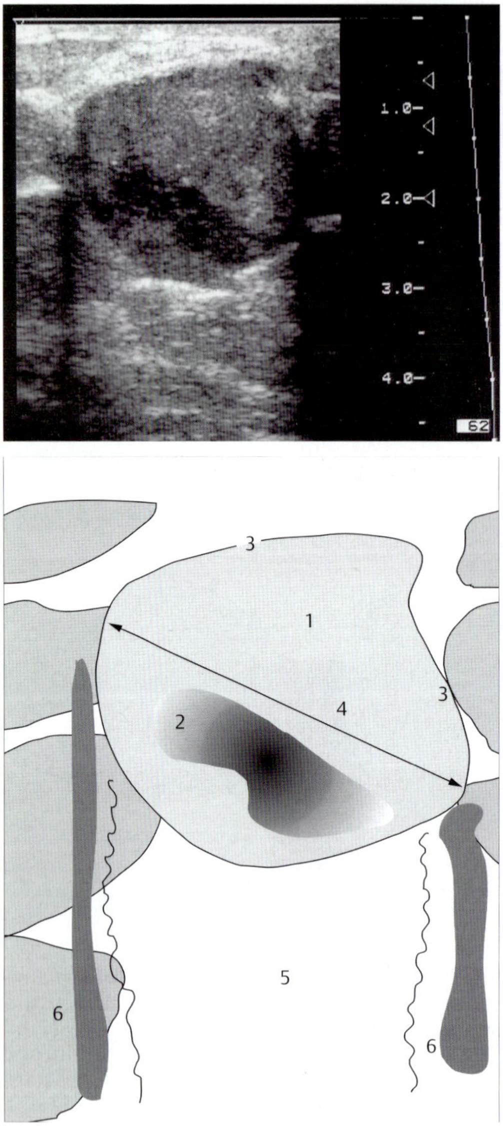

Fig. 6.**3a** Sonographic features of an intracystic papilloma with elements of invasive ductal carcinoma. The mass appears slightly hypoechoic to its surroundings (papilloma) and has an anechoic center (intracystic fluid). The borders are narrow and smooth, and the main axis of the mass is oriented transversely. Posterior enhancement and bilateral edge shadows are also seen. **b** Corresponding diagram.
1 Papilloma, 2 intracystic fluid, 3 border, 4 axial orientation, 5 posterior enhancement, 6 bilateral edge shadows.

textured, they may appear as a mural or papillary mass, or they may have a sediment-like appearance. Various internal echo patterns are illustrated in Fig. 5.**3** and Figs. 6.**3**–6.**8.**

Usefulness in Differential Diagnosis

It is not unusual to find relatively high-level internal echoes within hypoechoic breast masses. In the study in Table 6.**2,** for example, internal echoes were found in 81 of 213 patients with benign lesions and in 29 of 97 patients with breast carcinoma. When internal echoes are discovered, there is a slightly reduced risk that the lesion is malignant (OR 0.69). However, there is no significant difference between benign and malignant lesions in the occurrence of this feature.

Internal echoes, particularly in a small mass (< 1 cm), cannot be consistently identified when located deeper than 3 cm in the breast parenchyma due to excessive attenuation of the sound beam. Thus, the determination of whether internal echoes are present or absent cannot significantly advance the differential diagnosis.

The nature of the internal echoes may provide additional information, however. Fibroadenomas typically contain a fine network of high-level internal echoes (Fig. 6.**6**). Some cysts exhibit wall irregularities (Fig. 6.**5**). Intraductal lesions can be detected by ultrasound when they produce bright internal echoes within the lactiferous ducts (Fig. 6.**4**). Internal echoes appearing as a granular sediment may represent pus within an abscess (Fig. 6.**8**). Coarse internal echoes are suggestive of malignancy (Fig. 6.**7**).

Axial Orientation

Definition

The axial orientation of a mass in breast ultrasound refers to the alignment of the longest diameter of the mass in relation to the chest wall. Some researchers quantitate

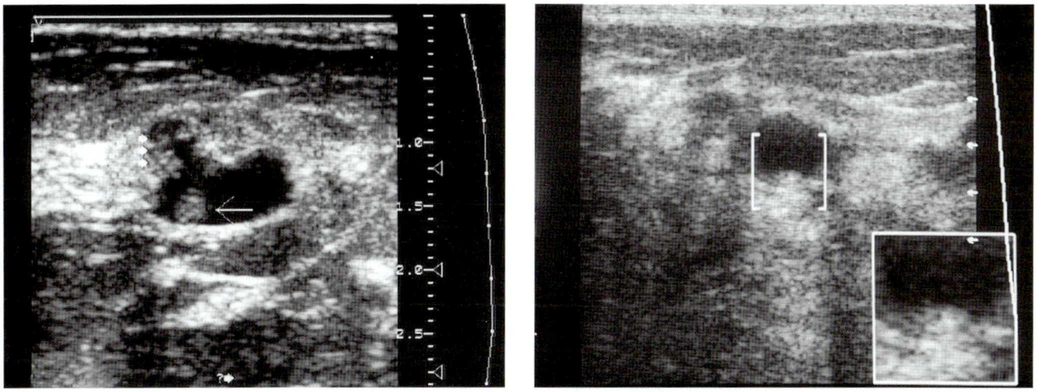

a b

Fig. 6.4a Sonographic appearance of an intracystic papillary carcinoma. The lesion is predominantly anechoic, and contains a coarse papillary mass (large arrow). Fine intraductal papillary projections (short, broad arrows) correlated histologically with sites of tumor invasion. **b** Appearance of a small, benign intracystic nodule.

this feature by calculating the L/T ratio, or the ratio of the longitudinal and transverse diameters. An L/T ratio less than 1 indicates a "taller than wide" or vertical tumor axis (Fornage et al. 1990, Leucht 1992, Radmann and Heinrich 1993).

Usefulness in Differential Diagnosis

After the interior appearance of the mass has been scrutinized, its orientation is assessed by noting the relation of its longest diameter to the chest wall. If the major axis is perpendicular to the chest wall (vertical orientation) or if the mass is round, the risk of carcinoma is increased by a factor of 4 (OR 4.4). Fibroadenomas, cysts, and medullary and mucinous (colloid) carcinomas typically show a transverse orientation.

Thus, a transverse orientation (parallel to the chest wall) is suggestive of a benign mass (Figs. 6.**5**, 6.**6**, 6.**8**), except for the rare instances of a mucinous or medullary carcinoma, which also tends to show a transverse alignment (see Figs. 8.**36,** 8.**37**).

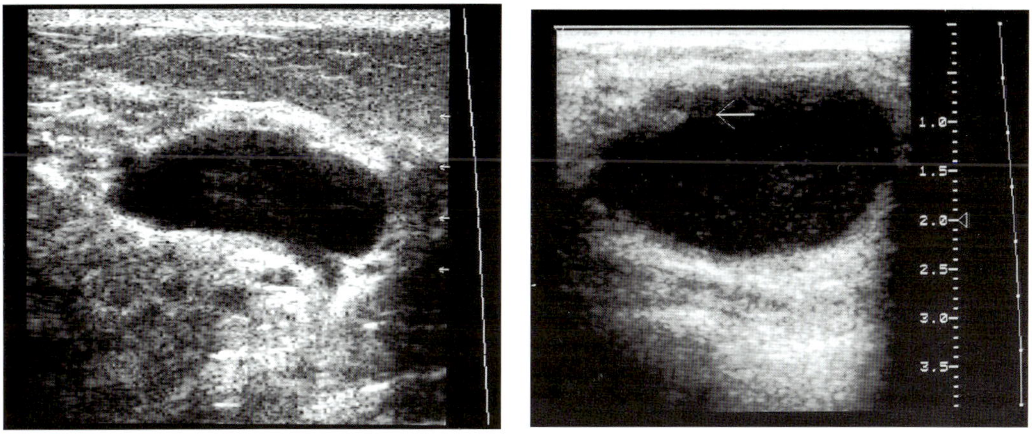

a b

Fig. 6.**5a** Typical sonographic appearance of a breast cyst. The cyst has an anechoic center and smooth, narrow borders. Its main axis is oriented transversely, and there is marked posterior enhancement. **b** The arrow marks a slight wall irregularity within the cyst.

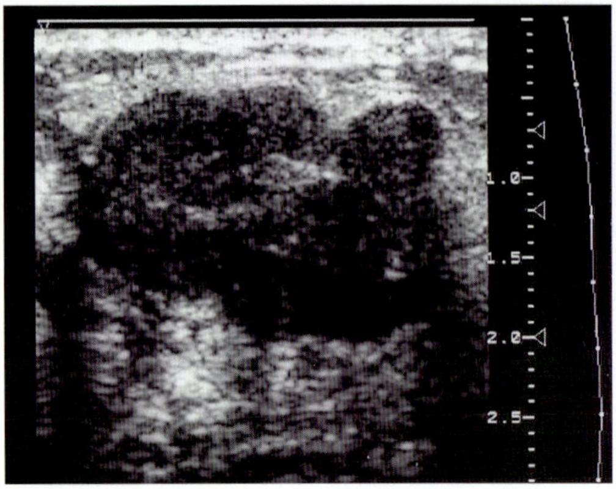

a

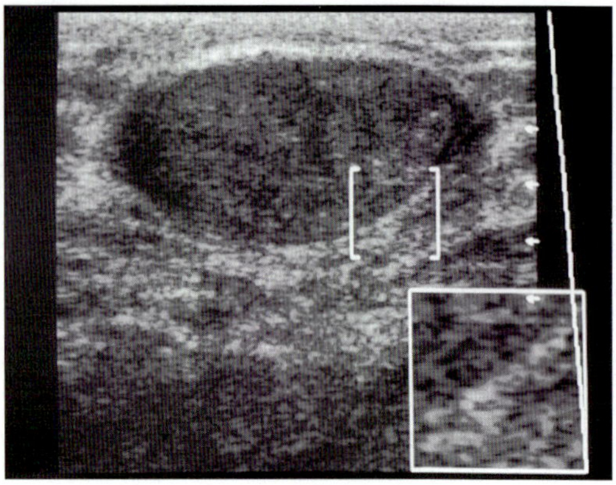

b

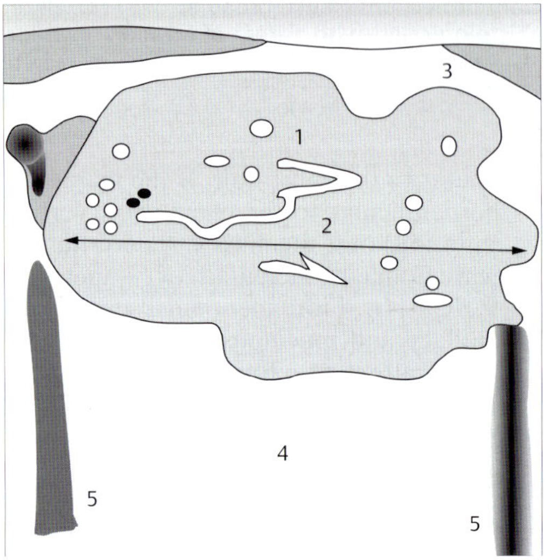

c

Fig. 6.**6a** Typical sonographic appearance of a fibroadenoma. The mass is hypoechoic, and contains fine internal echoes. Its main axis is oriented transversely, and its borders are narrow but not completely smooth. There are bilateral edge shadows and posterior enhancement.
b Corresponding diagram. 1 Internal echoes, 2 transverse tumor axis, 3 border, 4 posterior enhancement, 5 bilateral edge shadows. **c** Typical sonographic appearance of fibroadenoma.

A round or vertically oriented and "taller than wide" mass is strongly suggestive of carcinoma (Fig. 6.**9**). Exceptions are possible, of course (Fig. 6.**10**), but cancers with an atypical orientation will usually show other sonographic criteria of malignancy such as wide, jagged borders.

The axial orientation of small breast lesions (< 5 mm) cannot be evaluated. This criterion is therefore of limited value for the sonographic differential diagnosis of small focal lesions in the female breast.

It is noteworthy that Adler et al. (1991) could find no significant difference between carcinomas and benign solid masses in the ratio of length to anteroposterior diameter as determined by sonography.

Borders

Definition

The border of a mass is defined sonographically as the area that is located between the central core of the mass and the surrounding tissue and whose echogenicity contrasts with that of the mass and the surrounding region. An abrupt transition of echogenicity between the mass and surrounding tissue (signifying an abrupt change in impedance) results in a narrow border. This is typical of cysts, for example, where a low impedance in the fluid-filled interior of the cyst contrasts sharply with a high impedance in the surrounding breast parenchyma. With an invasive carcinoma, however, the tumor tissue and the surrounding edema or lymphocyte rim produce a more gradual transition to healthy surrounding tissue, resulting in a wide border.

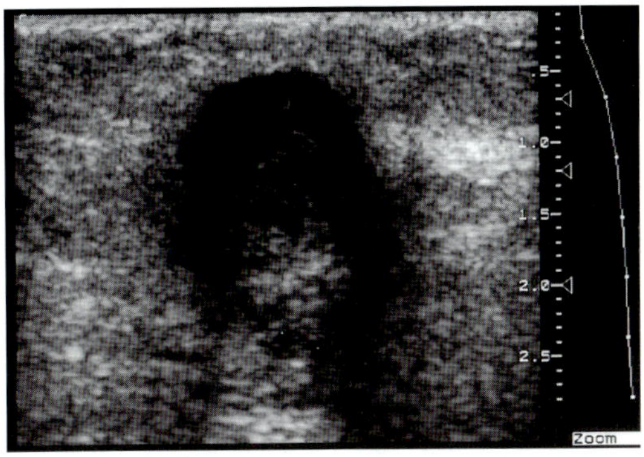

a

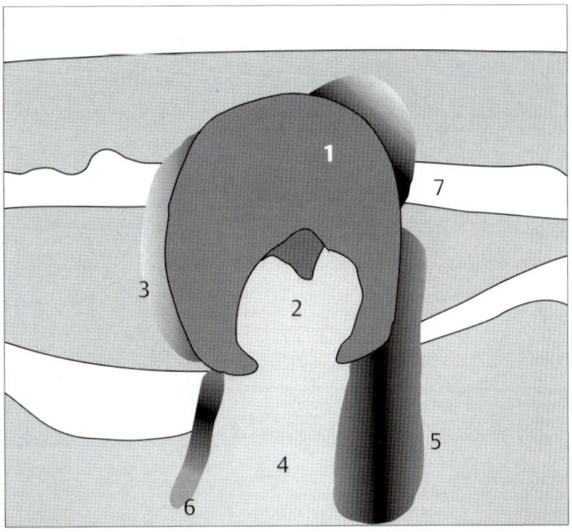

b

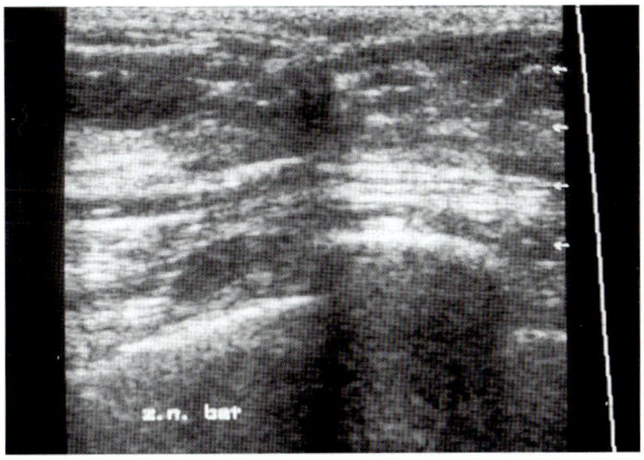

c

Fig. 6.**7a** Sonographic appearance of recurrent carcinoma in the axilla. The mass is hypoechoic and contains a nodular internal projection. Its borders are indistinct, and there is posterior enhancement deep to the mass. A very broad edge shadow appears on the right side and a straight, narrow edge shadow on the left. The mass disrupts the continuity of the superficial fascia. **b** Corresponding diagram. 1 Hypoechoic mass, 2 nodular internal mass, 3 ill-defined border, 4 faint posterior enhancement, 5 broad edge shadow, 6 narrow edge shadow, 7 disruption of superficial fascia. **c** Recurrence in the axillary tail after breast-conserving surgery for breast carcinoma.

Usefulness in Differential Diagnosis

After the interior appearance and orientation of a mass have been evaluated, attention is turned to the border, or the area between the center of the mass and the surrounding tissue. If the border is wide and irregular, the risk of malignancy is very high (odds ratio 378); this criterion was found in only 3.3 % of benign focal lesions vs. 93 % of breast carcinomas (Table 6.**2**).

Thus, the borders of a breast mass provide a very useful criterion for the sonographic differentiation of benign and malignant lesions. A smooth, narrow border is consistent with a benign lesion (Figs. 5.**5**, 6.**5**), while a wide, irregular border is a probable sign of malignancy (stage I scirrhous carcinoma, Fig. 6.**9**). Narrow but jagged borders may be seen with fibroadenoma (Fig. 6.**6**), an advanced or cellular carcinoma (Fig. 6.**10**), fibrosis (Fig. 6.**2**), or an abscess (Fig. 6.**8**).

Central echogenicity, internal echoes, axial orientation, and borders are among the *primary acoustic phenomena* that relate directly to the mass itself (Hackelöer et al. 1986).

Edge Shadows

Definition

Shadows emanating from the edges of a mass are among the *secondary acoustic phenomena* that may be observed deep to a focal lesion. Edge shadows are anechoic bands, visible in every plane of the lesion, that extend posteriorly (toward the chest wall) from the borders of the lesion (Fig. 6.**6**). Edge shadows may be unilateral, bilateral, broad (> 3 mm), or narrow

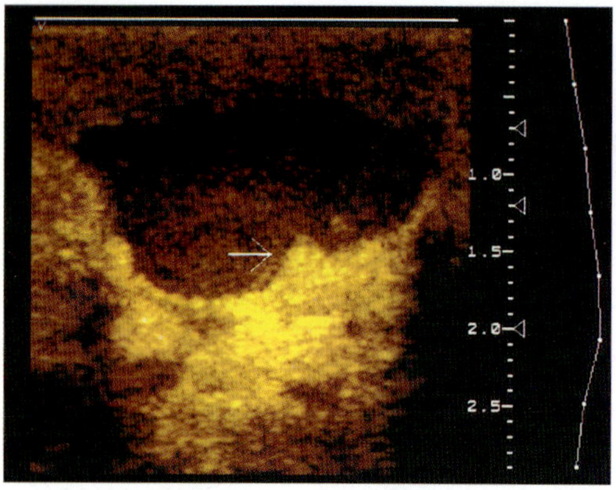

a

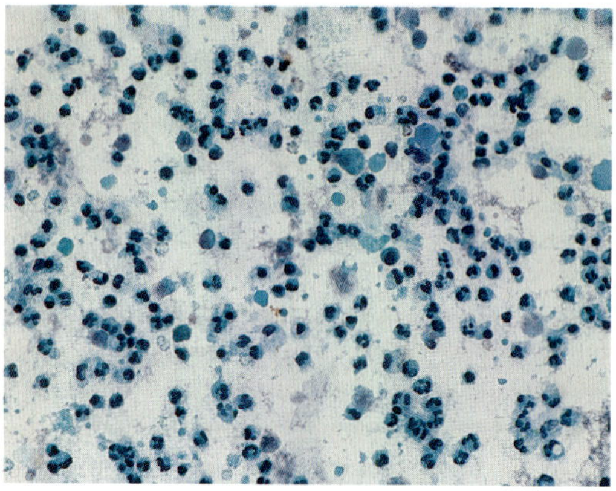

b

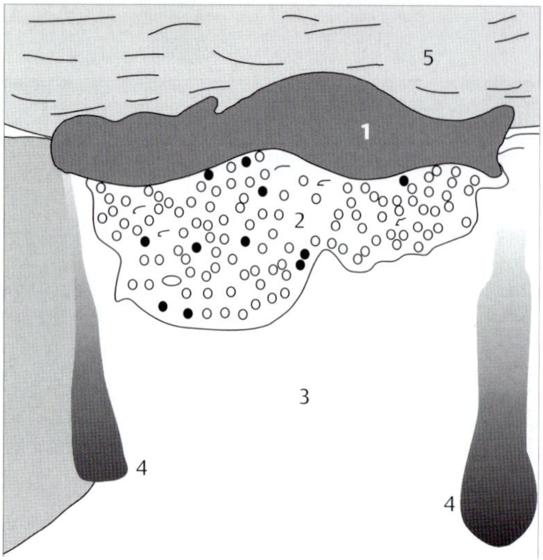

c

Fig. 6.**8a** Color B-mode image of an abscess in nonpuerperal mastitis. The borders of the abscess are narrow and irregular (arrow). Pus forms a finely granular, relatively echogenic layer inside the hypoechoic mass. There is posterior enhancement and bilateral edge shadowing. The skin shows inflammatory thickening. **b** Corresponding diagram. 1 Hypoechoic center of mass, 2 internal echoes, 3 posterior enhancement, 4 edge shadows, 5 thickened skin.
c Cytological examination of the abscess contents (Papanicolaou, 400 ×). Leukocytes dominate the cytological picture.

(< 3 mm). Their cause is not fully understood, but it presumably relates to the diffraction of sound waves encountering a change in acoustic impedance. The degree of diffraction is relatively constant at the smooth borders of benign masses (expansile growth) and their homogeneous contents (cysts, fibroadenomas), resulting in the formation of narrow, bilateral shadows.

Usefulness in Differential Diagnosis

If high-resolution sonography does *not* demonstrate *narrow* bilateral shadows deep to a mass, there is a markedly increased risk that histological examination will reveal carcinoma (odds ratio 49; Table 6.**2**). Thus, 97 % of the carcinomas (Fig. 6.**9**) and 39 % of the benign masses in the study were *not* associated with the narrow bilateral shadows that are typical of benign lesions (Figs. 6.**5**, 6.**6**). Carcinomas may be associated with broad edge shadows that are sometimes bilateral (Figs. 6.**1**, 6.**3**, 6.**7**). These effects are associated with cellular, spherical, or mucinous carcinomas, or with tumor recurrences, which often present with atypical sonographic features.

The phenomenon of edge shadowing is very useful for the differential diagnosis of focal sonographic lesions. Narrow, bilateral edge shadows are strongly suggestive of a benign lesion. If only a single, broad edge shadow is found, additional differentiating criteria should be applied.

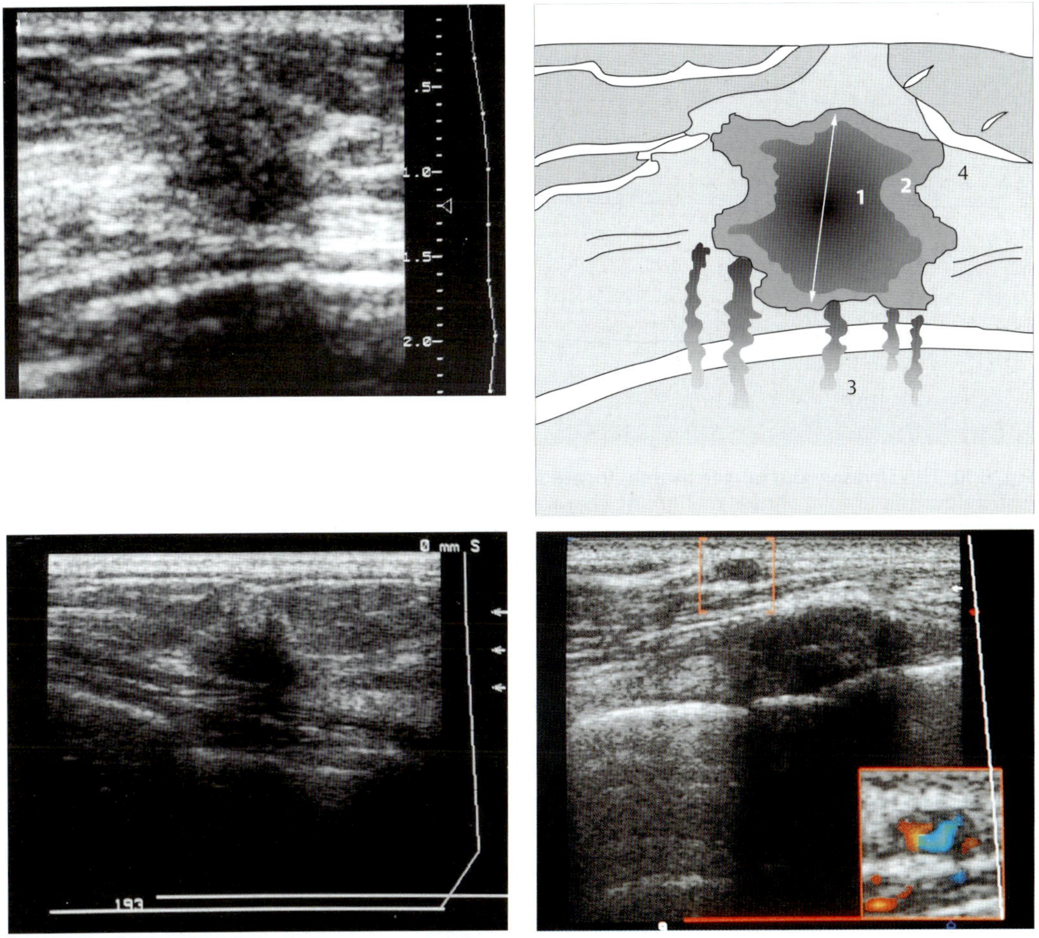

Fig. 6.9a Typical sonographic appearance of a scirrhous invasive ductal carcinoma. **b** Corresponding diagram. 1 Vertical orientation of mass; 2 wide, indistinct border; 3 diffuse posterior acoustic effects; 4 disruption of superficial fascia. **c** Breast carcinoma abutting the pectoral fascia. **d** A very small breast mass, identified as a carcinoma by its high blood flow.

Posterior Acoustic Phenomena

Definition

The phenomena of posterior acoustic enhancement (white area behind the structure of interest), acoustic attenuation (gray area behind the structure), and acoustic shadowing (black area behind the structure) are classified as secondary acoustic criteria, as they occur behind or deep to the mass lesion (Hackelöer et al. 1986). Posterior enhancement behind cysts and other structures is a relative phenomenon that is noted by comparison with areas that appear darker due to absorption, reflection, scattering, and other attenuating processes in the surrounding tissues. By contrast, sound waves that pass through a fluid-filled cyst lose very little energy to absorption and scattering, and the signals returned from this area of "increased through-transmission" are assigned correspondingly brighter gray-scale values in the sonographic image.

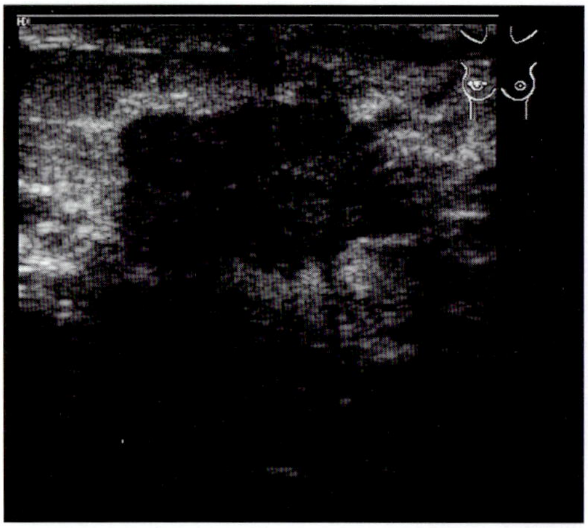

Fig. 6.**10** This invasive ductal carcinoma, located just below the areola, shows malignant characteristics similar to those in Fig. 6.**9**, except for its transverse orientation and lack of penetration of the superficial fascia. Nevertheless, architectural distortion is apparent in the altered course of the central duct (right side of image; see also Fig. 8.**48**).

Usefulness in Differential Diagnosis

The observation of acoustic attenuation or shadowing behind a mass is of little help in the differential diagnosis of focal sonographic lesions in any specific case, despite the fact that the odds ratio is 10 (Table 6.**2**) and the difference between groups is significant. Posterior attenuation or shadowing is typical of carcinomas (74 of 97 cases), but 50 of the 213 benign lesions in Table 6.**2** also displayed this feature.

Posterior enhancement is characteristic of large or superficial breast cysts (Fig. 6.**5**). Fibroadenomas may cause enhancement or attenuation (Fig. 6.**6**). Gerlach and Holzgreve (1993) note that heavy calcification in a fibroadenoma may produce a central shadow like that commonly seen with carcinomas. Enhancement can occur behind a breast abscess (Fig. 6.**8**), and attenuation can occur behind a circumscribed area of fibrosis (Fig. 6.**2**). Predominantly stromal (scirrhous) carcinomas typically cause posterior attenuation with a central shadow (Fig. 6.**11**), while other types of carcinoma

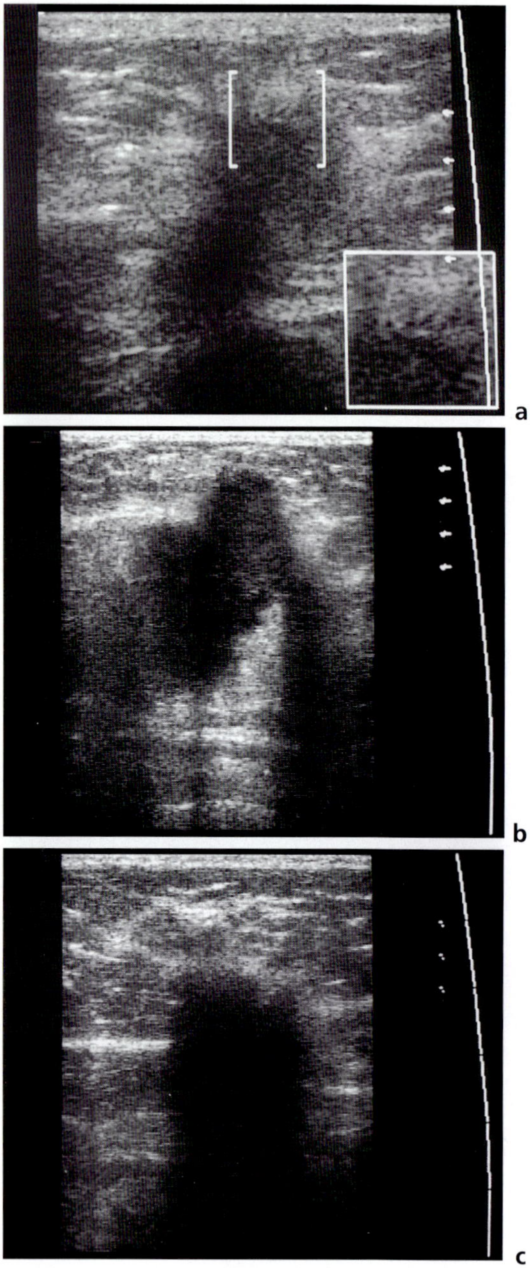

Fig. 6.**11a** Typical sonographic appearance of a scirrhous invasive ductal carcinoma. Posterior attenuation is common with this type of tumor. **b** Typical vertical orientation of an invasive cancer. **c** Carcinoma causing an abrupt architectural disruption.

may be associated with any of the secondary acoustic phenomena (Figs. 6.**1**, 6.**3**). As a result, these phenomena are considered to have little practical significance in the sonographic differential diagnosis of breast masses.

It is difficult to evaluate the secondary acoustic phenomena produced by small focal lesions (< 5 mm) and deeply situated lesions (> 3 cm), particularly in glandular tissue that is highly echogenic.

Compressibility and Mobility

Definition

By applying pressure on the transducer, the examiner can compress the breast tissue to determine whether the pressure alters the shape of a detected mass or changes its anteroposterior and mediolateral dimensions. If so, the mass is compressible (Fig. 4.**11**).

When a carcinoma infiltrates surrounding tissues and reaches the Cooper ligaments or pectoral fascia, its position within the breast tissue becomes fixed. Since mobility is related to compressibility and an absence of architectural disruption, it is a useful criterion for differentiating benign and malignant breast lesions by physical examination.

Usefulness in Differential Diagnosis

After a focal lesion has been scrutinized and evaluated for posterior acoustic phenomena, attention is turned to its surroundings. If the lesion is noncompressible and immobile, the odds ratio is 31 (Table 6.**2**), signifying a 31-fold increase in the risk that the lesion is malignant. Ninety of the 97 carcinomas in the study were noncompressible (Table 6.**2**), but so were 63 of the 213 benign lesions (fibroadenomas and fibrosis).

Under optimum conditions, compressibility offers a reasonable degree of confidence that the lesion is benign (cyst).

Only seven carcinomas in the study were compressible (mucinous carcinomas, medullary carcinomas, and cellular invasive ductal carcinomas). Fibrosis was never compressible, and fibroadenomas could rarely be compressed.

Compressibility also depends on the size of the lesion (size and shape changes are very difficult to appreciate in lesions smaller than 5 mm), the depth of the lesion in the breast, and the nature of the surrounding tissue. Masses located at a depth of 3 cm in fibrotic breast tissue show little if any response to compression, regardless of whether they are benign or malignant.

The inability to demonstrate the mobility of a breast mass with ultrasound implies a high risk of carcinoma. Benign masses are almost invariably mobile in relation to surrounding tissues.

Architectural Disruption

Definition

Disruption of the breast architecture is present in cases in which a tumor has penetrated the Cooper ligaments or mammary fascia (Nishimura et al. 1992). The continuity of these echogenic tissue planes is disrupted at the site of the carcinoma and is otherwise intact. The carcinoma, which may be of the mucinous or medullary type, appears to have been "punched into" that region of the glandular tissue (Figs. 6.**3**, 6.**9**–6.**11**). An inflammatory reaction or edema may be observed in surrounding tissues (p. 73). The lesion may exert traction on the Cooper ligaments, causing skin retraction or dimpling.

Usefulness in Differential Diagnosis

Architectural disruption is a characteristic feature of breast carcinoma. The odds ratio is 230 (Table 6.**2**), signifying a 230-fold increase in the risk that breast cancer is present when this sign is observed. Architectural changes were seen in 89 % of the breast cancer patients reviewed by Blohmer et al. (1995b).

Benign lesions grow in an expansile fashion. They may elevate the adjacent Cooper ligaments, but they do not disrupt their continuity (Figs. 6.**5,** 6.**6**). Circumscribed fibrosis develops as a component of the Cooper ligaments (Fig. 6.**2**).

Summary

The *best sonographic criteria* for the presence of breast carcinoma are summarized in Table 6.**3.** Since there is no "typical breast cancer" from a histological standpoint (Chapter 7), there is no typical sonographic presentation that is valid for every carcinoma.

Even the advent of high-resolution ultrasound has not significantly altered these "classic" criteria for a scirrhous invasive ductal carcinoma (Marquet et al. 1993, Venta et al. 1994). It is rare to find all the criteria in one carcinoma, and architectural change may be the only remarkable feature of cellular tumors or of mucinous or medullary carcinomas (see Figs. 8.**36,** 8.**37**). Ishii (1993) devised a scoring system for the evaluation of focal sonographic lesions. But given the odds ratios of 378 for wide, jagged borders and 230 for architectural change, either of these criteria should be sufficient to classify a lesion as malignant based on sonographic characteristics. Also, when we consider that Blohmer et al. (1995b) calculated a sensitivity of 93 % and a specificity of 95 % for wide, jagged borders, this parameter alone would dominate a scoring system.

When the various sonographic criteria for the benign or malignant nature of a lesion are known and applied, even carcinomas smaller than 1 cm^3 can be detected (Fornage et al. 1990). These criteria also permit the sonographic differentiation of fibroadenoma and carcinoma, even when both lesions are juxtaposed in the same image (see Fig. 8.**33**).

A recent paper by Stavros et al. (1995) assesses the role of ultrasonography in distinguishing benign solid breast nodules from indeterminate or malignant lesions, thus obviating the need for biopsy. Benign histological features in their series included intense hyperechogenicity of a lesion, ellipsoid shape, a thin echogenic pseudocapsule, and gentle bilobulations or trilobulations. Malignant characteristics included spiculation and angular margins, corresponding to a thick echogenic "halo," marked hypoechogenicity, shadowing lesions, lesions that were "taller than wide," punctuate calcifications, a branch pattern (= multiple projections from a nodule), or microlobulations. Indeterminate criteria included isoechogenicity or mild hypoechogenicity of lesions, normal or enhanced sound transmission, and a heterogeneous or homogeneous echo texture. If even a single malignant feature was encountered, the nodules were excluded from classification as a benign lesion. If no malignant characteristics were found in a lesion, one of the three combinations of benign characteristics was sought and, if present, the lesion was classified as benign. If no malignant characteristics were present and none of the combinations of benign characteristics were found, the lesions were by default classified as indeterminate. In Stavros's series, benign histological features were found in 83 % of lesions, and malignant histological features were found in 17 %. Using their classification scheme, the authors found a negative predictive value of 99.5 % for a solid benign classification. Of the 125 malignant lesions, 123 were correctly

Table 6.**3** The best sonographic criteria for breast carcinoma.

- Wide, jagged borders
- Architectural disruption (Cooper ligaments)
- Lack of compressibility
- Vertical orientation

Note:

> The criteria are uncertain in masses smaller than 5 mm.
> The criteria are difficult to evaluate in deeply situated masses.
> There are many types of carcinoma.

classified as indeterminate or malignant. When any nodule with even a single finding of malignancy was excluded from the benign category, the sensitivity for cancer was 98.4%. The sonographic finding of malignancy with the highest positive predictive value was spiculation, also reported in the literature as "thick echogenic halo." Stavros' series agreed with previously published reports showing a substantial overlap in sonographic characteristics between benign and malignant lesions, but it disagreed with previous assessments that because of this overlap, sonography should not be used to determine whether a lesion is benign or malignant. Their study demonstrates that sonography is useful in the characterization of certain solid breast masses and may identify a subgroup of lesions in which the certainty of malignancy is low enough to avoid biopsy, resulting in improved patient care with a reduction in patient discomfort, morbidity, mortality, and the cost of health care.

7 Pathology of Breast Lesions

It is helpful for the physician diagnosing focal breast abnormalities to be familiar with the frequency of the various breast diseases, their peak incidence, and their main histological variants. This allows one to look more selectively for specific disorders and gain an awareness of their diverse sonographic and mammographic appearances. While radiologists tend to make fewer misinterpretations as they grow more experienced with a modality, many errors of differential diagnosis can be avoided at the outset by learning important facts about the pathology of benign and malignant breast disorders.

In keeping with the subject matter and scope of this book, we shall limit our consideration of breast pathology to a brief overview. A more detailed discussion can be found in textbooks of breast pathology.

Nonhomogeneity is a characteristic of breast diseases, and particularly of carcinomas. It is common for various types and forms of lesions to coexist in the same breast. This should be borne in mind while reviewing this outline of breast pathology.

Malignant Breast Lesions

Noninfiltrating Carcinomas

Prevalence: 3–5 % of all palpable breast carcinomas and 15–20 % of breast carcinomas in a mammographically screened population.

Types:
- Ductal carcinoma in situ (DCIS) and subtypes (comedocarcinoma, solid, cribriform, papillary, and micropapillary types), grades I–III with or without necrosis (Silverstein et al. 1995).
- Lobular carcinoma in situ (LCIS).

Comments: DCIS is multicentric in 35 % of cases. LCIS is multicentric in 70–80 % of cases and is bilateral in 20–70 %. Thirty percent of patients with LCIS will develop infiltrating carcinoma. The invasive cancer which develops is usually ductal, not lobular. The risk applies to both breasts.

Invasive Ductal Carcinoma ("Typical Solid Breast Carcinoma")

Prevalence: 70–80 % of all breast carcinomas.

Peak incidence: around 50 years of age.

Types:
- Scirrhous (predominantly stromal composition).
- Cellular (relatively smooth borders; about 20 % of invasive ductal carcinomas).
- Transitional forms between scirrhous and cellular carcinomas.
- Ductal carcinoma with an extensive intraductal component (EIC; about 70 % are multicentric).

Invasive Lobular Carcinoma

Prevalence: 8–15 % of all breast carcinomas.

Peak incidence: 55 to 70 years of age.

Comments: invasive lobular carcinoma infiltrates diffusely without altering the surrounding tissue. This explains the frequent discrepancy between mammographic and histological tumor size. The tumor is multicentric in about 70 % of cases (including LCIS).

Mucinous Carcinoma—Colloid Carcinoma

Prevalence: 2 % of all breast carcinomas.

Peak incidence: 60–70 years of age.

Comments: good prognosis (may have the best prognosis of the invasive ductal cancers). A soft, sticky tumor with carcinoma cells suspended in a mucinous material. Sharply demarcated from surrounding tissue. Lacks typical clinical stigmata of breast cancer (skin dimpling, nipple retraction).

Medullary Carcinoma

Prevalence: 4–9 % of all breast carcinomas.

Peak incidence: premenopausal.

Comments: good prognosis. Characterized by circumscribed margins and lymphoplasmatic infiltration. Types I–III (type III: medullary component in an invasive ductal carcinoma).

Other Infiltrating Epithelial Carcinomas

Prevalence: each accounts for 1–2 % of all breast carcinomas.

Types: papillary carcinoma, tubular carcinoma, Paget‘s disease.

Nonepithelial Malignant Tumors

Sarcomas

Prevalence: 1–2 % of all malignant breast tumors.

Types: fibrosarcoma, liposarcoma, leiomyosarcoma, etc.

Comments: poor prognosis; 30 % of tumors have already metastasized when diagnosed. A special form is malignant phyllodes tumor (polymorphocellular variant of stromal sarcoma), along with a benign form (proliferative fibroadenoma) and a borderline form.

Lymphomas of the Breast

Breast lymphomas are symptomatic of a more generalized disease (see textbooks of internal medicine).

Manifestations of Invasive Breast Carcinoma

Paget's Disease

Prevalence: 1–3 % of all breast carcinomas.

Description: metastatic manifestation of an intraductal or invasive ductal carcinoma involving the epidermis of the nipple and areola.

Inflammatory Carcinoma

Prevalence: 1 % of all breast carcinomas.

Description: not a histological entity. Presents clinically as erysipelas. The cause is a cutaneous carcinomatous lymphangitis arising from a poorly differentiated carcinoma.

Comments: Poor prognosis. The prognosis is worse than infiltrating ductal carcinoma with skin involvement.

Prognostic Factors

Grading: Bloom and Richardson grade 1–3.

Staging: TNM (tumor size, lymph-node involvement, distant metastases).

Hormone receptor status: progesterone-receptor and estrogen-receptor positive or negative.

Other indicators: DNA content, degree of aneuploidy, growth factors such as Ki-67, expression of p53 protein, cathepsin D, etc.

Multifocality

Multifocality denotes the presence of additional carcinoma cells outside the boundary of the primary carcinoma but within the same breast segment or quadrant or within a 2-cm radius of the primary tumor.

There is about a 25 % incidence of multifocal growth in the same quadrant with T1 carcinomas and about a 40 % incidence with T2 carcinomas (Rosen et al. 1975).

Multifocal carcinomas may also be multicentric in about 50 % of cases (Tulusan et al. 1989).

Multicentricity

Multicentricity refers to additional foci of invasive or noninvasive carcinoma outside the quadrant or segment bearing the primary cancer, or foci occurring more than 2 cm from the primary tumor.

From 21 % to 75 % of all breast carcinomas may be multicentric, depending on the examination method, tumor size, growth pattern, and histological type (Holland et al. 1985, Tulusan et al. 1989).

Bilaterality

It is estimated that approximately 45 % of patients with multicentric breast carcinoma have bilateral disease, i.e., cancer in both breasts (Tulusan et al. 1989).

Benign Breast Lesions

Fibroadenoma

Prevalence: 30 % of all women.

Peak incidence: 20–25 years, followed by a plateau until age 45.

Comments: carcinoma develops in a fibroadenoma in 1–2 % of cases. Proliferative fibroadenoma phyllodes (benign) is present in about 3 % of all fibroadenomas and may recur after complete excision.

Fibrocystic Change (Fibrocystic Disease)

Prevalence: 40–50 % of all women.

Peak incidence: 45–55 years.

Description: fibrocystic change (FCC) is a generic term covering all nonneoplastic structural alterations in the breast parenchyma.

Types:
- Microcystic and fibrous mastopathy due to involutional change;
- Focal fibrosis (in young women, also fibrous mastopathy);
- Fibrocystic lesions (duct ectasia, cysts, fibrosis, adenosis, ductal epithelial proliferation).
  Ductal or lobular epithelial hyperplasia (ordinary, proliferative, atypical).

Mastitis

Types and prevalence: 70 % of mastitis cases are puerperal. The remaining 30 % are nonpuerperal: chronic, purulent, granulomatous, or specific-tuberculosis, sarcoidosis, syphilis, mycosis, actinomycosis.

Peak incidence: 30 and 50–60 years of age.

Other Benign Breast Lesions

Pure adenoma, ductal papilloma (intraductal or intracystic; juvenile papillomatosis as a precancerous lesion), lipoma, hamartoma (dysontogenetic tumors such as fibroadenolipomas), fibromatosis.

Gynecomastia

Prevalence: 40 % of all disorders of the male breast.

8 Sonography of Breast Carcinoma

Carcinoma in situ (Figs. 8.1–8.23)

Carcinoma in situ (CIS) is a preinvasive lesion that does not alter the surrounding breast tissue, and there are therefore no associated changes in tissue echogenicity. Microcalcifications are a typical feature of CIS on mammograms, but even high-resolution ultrasound often cannot define them due to insufficient lateral resolution. As a result, breast ultrasound is rarely able to detect the lesions of CIS.

Sonographically visible lesions such as fibroadenoma, ductal ectasia, and cysts (particularly those with complex internal structures), however, may harbor preinvasive changes that are not detected until histological evaluation. Likewise, ultrasound imaging of a mammographically suspicious region may reveal dilated ducts or cysts with internal echoes (Figs. 8.**1**, 8.**23**). Similarly, histological examination may show elements of DCIS or LCIS occurring at the periphery of sonographically visible invasive carcinoma (Chapter 7) (Fig. 8.**2**). CIS is found unexpectedly in 3–5 % of palpable masses, accounting for the various reports about the (incidental) detection of CIS. Harper (1985), for example, observed thickened Cooper ligaments as an associated feature of CIS on breast sonograms. Madjar (1991) and Teboul (1988) describe intraductal or intracystic structures and dilated peripheral ducts as sonographic findings that may be suggestive of CIS.

Mammography is still the modality of choice for the detection of CIS. Preinvasive lesions are found in 15–20 % of excised breast masses in a mammographically screened population (Dongen et al. 1989).

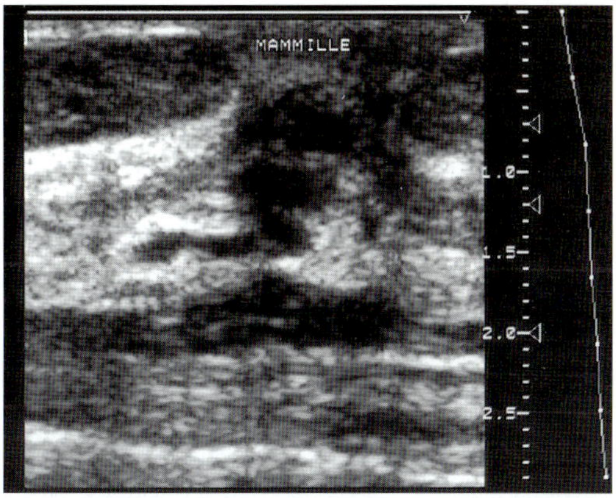

Fig. 8.**1** Sonographic appearance of central duct ectasia. The dilated (here, to 3 mm) and tortuous lactiferous duct is visible below the nipple. A cytologically suspicious nipple discharge (see Fig. 8.**40c**) necessitated excision of the central ducts. The histological examination revealed a papillary type of intraductal carcinoma. The papillary lesion was not demonstrated by mammography.

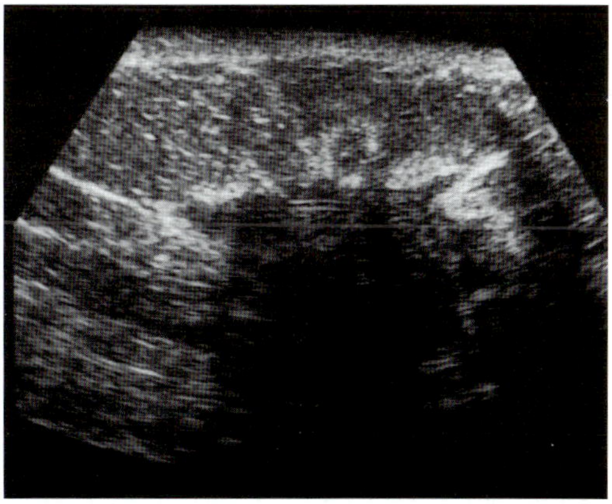

Fig. 8.**2** Breast carcinoma, showing typical wide, jagged borders and peripheral foci of DCIS.

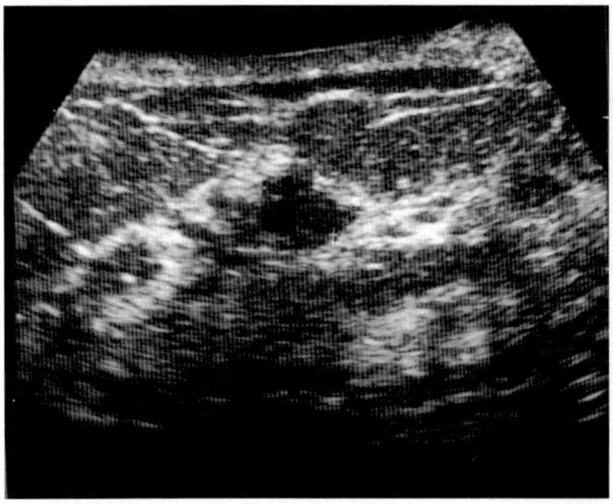

Fig. 8.3 Small breast carcinoma. The wide border is poorly demarcated from the echogenic breast parenchyma.

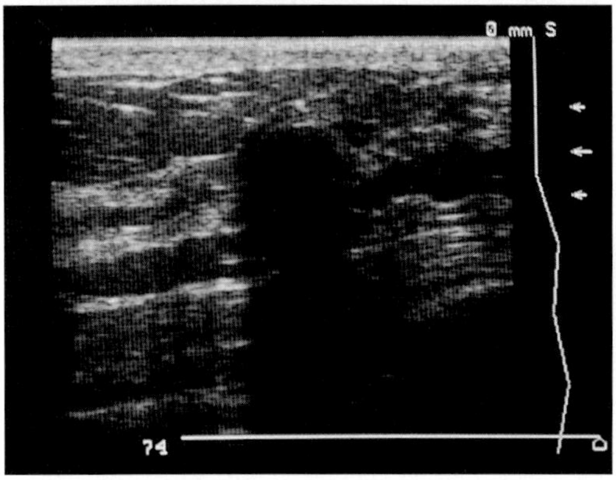

Fig. 8.4 An acoustic shadow is the only sonographic manifestation of this breast carcinoma. There is no apparent tissue reaction.

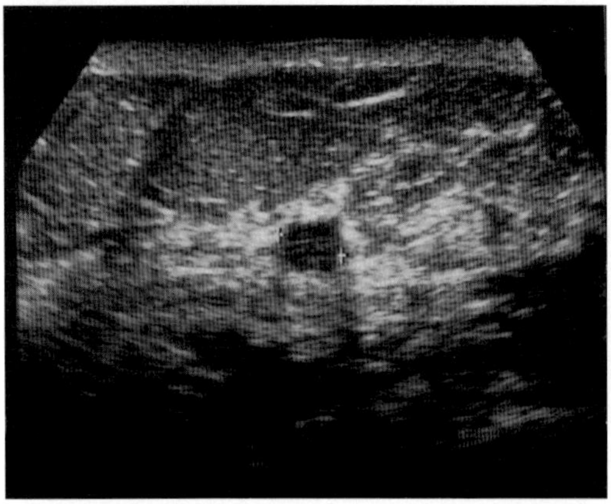

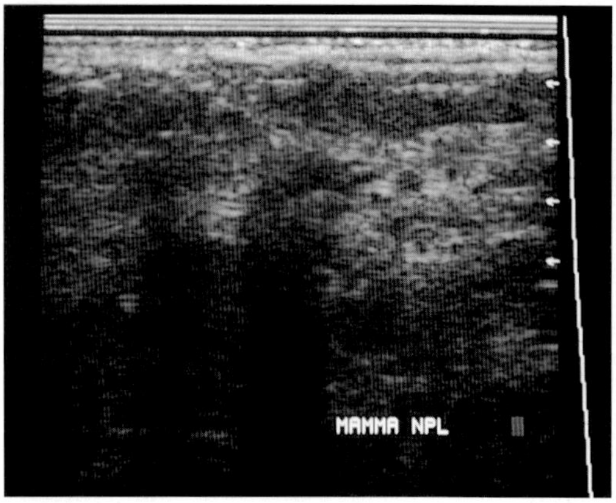

Fig. 8.6 This breast carcinoma is not defined as a discrete mass, but is manifested only by an acoustic shadow and architectural disruption of the breast parenchyma.

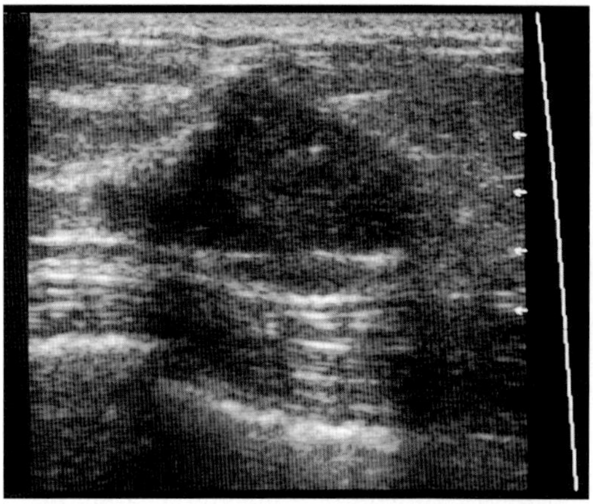

Fig. 8.7 Breast carcinoma, showing architectural disruption and mixed areas of posterior enhancement and attenuation.

◀ Fig. 8.5 This 4.5-mm breast carcinoma demonstrates bilateral edge shadows, a sign usually seen with benign lesions.

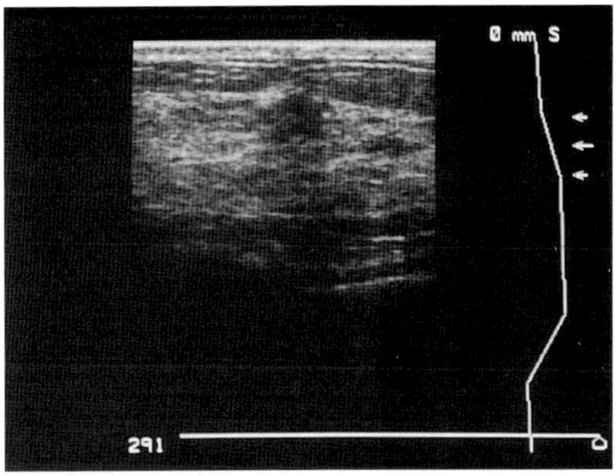

Fig. 8.**8** Small breast carcinoma, appearing as a hypoechoic mass disrupting the more echogenic breast parenchyma.

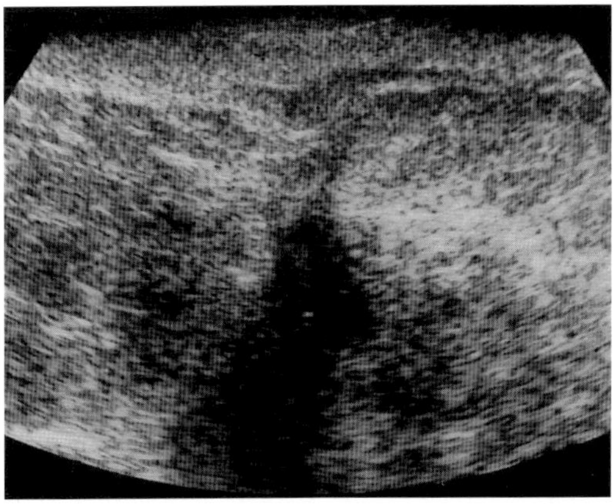

Fig. 8.**9** Small breast carcinoma, conspicuous by its vertical orientation: "taller than wide."

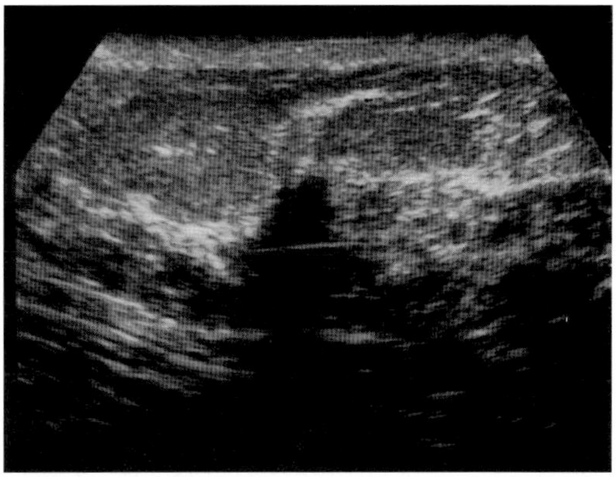

Fig. 8.**10** Small breast carcinoma with a predominantly vertical orientation and posterior shadowing.

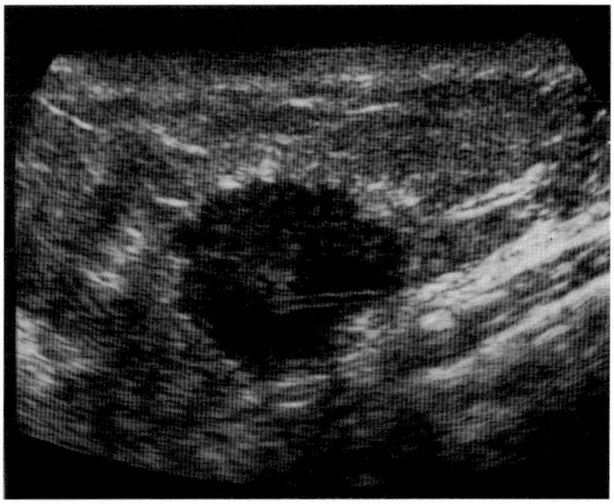

Fig. 8.**11** Jagged border surrounding a breast carcinoma.

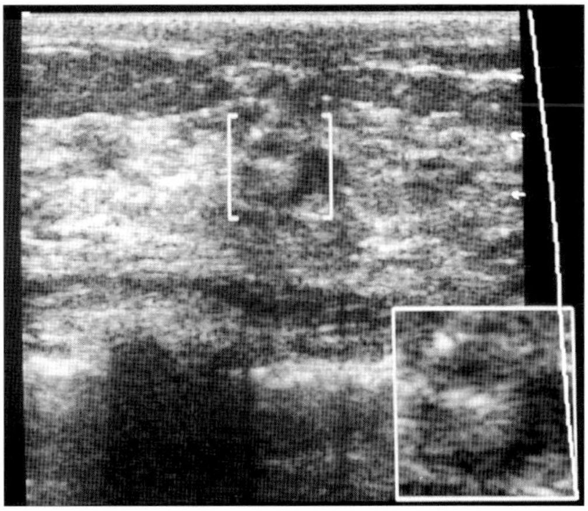

Fig. 8.**12** Small, hyperechoic breast carcinoma, manifested by architectural disruption.

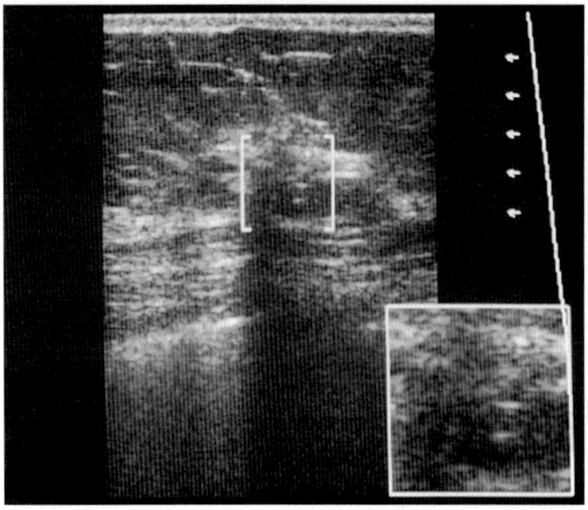

Fig. 8.**13** Small breast carcinoma with mixed hypoechogenicity and hyperechogenicity disrupting the glandular architecture.

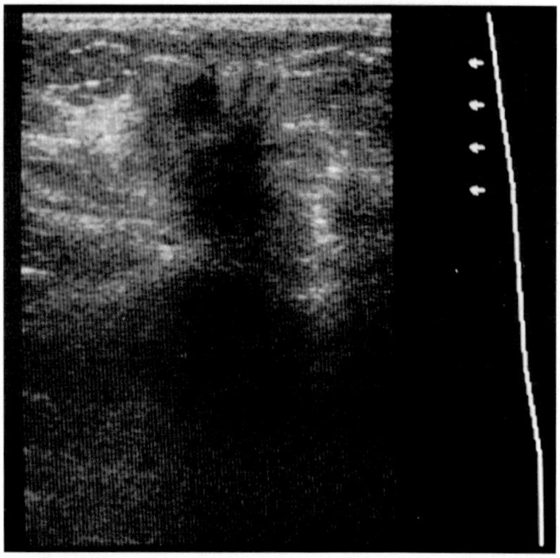

Fig. 8.**15** Breast carcinoma with indistinct borders and a posterior acoustic shadow.

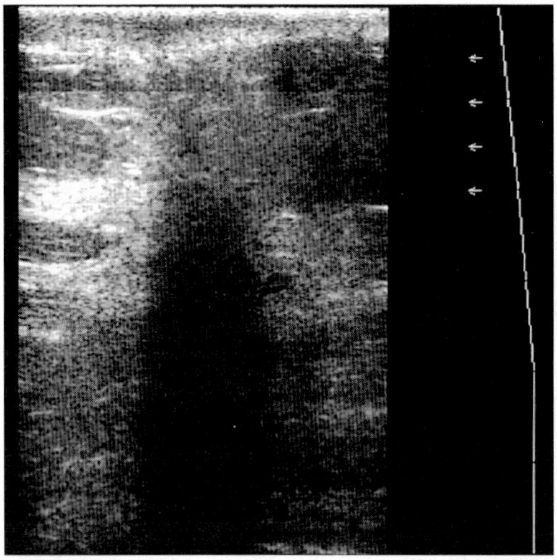

Fig. 8.**14** Breast carcinoma, the only ultrasound manifestation of which is a posterior acoustic shadow.

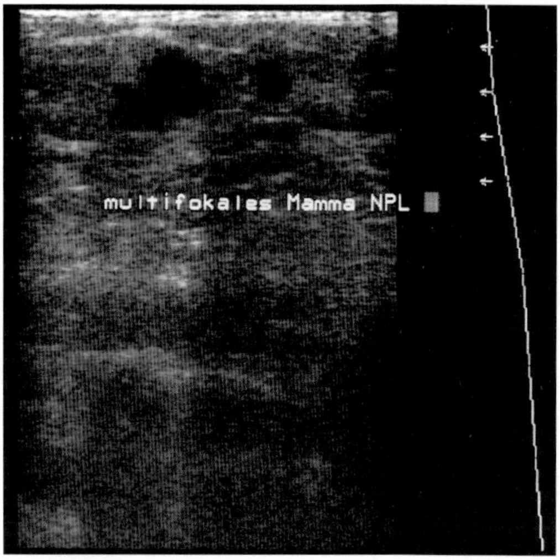

Fig. 8.**16** Multifocal breast carcinoma, manifested by several hypoechoic foci.

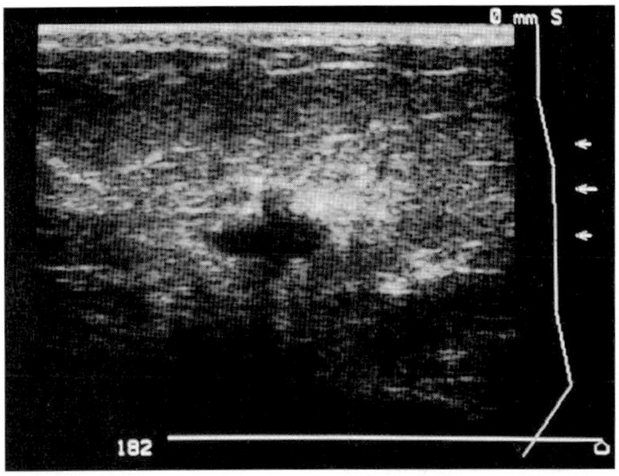

Fig. 8.17 Breast carcinoma exhibiting a marked horizontal and vertical growth axis.

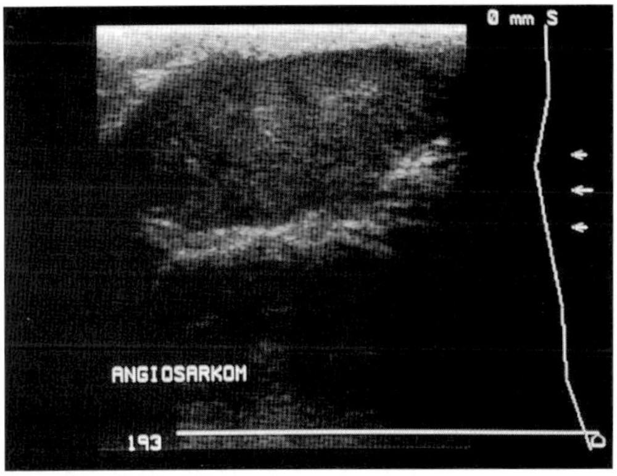

Fig. 8.18 Angiosarcoma, a rare type of breast tumor.

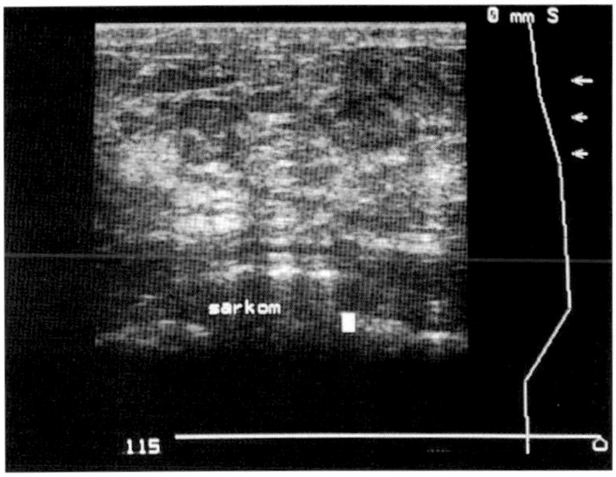

Fig. 8.19 A rare mammary sarcoma, poorly defined by ultrasound.

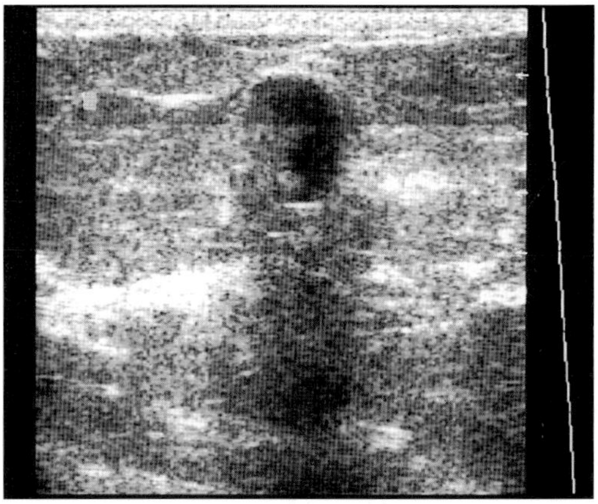

Fig. 8.20 Intracystic breast carcinoma.

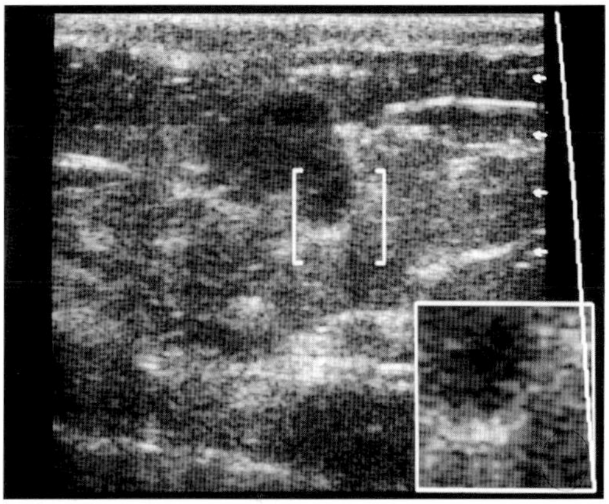

Fig. 8.21 Area of fibrocystic change, exhibiting wide borders but no other suspicious features.

Fig. 8.22 Breast carcinoma, appearing only as a hypoechoic focal lesion. There is no shadowing or peripheral tissue reaction.

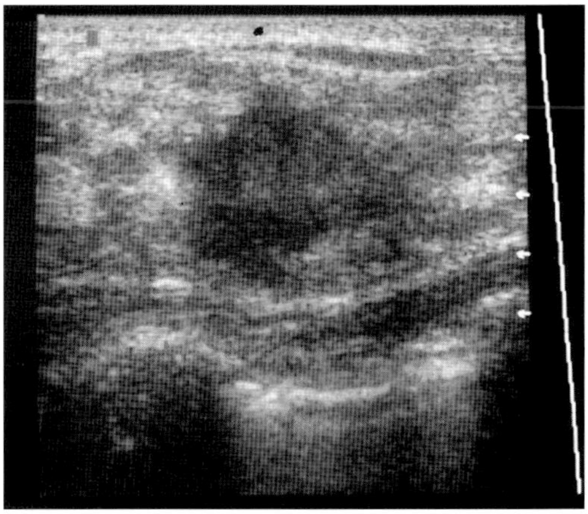

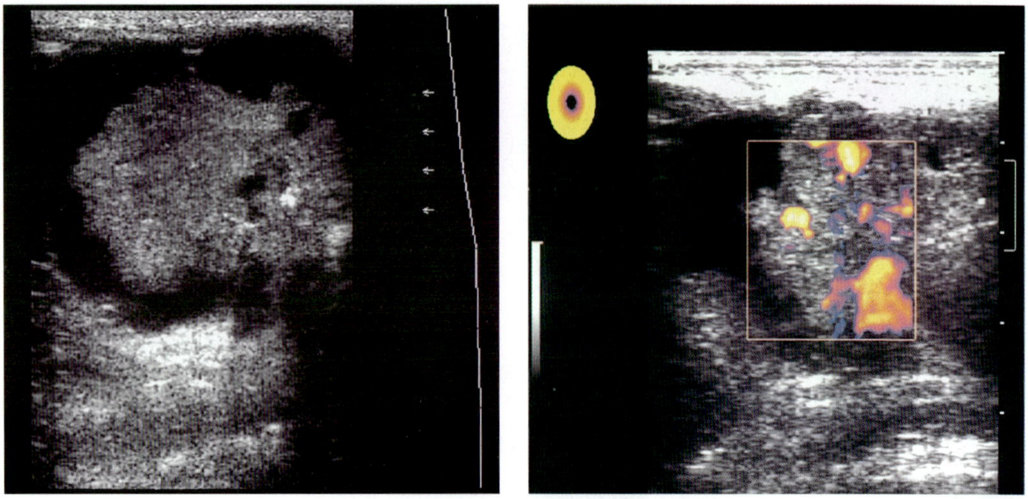

a b

Fig. 8.**23a** Large intracystic carcinoma. **b** Power Doppler image demonstrating intratumoral vascularity.

Invasive Ductal and Lobular Carcinomas

The sonographic features of these most common breast carcinomas, and their mammographic features (Barth and Prechtel 1990), depend on the relative amount of tumor cells and stroma. In many cases the early stage of invasive lobular carcinoma is not associated with histological changes in surrounding tissues (Chapter 7), making the lesion difficult to detect with ultrasound. It is common to underestimate both the extent of the lesion and its potential multicentricity.

Scirrhous Carcinomas

The "typical" breast cancers demonstrated by sonography and mammography are predominantly stromal tumors that contain few neoplastic cells. Ultrasound typically shows a mass with a hypoechoic or anechoic center. The central structures of the mass have a relatively homogeneous composition (fibrohyalinosis with scant tumor cells). Since these structures cause little scattering of ultrasound, they appear anechoic (Teubner 1985b). The periphery of the carcinoma, where tumor is infiltrating healthy tissue, has a heterogeneous composition. The variations of tissue density and consistency at the tumor periphery create impedance mismatches on a microscale that cause heavy scattering of ultrasound. As a result, the borders of the carcinoma show some degree of echogenicity (Teubner 1985b). Whether they are hyperechoic or hypoechoic depends on the echogenicity of the surrounding infiltrated tissue. If the carcinoma and surrounding breast parenchyma are both hyperechoic, the border will appear hypoechoic (Fig. 8.**24**). If the carcinoma infiltrates surrounding fat, the border will appear hyperechoic as a result of scattering and reflection (Fig. 8.**25**).

The sonographic and mammographic contours of these lesions appear jagged or spiculated due to infiltration of the surrounding glandular and fatty tissue by the fibrous carcinoma (Figs. 8.**26,** 8.**27**). Attenuation and central shadowing usually occur behind the sonographic mass (Figs. 8.**25,** 8.**26,** 8.**28**). These effects are caused by very heavy scattering of the ultrasound beam within the tumor and at its rough surface. Some tumors cast a unilateral edge shadow (Fig. 8.**27**) caused by strong refraction of the sound waves at the interface with sur-

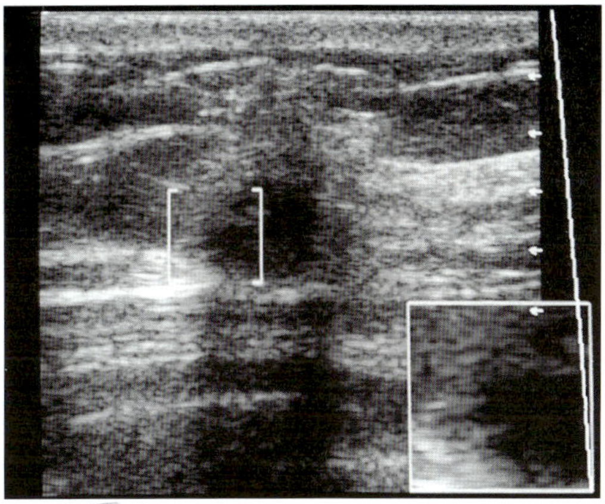

Fig. 8.24 T2 carcinoma displaying an anechoic center, wide hypoechoic borders, and disruption of the superficial mammary fascia.

rounding tissue. A typical carcinoma penetrates fascial planes within the fat and disrupts the continuity of the connective tissues surrounding the mammary lobe. This architectural disruption, along with acoustic shadowing, is often the first sign that directs attention to breast cancer in the survey scan (Figs. 8.**24**–8.**26**). Zoom images can then be used to investigate other sonographic criteria for benign/malignant differentiation (Chapter 6).

The overall appearance of the carcinoma may be that of a foreign body that has been "punched into" the healthy breast tissue (Fig. 8.**29**).

A sonographic mass that is suspicious for malignancy is noncompressible – i.e., it does not change its shape when transducer pressure is applied to that region of the breast. The lesion is immobile relative to its surroundings.

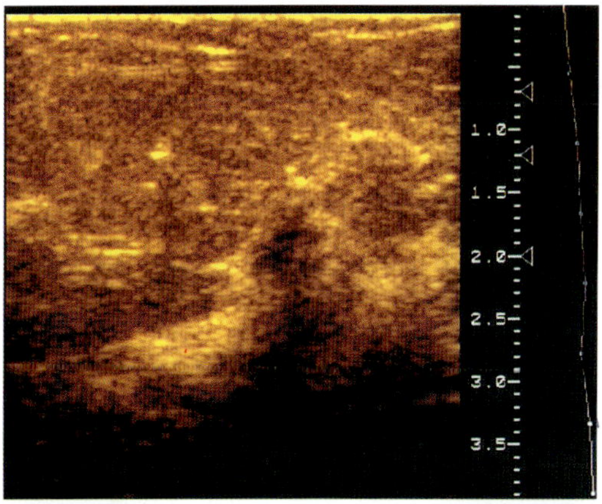

a

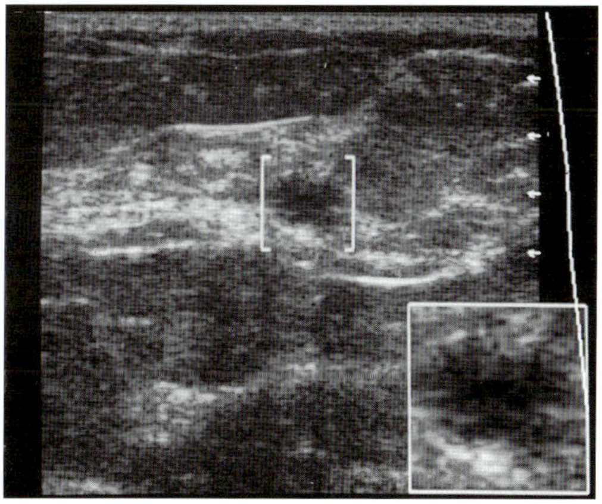

b

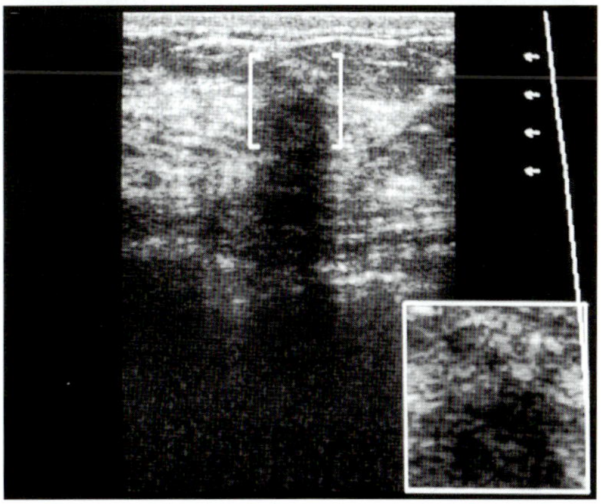

c

Fig. 8.**25a** Color B-mode image shows an 8-mm breast carcinoma deep to a thick layer of subcutaneous fat. The tumor has a hypoechoic center and broad, hyperechoic borders. **b** Small carcinoma (3–4 mm) with indistinct borders. **c** A small breast carcinoma, the most conspicuous feature of which is a posterior acoustic shadow.

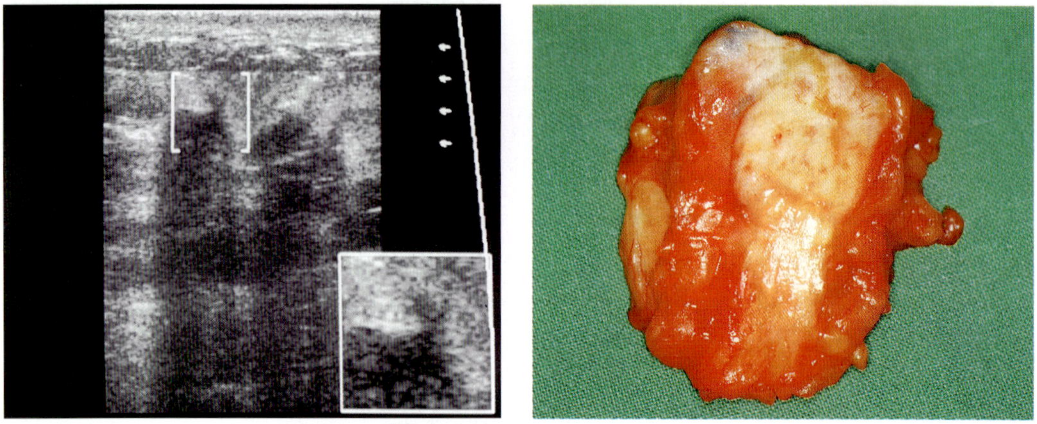

Fig. 8.**26a** Sonographic appearance of an invasive ductal carcinoma 3 cm in diameter. Note the typical wide, jagged borders and vertical orientation. **b** Part of the excised specimen. Infiltration is grossly apparent.

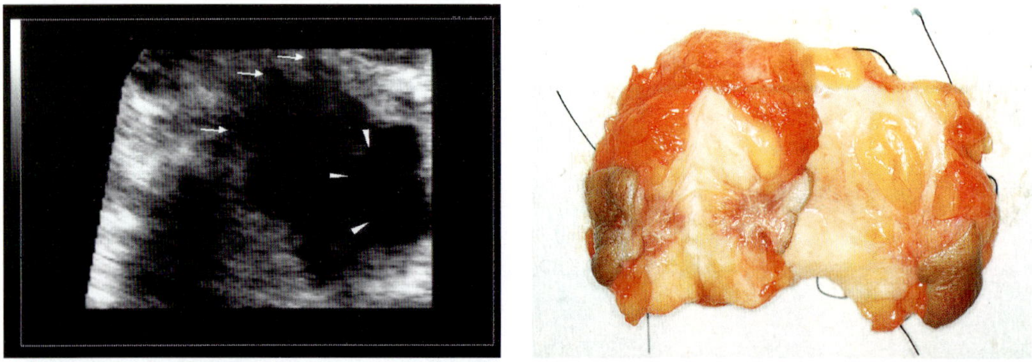

Fig. 8.**27a** Three-dimensional sonography shows finger-like spicules radiating from the breast carcinoma into surrounding tissue (large arrows). Broad borders surround an anechoic center (arrowheads). **b** Excised retroareolar carcinoma.

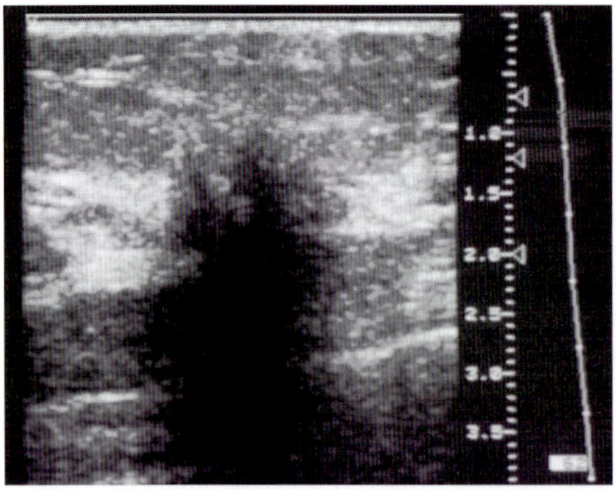

◀ Fig. 8.**28** Typical sonographic features of breast carcinoma: wide borders, posterior acoustic shadow, and architectural disruption.

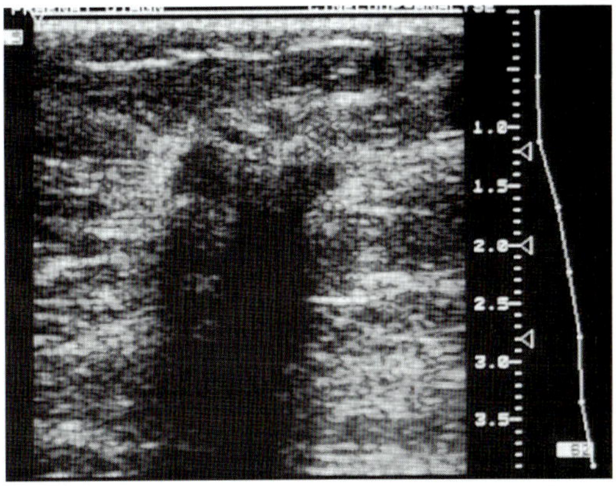

Fig. 8.**29** The carcinoma appears to have been "punched into" the glandular breast tissue, disrupting its architecture. Note the central acoustic shadow and peripheral attenuation.

Table 8.**1** Typical sonographic features of scirrhous invasive ductal and lobular carcinomas.

Acoustic phenomena	Description
Central echogenicity	Hypoechoic to anechoic
Borders	Wide, jagged, hypoechoic
Orientation of major axis	Vertical
Posterior acoustic phenomena	Attenuation, central shadow
Edge shadows	Rarely observed
Compressibility	Noncompressible
Architectural change	Disruption of septa and tissue surfaces

The sonographic features described above are characteristic of scirrhous invasive ductal and lobular carcinomas, particularly T1 lesions (Table 8.**1**). They are rarely mistaken for a benign breast mass.

Cellular Carcinomas

These invasive ductal and lobular carcinomas contain scant fibrous tissue, and the alteration of surrounding tissues is a late event (Chapter 7). Generally these tumors must reach a considerable size before affecting the echogenicity of adjacent structures. In addition, they are not suspicious on palpation in their early stages, as they are well circumscribed, and do not cause skin dimpling (Chapter 7). Cellular carcinomas are difficult to distinguish mammographically from benign solid tumors (Barth and Prechtel 1990).

Thus, it is not unusual for radiologists to misinterpret the nature of these lesions based on imaging studies. Cellular carcinomas are, however, less common than scirrhous cancers.

The typical sonographic features of these tumors are listed in Table 8.**2**; their sonographic appearance is illustrated in Figures 8.**30** and 8.**31**. As the figures show, cellular carcinomas may have narrow borders rather than the wide borders that are typical of scirrhous breast cancers (Harper 1985). Posterior acoustic enhancement may occur and the tumor also may contain coarse internal echogenic regions (Fig. 8.**32**). Typically, the mass is noncompressible and has the appearance of a "foreign body" embedded in the glandular breast tissue.

Disruption of continuity, particularly in the superficial fascia, aids in the sono-

Table 8.**2** Typical sonographic features of cellular invasive ductal and lobular carcinomas and of carcinomas higher than stage T1.

Acoustic phenomena	Description
Central echogenicity	Hypoechoic with high-level internal echoes
Borders	Narrow, jagged, hyperechoic
Orientation of major axis	No particular orientation
Posterior acoustic phenomena	Mixed enhancement and attenuation
Edge shadows	Rare; when present, broad and unilateral
Compressibility	Noncompressible
Architectural change	Distortion with septal displacement

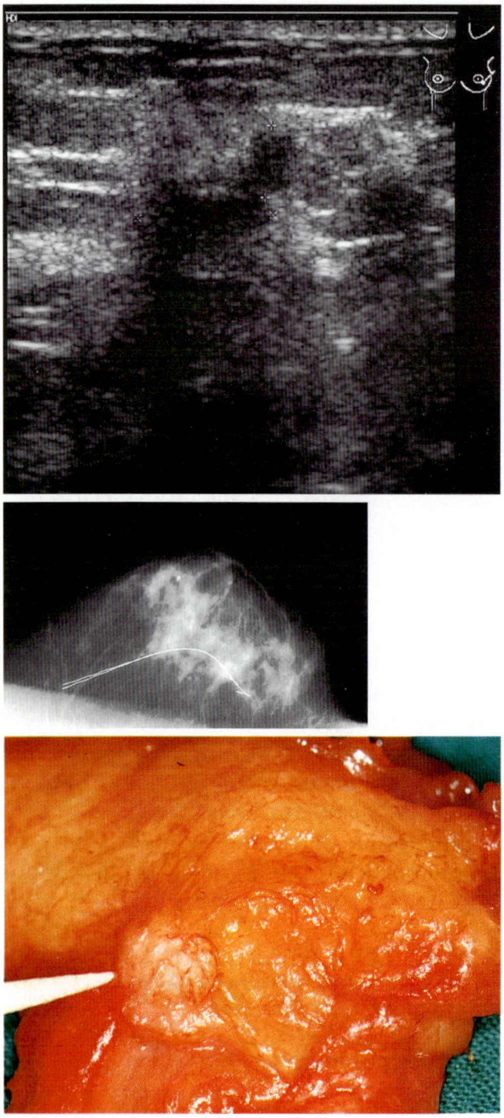

a

b

c

Fig. 8.**30a** Sonographic appearance of a cellular invasive lobular carcinoma: relatively narrow borders and a lobulated contour with streaky posterior attenuation. Fascial planes are disrupted in the hyperechoic breast parenchyma. **b** Mammography demonstrates a relatively smooth-bordered focal lesion. (The wire is marking the nonpalpable mass.) **c** The excised specimen shows a relatively well-circumscribed solid tumor with a lobulated growth pattern.

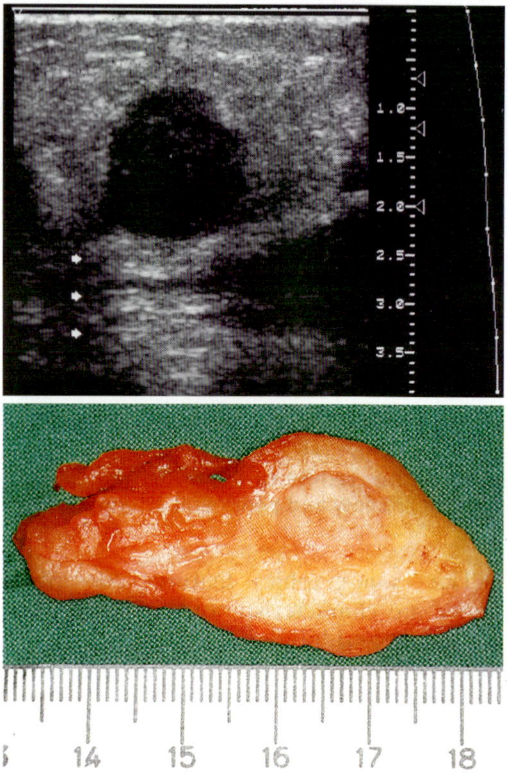

a

b

Fig. 8.**31a** Sonographic appearance of a cellular invasive ductal carcinoma: smooth, narrow borders with heterogeneous internal echoes, a vertical orientation, and posterior enhancement (arrows). **b** Excised specimen shows relatively well-circumscribed tumor margins.

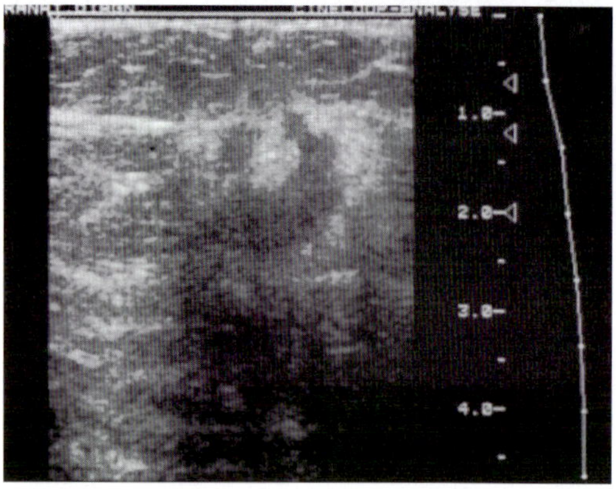

Fig. 8.**32** Sonographic appearance of a cellular breast carcinoma. A bright, mass-like internal echo is visible within the hypoechoic center of the tumor. There is marked disruption of the superficial fascia and streaky posterior attenuation.

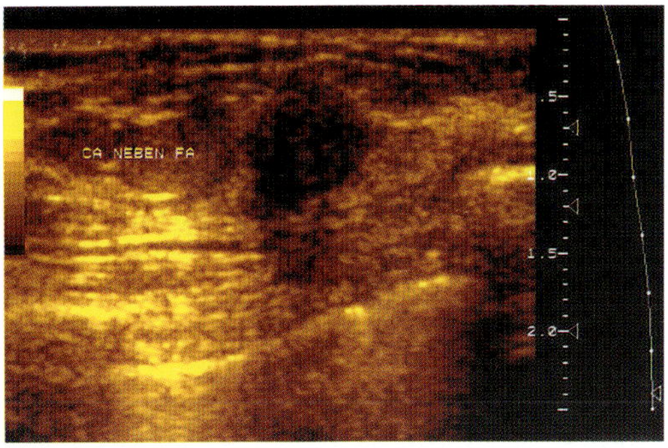

Fig. 8.**33** Color B-mode image of a cellular invasive lobular carcinoma (right side of the image). The cancer appears as a hypoechoic mass with a vertical orientation and disruption of the superficial fascia. Adjacent to the carcinoma is a fibroadenoma (left side of the image). This lesion is hyperechoic, shows a transverse orientation, and lies deep to the superficial fascia.

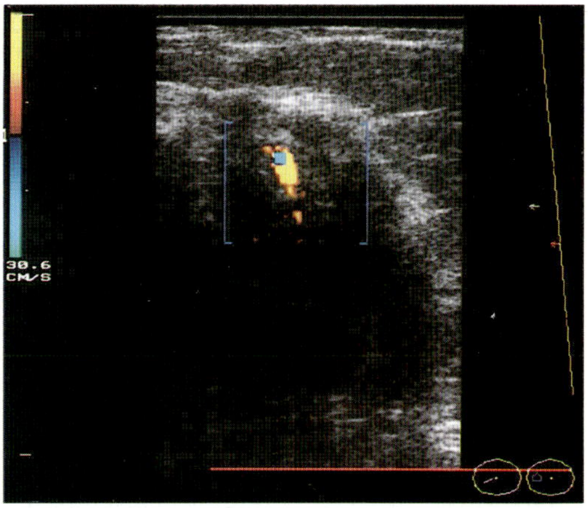

Fig. 8.**34** Invasive ductal carcinoma, only partially imaged because of its large size (5 cm). It displays an anechoic center with hyperechoic peripheral internal structures and a narrow border. Color Doppler demonstrates central blood flow (of high velocity).

graphic differential diagnosis of these lesions. Vertical orientation of the tumor ("taller than wide") is another typical sign of cancer (Chapter 6) and can help distinguish a cellular invasive lobular carcinoma, for example, from an adjacent fibroadenoma (Fig. 8.**33**).

Advanced stages of cellular and scirrhous breast carcinomas have a similar sonographic appearance – that of a lobulated, relatively smooth-bordered mass. The center of these advanced tumors consists of homogeneous stroma or necrosis and may appear hypoechoic with scattered high-level internal echoes. Sound waves are transmitted through the tumor core without significant energy loss, causing posterior enhancement. With a very fast-growing cancer,

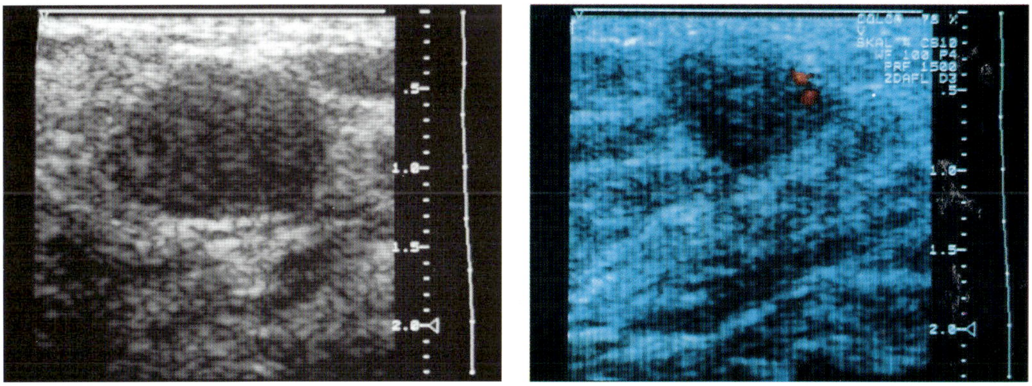

a b

Fig. 8.**35** Appearance of an invasive ductal carcinoma about 3 cm in diameter. **a** The smooth borders, homogeneous internal echoes, and transverse orientation seen on this plane could easily suggest a fibroadenoma. However, there is an absence of posterior enhancement with narrow, bilateral edge shadows. **b** Shifting the image plane reveals penetration of the superficial mammary fascia, raising a suspicion of carcinoma. Color Doppler imaging indicates blood flow at the periphery of the mass.

changes in the surrounding tissues may cause a smooth-bordered pseudocapsule of uniformly low echogenicity to develop around the tumor (Figs. 8.**34,** 8.**35**).

Other Types of Breast Cancer

The diagnosis of less common types of breast cancer is difficult to obtain by ultrasound. These lesions often lack the typical sonographic criteria allowing differentiation between benign and malignant tissue – criteria that best describe the features of "scirrhous" invasive ductal carcinomas, i.e., tumors that have a high stromal content and little cellularity (Chapter 6 and p. 63).

Medullary and Mucinous Carcinoma

These histologically distinct tumors are discussed under a common heading because of their similar sonographic features. With their smooth margins and narrow, echogenic walls, medullary and mucinous carcinomas are virtually indistinguishable by ultrasound from fibroadenomas. Posterior enhancement is common, and refractive

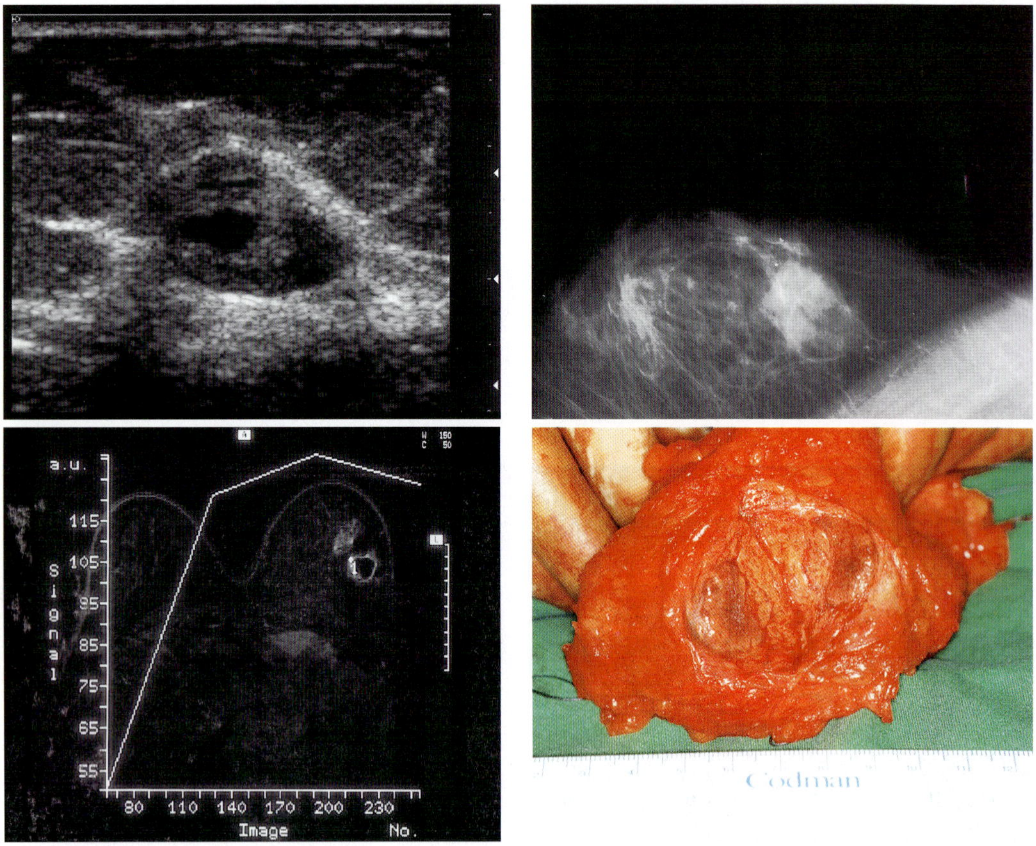

Fig. 8.**36a** Sonographic appearance of a medullary carcinoma. The coarse internal echoes are a conspicuous feature and are the only sign suggestive of malignancy. **b** Corresponding mammographic density. **c** The T1-weighted magnetic resonance image shows an enhancing tumor margin. The graphic display represents the inflow, plateau, and washout of the contrast medium (image courtesy of Dr. Oellinger, Rudolf Virchow University Medical Center, Berlin). **d** The excised specimen is well circumscribed and presents a glassy cut surface.

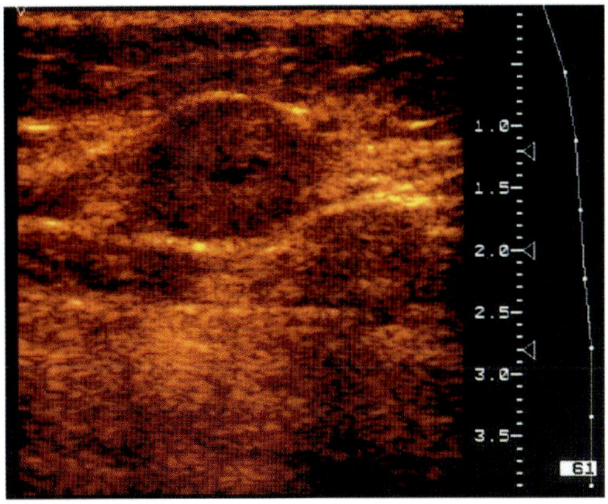

Fig. 8.**37** Color B-mode image of medullary carcinoma. The anechoic center and almost circular shape of the solid mass are consistent with a malignant tumor.

effects at the smooth surface of the tumor may cause bilateral edge shadows. These focal sonographic lesions may be round or show a transverse orientation (Figs. 8.**36,** 8.**37**).

Because of these features, medullary and mucinous carcinomas are easily mistaken for fibroadenomas (Harper 1985). Malignancy may, however, be suggested by the anechoic center of the tumor, which may represent central necrosis, or by its nonhomogeneous internal structure, which has a generally suspicious or abnormal appearance (Chapter 7) (Figs. 8.**36,** 8.**37**). Like fibroadenomas, these cancers show little if any compressibility. Architectural change may be noted in surrounding tissues. If sonographic follow-up demonstrates enlargement of the mass, prompt referral for biopsy or surgical removal of these prognostically favorable carcinomas is recommended. If the nature of the lesion is indeterminate, core biopsy or excision of the lesion is usually performed. If a lesion is thought to represent a fibroadenoma on the basis of sonographic appearance, subsequent sonographic or mammographic follow-ups can be scheduled at 6-month to 12-month intervals. Of course, excision or biopsy is appropriate if the nature of the lesion is indeterminate.

Papillary Carcinoma

Intracystic and intraductal structures may be visible with high-resolution ultrasound, especially when three-dimensional technology is employed (Figs. 8.**38,** 8.**39**). Ultrasound cannot distinguish the early stages of papillary carcinoma from benign papillomas. This particularly applies to papillary carcinoma in situ, which has both an intracystic and an intraductal form. Reportedly, the intracystic form is more apt to become

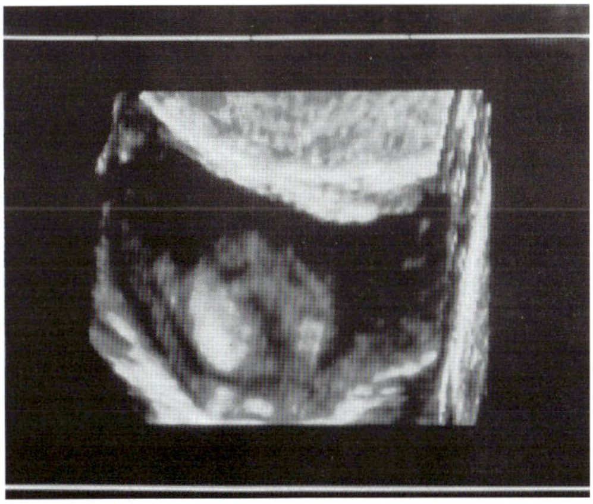

Fig. 8.**38** Three-dimensional sonogram of an intracystic papilloma. The observer is looking into the cyst, which contains a hyperechoic mural mass with irregular borders.

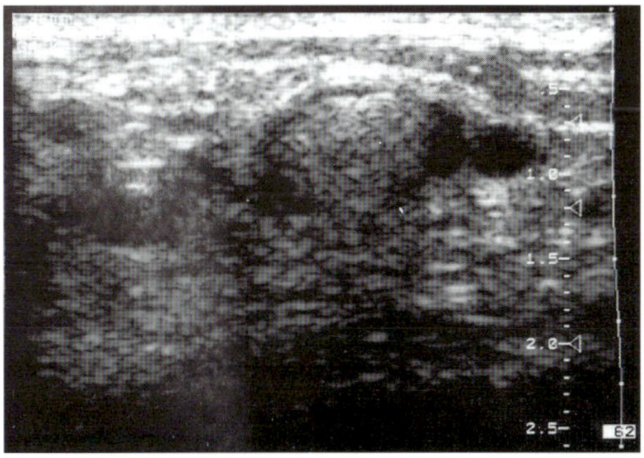

Fig. 8.**39** This ductal papilloma appears as a smooth-bordered, solid mass of uniformly high echogenicity within the dilated central ducts.

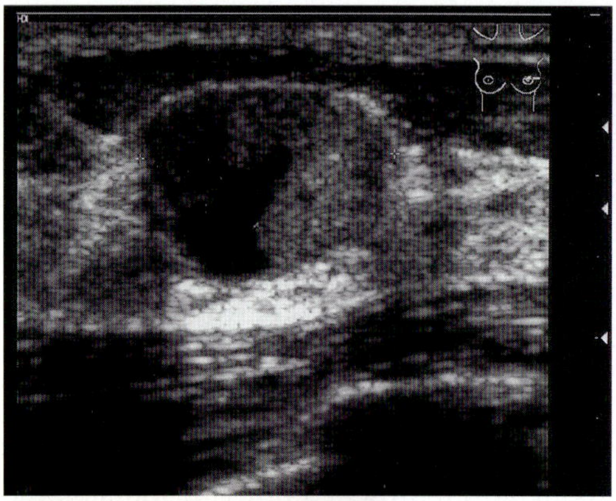

a

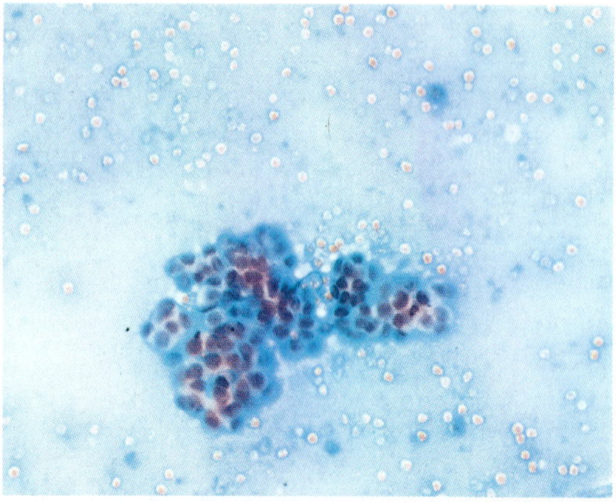

b

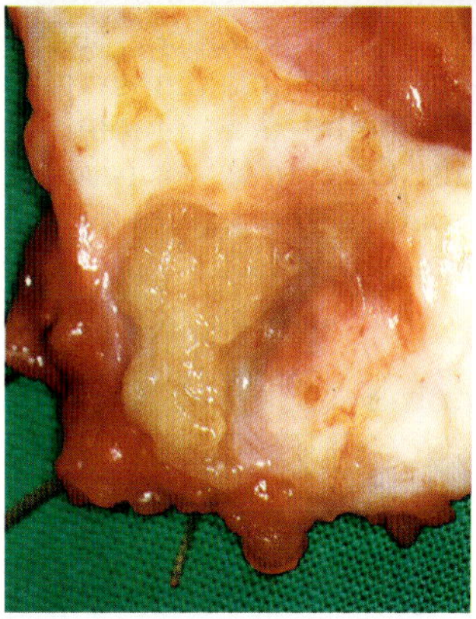

c

Fig. 8.**40a** Breast ultrasound demonstrates an intracystic, hyperechoic papillary mass within a smooth-bordered, anechoic to hypoechoic structure (papilloma occupies right half of cyst). **b** Excised specimen. The yellowish, grape-like mass is visible within the otherwise smooth-walled cyst. **c** A cytological specimen prepared from the abnormal discharge (Papanicolaou stain, 100 x) shows the papillary arrangement of the cells with a slightly altered nuclear-cytoplasmic ratio and erythrocytes in the background. Histological diagnosis: intraductal carcinoma of the papillary type.

invasive than the intraductal form (Soo et al. 1995). Intraductal lesions are usually detected at mammography by the presence of clustered microcalcifications. The intracystic form appears mammographically as a smoothly marginated mass, while ultrasound may reveal solid intracystic structures that prompt referral for histological evaluation (Soo et al. 1995) (Fig. 8.**39**). In some cases, aspiration cytology of the cyst or the dilated duct containing the papillary fronds will advance the diagnosis (Fig. 8.**40**). Matsuo et al. (1993) recommend measurement of carcinoembryonic antigen (CEA) in the aspirated cystic fluid as a simple and reliable method for diagnosing intracystic carcinoma.

If the carcinoma has become invasive, ultrasound can demonstrate changes in the architecture and echogenicity of the infiltrated tissues (Fig. 8.**41**).

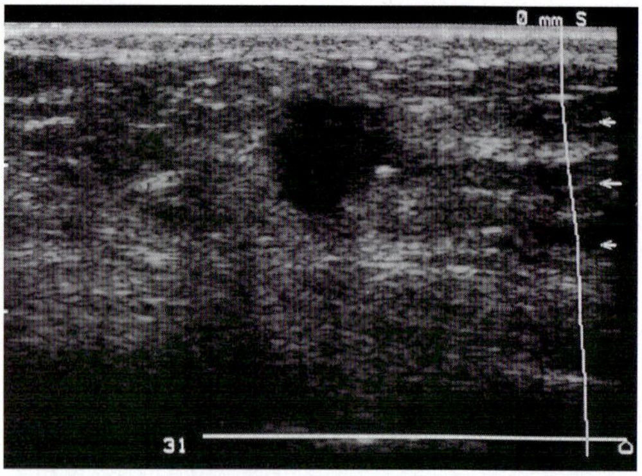

Fig. 8.**41** Intracystic carcinoma. The cyst has a typical sonographic appearance, except for a papillary structure projecting into the cyst lumen (lower right). The altered echogenicity of the adjacent breast tissue may represent the site of invasion.

Malignant Phyllodes Tumor

Phyllodes tumor is a type of sarcoma that is distinguished clinically by its rapid growth, particularly in younger women. It presents as a mobile, well-circumscribed palpable mass (Fig. 8.**42**). Patients‘ descriptions of enlargement of a mass are often unreliable, since most patients subsequently found to have a fibroadenoma also seek medical attention for a "rapidly enlarging" breast mass. Thus, many young women still undergo surgical removal of fibroadenomas, despite clear-cut radiological findings, for fear that the lesion may be a malignant phyllodes tumor or a borderline form.

The ultrasound appearance of a phyllodes tumor is that of a hypoechoic mass with smooth, narrow borders and low-level internal echoes. The mass is oriented transversely and is compressible. These features are identical to those of fibroadenoma, and only the size of the mass (> 5 cm) and its growth (doubling time) are suggestive of cystosarcoma phyllodes. Surgical excision is imperative (Schön et al. 1994).

Pulsed and color Doppler may demonstrate a rich vascular supply that is unusual for a fibroadenoma. However, proliferating fibroadenomas can also be very vascular, therefore limiting the specificity of Doppler ultrasound in evaluating these lesions (Chapter 13).

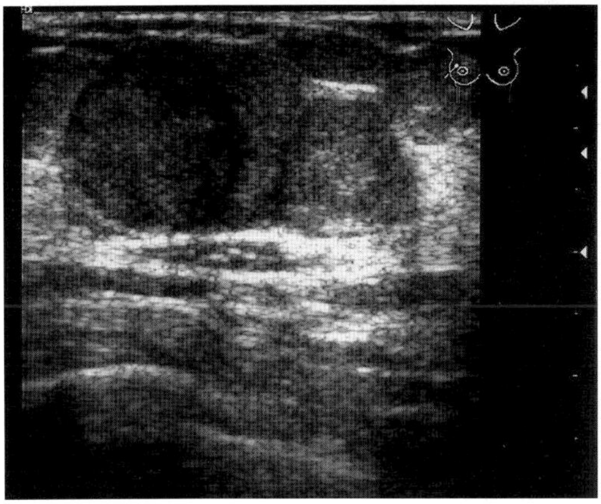

Fig. 8.**42** A sonographic mass suspicious for a malignant phyllodes tumor. Differentiation is required from a proliferating fibroadenoma. The rapidly enlarging mass contains nonhomogeneous central echoes and several anechoic areas (necrosis). There is possible penetration of the superficial fascia.

Lymphoma

Lymphomas should be included in the differential diagnosis of solid breast masses. Intramammary lymph nodes are detected more frequently at mammography than at breast ultrasound.

Lymphomas do not have a specific mammographic or sonographic appearance. The histopathological subtypes of malignant lymphoma cannot be differentiated by ultrasound (Libermann et al. 1994).

The sonographic appearance of *intramammary lymph nodes* is identical to that of axillary lymph nodes (Fig. 8.**43**; see Chapter 11).

Lymph-node metastases in the breast often have smooth contours and show the typical reniform shape of lymph nodes, but most are uniformly hypoechoic and lack the corticomedullary structural differentiation ("fatty hilum") seen in healthy lymph nodes (Fig. 8.**44**). The sonographic appearance of these lesions is very similar to that of cellular breast carcinomas.

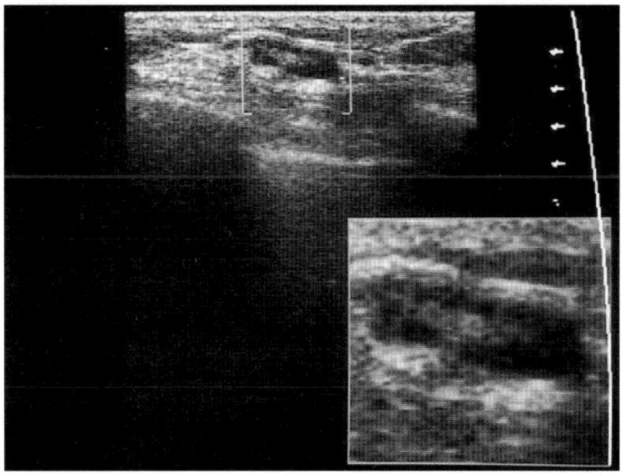

Fig. 8.**43** Sonographic appearance of an intramammary lymph node. The corticomedullary structures and lack of architectural disruption suggest the true nature of the mass.

Malignant lymphomas appear sonographically as hypoechoic, smooth-bordered, noncompressible masses with posterior enhancement, so they are indistinguishable from primary cellular breast carcinomas and metastases (Fig. 8.**45**). This pattern should prompt immediate referral for biopsy or excision of the breast mass.

Multicentric and Multifocal Carcinoma

Since it is common for additional foci of carcinoma to occur in proximity to a detected carcinoma (multifocal disease) or elsewhere in the breast (multicentric disease, Chapter 7) (Holland et al. 1985, Tulusan et al. 1989), a search for coexisting lesions should be made whenever a carcinoma is found. Even T1 carcinomas are associated with about a

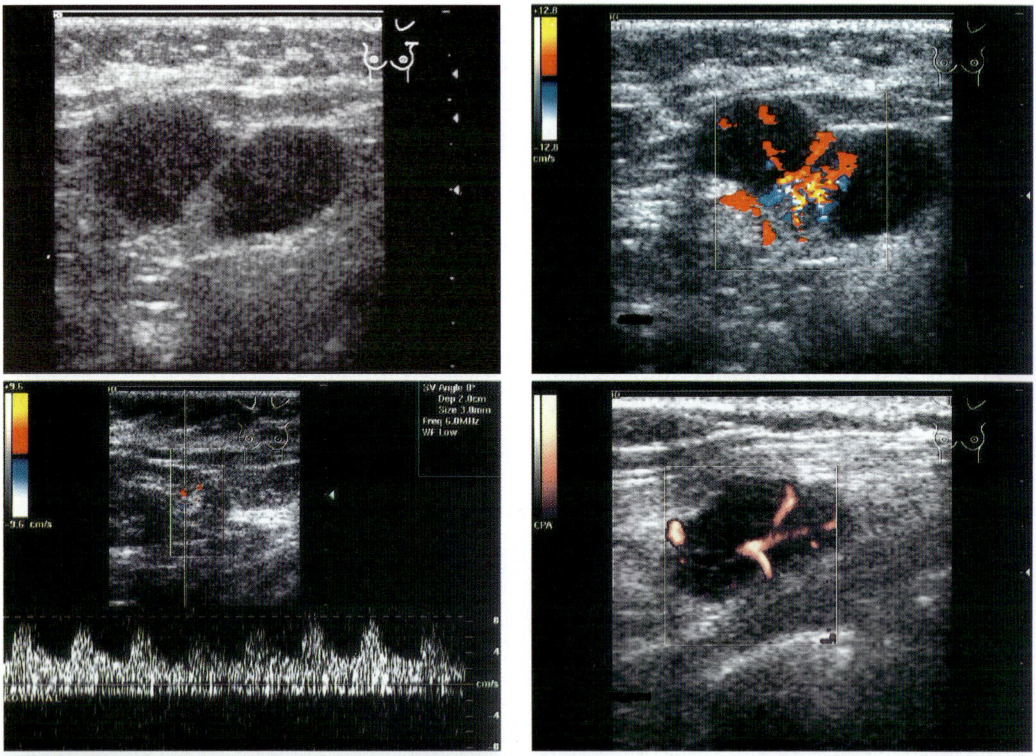

a b c d

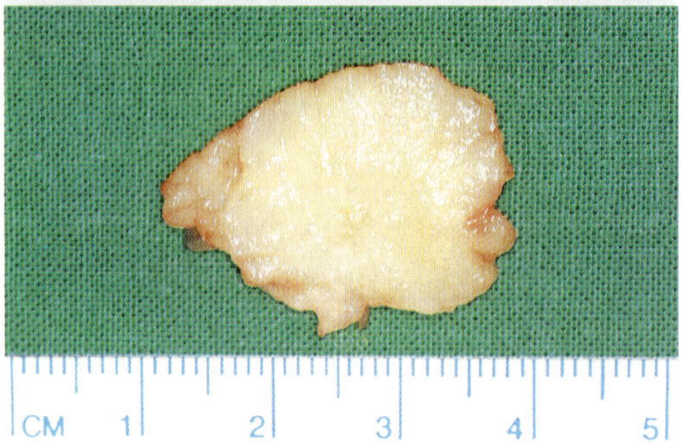

e

Fig. 8.**44a** A lymph-node metastasis in the pectoralis major muscle. The metastasis still has the typical reniform shape of a lymph node, but there is little evidence of medullary differentiation. **b** Color Doppler defines a vascular tree with high flow rates (turbulence) in the hilar area. **c** Color duplex shows a nonspecific Doppler waveform. **d** The power Doppler image, showing additional blood flow. **e** Excised lymph-node metastasis from a medullary carcinoma.

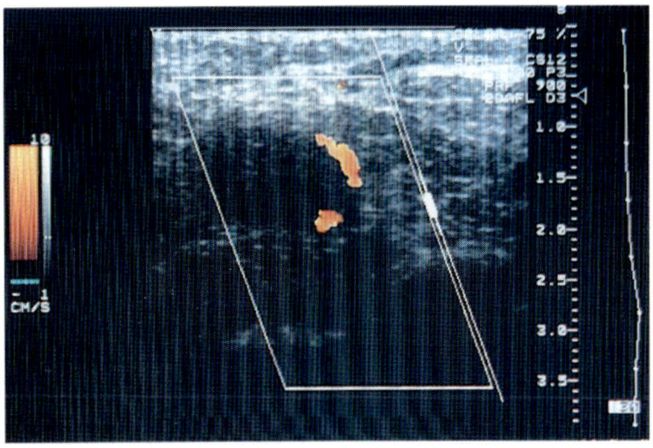

Fig. 8.**45** Color Doppler image of a malignant breast lymphoma shows a hypoechoic, smooth-bordered, noncompressible mass with peripheral blood flow.

25 % incidence of multifocal disease (Rosen et al. 1975).

Mammography can detect additional foci of breast carcinoma in only about 40 % of histologically confirmed cases (Ernst et al. 1986, Holland et al. 1983). There are limits to the efficiency of mammography in detecting additional small focal lesions, particularly in radiographically dense breasts. Sonography can be an effective alternative in these cases, leading Holland et al. (1983) to publish an early recommendation for breast ultrasound as a preoperative study. In the late 1980s, Madjar et al. (1989) correctly determined multicentricity in 87 % of women with multicentric carcinoma, and Ernst et al. (1986) did so in 20 of 29 cases.

Additional foci of carcinoma have much the same appearance as the initially detected lesion, but they are usually smaller (Fig. 8.**46**). Foci smaller than 5–8 mm have a nonspecific appearance, often presenting as simple hypoechoic masses showing no distinct signs to indicate whether they are benign or malignant (Figs. 8.**47**–8.**49**). Mammography should always be performed as part of the preoperative investigation. If mammograms show suspicious densities or suspicious microcalcifications, localization and excision should be performed in those areas. We have found magnetic resonance imaging (MRI) to be very helpful in the detection of multifocal and multicentric carcinomas (Fig. 8.**50**). At present, there is no established protocol for the MRI localization of breast masses, so these suspicious multicentric lesions often cannot be surgically evaluated. However, the development of adequate biopsy techniques with MRI guidance is currently under way. If multifocal disease is suspected, this problem can be solved by widely encompassing the suspicious area with an excision that also satisfies oncological requirements (Audretsch et al. 1995, Bostwick 1990, Silverstein et al. 1995).

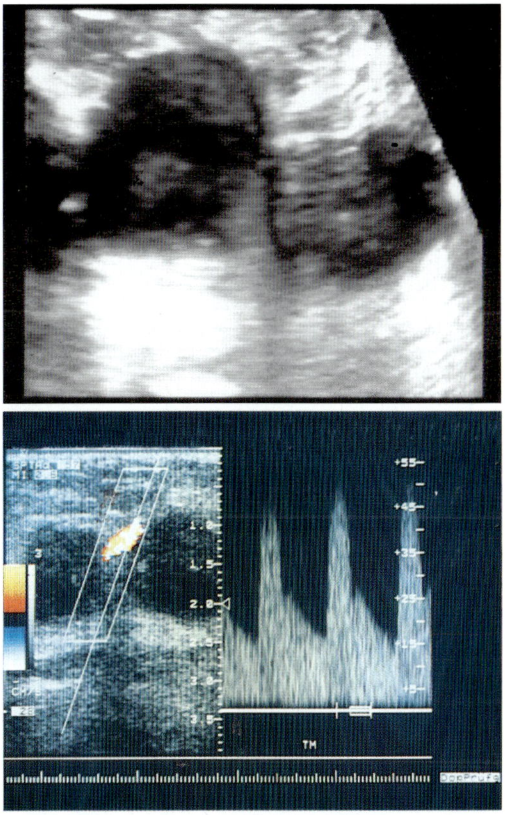

a

b

Fig. 8.**46a** Three-dimensional sonography of a bifocal breast carcinoma. This technique defines the contours of the mass more clearly than two-dimensional ultrasound (Fig. 6.**1**), demonstrating wide, indistinct borders, nonhomogeneous internal echoes, and the connection between the two foci. **b** Color Doppler and pulsed-wave (PW) Doppler appear to show an arterial vessel coursing between the two focal lesions. Notable features of the Doppler waveform are its high peak systolic velocity and low end-diastolic velocity.

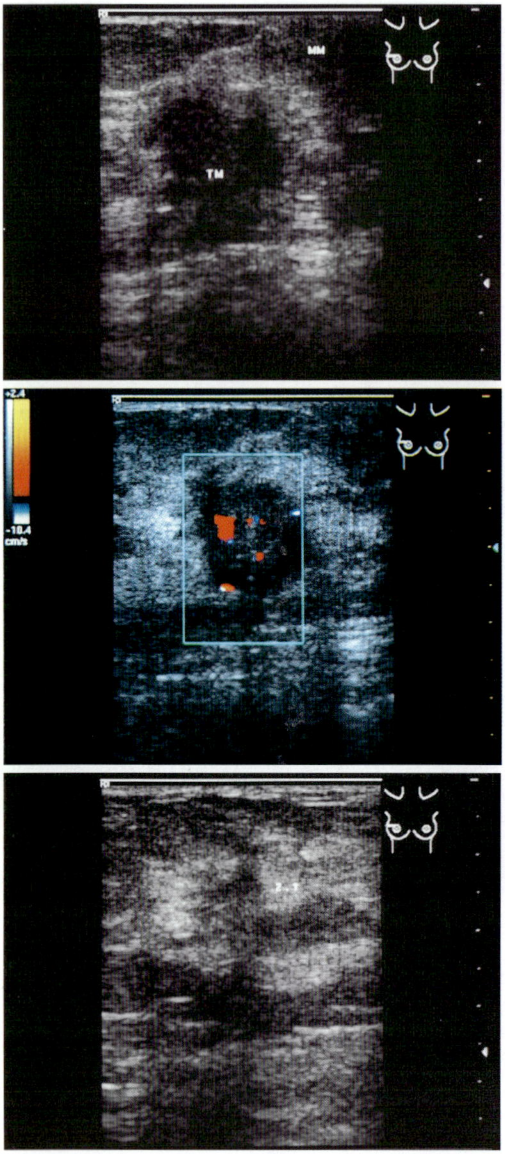

a

b

c

Fig. 8.**47a** The typical sonographic appearance of a primary focus of multicentric invasive ductal carcinoma. **b** Color Doppler imaging reveals central perfusion of the lesion. **c** The second focus appears only as a hypoechoic mass with posterior attenuation.

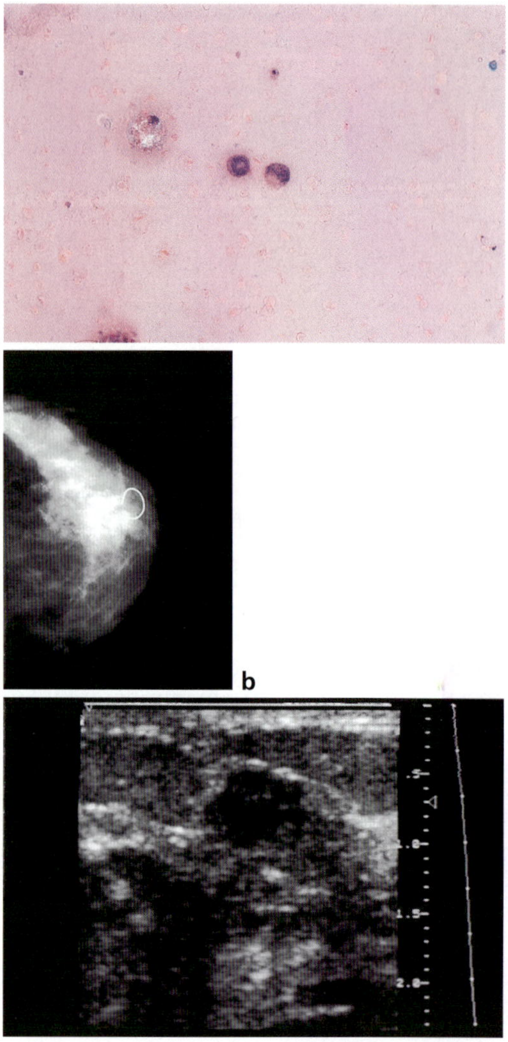

a

b

c

Fig. 8.**48** Multifocal and multicentric scirrhous invasive lobular carcinoma, with an extensive intraductal component. **a** Cytological examination of a unilateral bloody discharge from the left breast showed a hemorrhagic (neoplastic) background and two cells with an increased nuclear-cytoplasmic ratio. **b** Mammography shows multiple suspicious microcalcification clusters in the left breast. **c** At breast ultrasound, the disruption of the superficial fascia deep to the mass is typical of an invasive tumor, which otherwise shows no distinctive sonographic features. **d** Another focal sonographic lesion showing nonspecific features. **e** The cut surface of the excised specimen shows diffuse infiltration by the carcinoma.

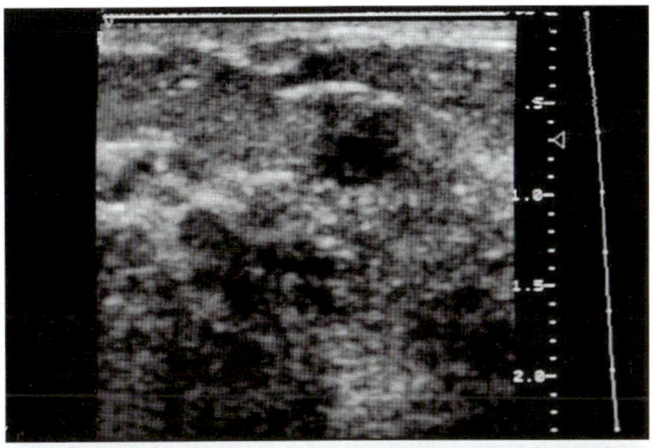

d

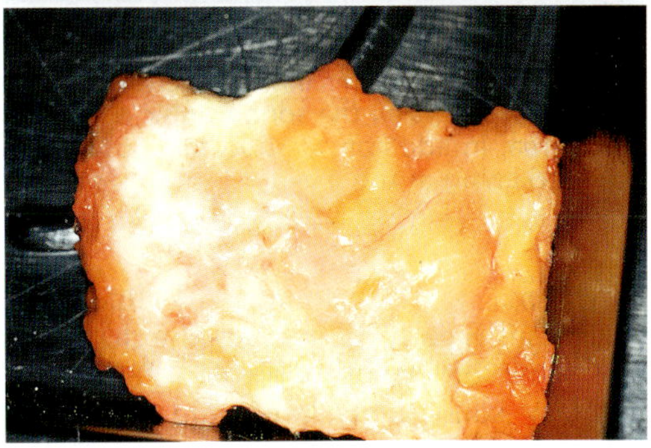

e

Fig. 8.**48 d, e**

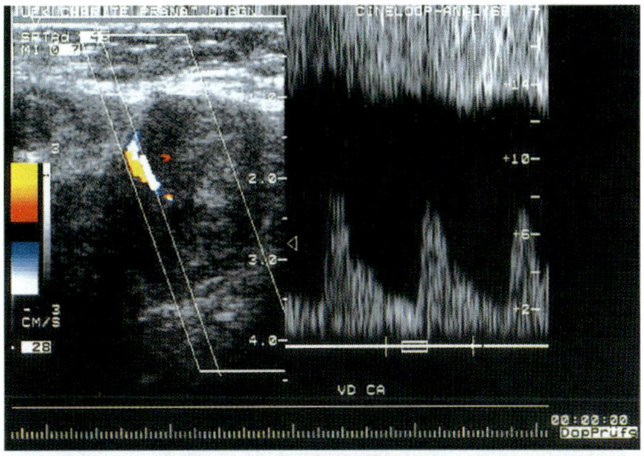

a

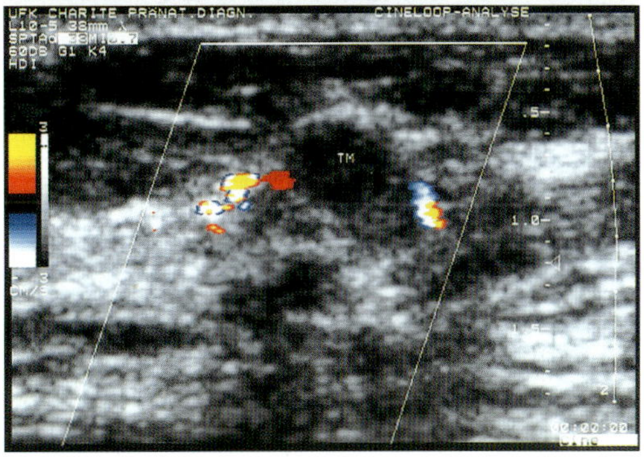

b

Fig. 8.**49 a** Pulsed color Doppler image of a multifocal invasive lobular breast carcinoma. The lesion is vertically oriented and noncompressible. Blood flow is demonstrated at the tumor periphery. The Doppler waveform shows a nonspecific pattern. **b** Another lesion in the same breast, representing a second focus of carcinoma, is not sonographically suspicious.

Inflammatory Carcinoma

Inflammatory carcinoma is not a separate histological entity. The reddish-brown discoloration and induration of the skin, caused by the infiltration of subcutaneous lymphatics, suggest the presumptive clinical diagnosis. Histological confirmation can be

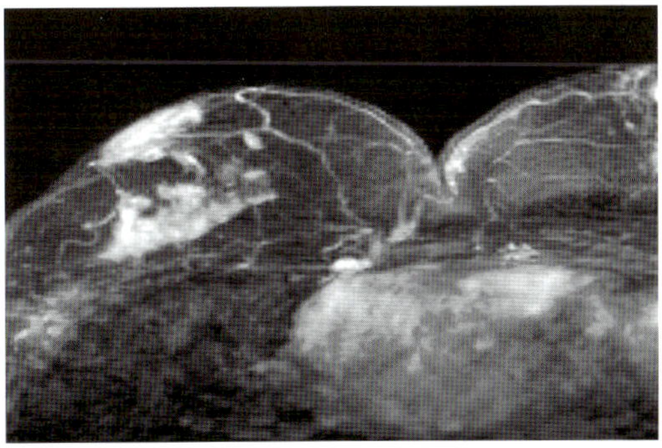

Fig. 8.**50** MRI appearance of multifocal breast carcinoma.

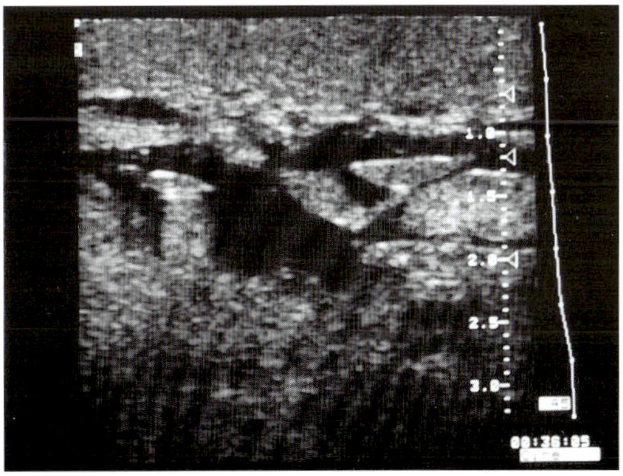

Fig. 8.**51** Sonographic appearance of inflammatory breast carcinoma.

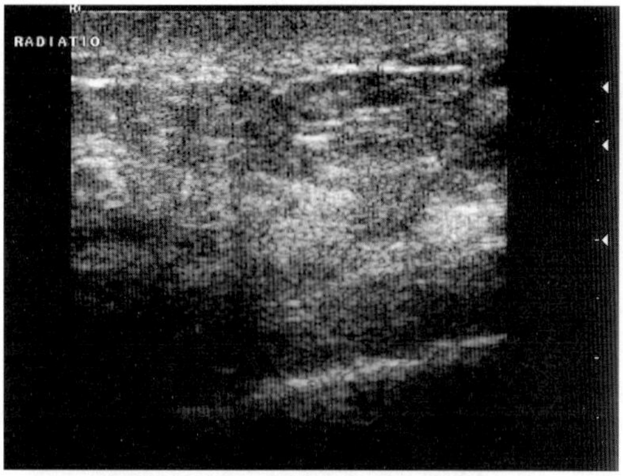

Fig. 8.**52** Breast sonogram of a patient on radiation therapy. The skin is thickened to more than 5 mm. There is gradual regression of the thin (anechoic) subcutaneous fluid layer.

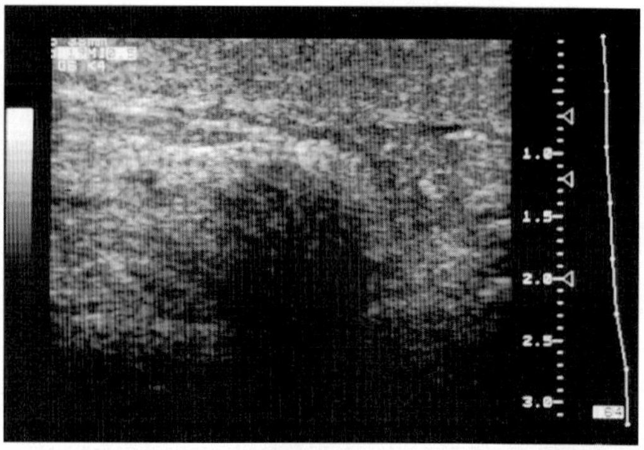

Fig. 8.**53** The typical sonographic appearance of inflammatory breast carcinoma. The central anechoic mass shows all the sonographic criteria of carcinoma, in addition to subcutaneous edema and thickening of the skin.

difficult to obtain in cases where a discrete lesion cannot be identified and excised. The affected region may yield a negative skin biopsy (Hermanek et al. 1992). The histological detection of axillary node metastasis is often helpful.

Breast ultrasound can demonstrate subcutaneous and interstitial edema and thickening of the skin (Harper 1985) (Fig. 8.**51**). These sonographic changes are not specific for malignancy, however, and may be seen after local irradiation following breast conservation surgery (Fig. 8.**52**) and in patients with mastitis (Chapter 10). The suspicion of carcinoma is strengthened by finding a malignant-type focal sonographic lesion in the same or opposite breast (Fig. 8.**53**). Axillary sonography can yield additional information in cases in which gross metastases have visibly altered the sonographic composition of the lymph nodes. If ultrasound still shows normal structural differentiation of the nodes (cortex, medulla, hilum), it is not possible to distinguish reactive inflammatory lymph-node enlargement from lymph-node metastases by ultrasound (Chapter 11).

9 Sonography of Benign Breast Lesions

The sonographic criteria for the differential diagnosis of breast masses are detailed in Chapter 7 above. The presence and prominence of the various criteria provide the key to the sonographic differentiation of benign and malignant breast lesions. It should be kept in mind, however, that the sonographic evaluation is not a histological diagnosis, and that there is an overlap between the sonographic appearances of benign and malignant lesions. Ultrasound can merely show a relationship between a known histological diagnosis and the sonographic appearance of a focal lesion.

Although posterior acoustic enhancement is suggestive of a benign lesion, it may also be seen with malignant tumors. Since both benign and malignant lesions can be hypoechoic, this criterion may not be helpful in the differential diagnosis. Similarly, the presence or absence of internal echoes is not a definite sign of the benign or malignant nature of a lesion; both malignant and benign lesions can be associated with internal echoes, depending on the stromal content. Narrow, bilateral edge shadows are a suggestive sign that the lesion is benign. Other benign criteria are the presence of smooth, narrow borders, a transverse orientation of the major tumor axis ("wider than tall"), compressibility, and mobility. A wide posterior shadow is more characteristic of a malignant tumor and may be its only distinctive sonographic feature. The criterion of axial orientation illustrates the relative nature of these tumor characteristics: a mass has to reach a certain size before it shows appreciable transverse extension due to expansile growth, or appreciable vertical extension due to infiltration.

It should be added that the major criterion in the differential diagnosis of a sonographically detected lesion is still the experience of the examiner, along with optimal machine and transducer characteristics, qualities that cannot always be evaluated in terms of definable criteria. The following examples and descriptions are intended to aid the examiner in recognizing various benign focal lesions in the breast.

Fibrocystic Changes and Breast Cysts

These benign conditions usually involve the entire breast, are very common, and are often found in premenopausal women, with varying degrees of prominence (Barth and Prechtel 1990). Fibrocystic change can be described histologically as a benign mammary dysplasia marked by the coexistence of cysts and fibrotic changes. Fibrocystic change is often used as a collective term for any nonneoplastic structural changes in the glandular breast tissue, although in the strict sense it refers to hormonally induced transformations of the breast parenchyma. Histological examination reveals interlobular and intralobular fibrosis, acinolobular hyperplasias with cysts and ductal ectasia, and ductal epithelial proliferation. Only the type that is accompanied by atypical epithelial proliferation (hyperplasia) is associated with an increased risk of carcinoma. Because this risk is demonstrated histologically and not by ultrasound, fibrocystic change is considered an indication for regular follow-up examinations.

The dividing line between a sonographically "normal" breast and a "fibrocystic"

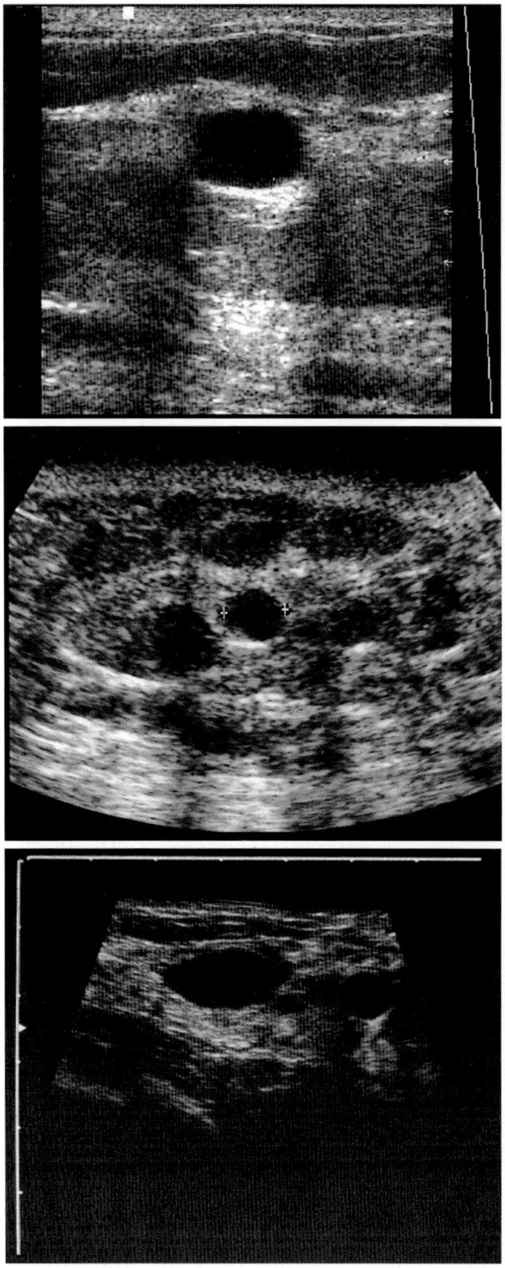

a

b

c

Fig. 9.1 Breast cysts. **a** A small, simple breast cyst about 1 cm in diameter. **b** A small, simple breast cyst about 4 mm in diameter. **c** Multiple cysts of varying size in a fibrocystic breast.

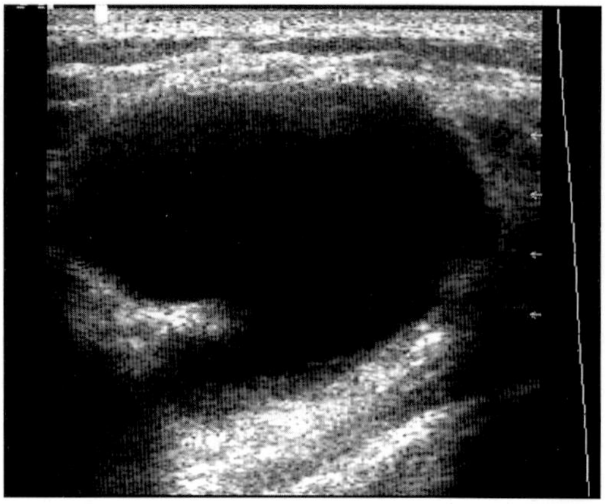

Fig. 9.2 A large breast cyst, several centimeters in diameter.

breast is undefined and depends largely on the subjective assessment of the examiner. It should be noted that nearly all women over age 30 have small breast cysts that can be detected mammographically and by ultrasound (Barth and Prechtel 1990). The cysts usually appear between 30 and 50 years of age and are very rare before age 20 and after age 60. The cysts range from a few millimeters to 5–6 cm in size (Figs. 9.**1**, 9.**2**).

The sonographic and mammographic evaluation of breast cysts is a good example of the way in which ultrasound and mammography complement each other in breast diagnosis. While mammography can define a focal lesion but cannot determine whether it is cystic or solid, ultrasound usually demonstrates signs that can definitely establish the cystic nature of a mass.

A *cyst* has typical acoustic properties that differentiate it from a solid lesion (Table 9.**1**). Because the ultrasound traverses the cyst with virtually no energy loss, the tissue behind the cyst appears more echogenic than adjacent tissues that are equidistant from the transducer. This phenomenon, termed "posterior acoustic enhancement," is typical of cysts (Fig. 9.**3**). A cyst located deep within the breast, and thus at some distance from the transducer, may show little or no posterior enhancement, and the eye may be unable to detect the enhancement caused by very small cysts. Typically, a

Table 9.**1** Typical sonographic features of breast cysts (> 1 cm).

Acoustic phenomena	Description
Central echogenicity	Anechoic
Borders	Narrow, hyperechoic
Orientation of major axis	Transverse
Posterior acoustic phenomena	Homogeneous enhancement
Edge shadows	Narrow, bilateral
Compressibility	Readily compressible
Architectural change	None

cyst will change its shape as variable amounts of transducer pressure are applied. The lateral borders of the cyst may cast a narrow edge shadow on each side. Most cysts are round and show a transverse orientation, i.e., their major axis is usually perpendicular to the axis of the ultrasound beam. Because cysts grow by expansion in preformed tissues such as the mammary glands and lactiferous ducts, they do not distort the surrounding breast architecture.

Cysts may be multilocular and generally have very thin walls (Fig. 9.**4**). These septa represent the atrophic walls of the lactiferous ducts that separate the cysts. Because cysts develop in the ducts and lobules, their shape conforms to these preexisting structures, creating figures on sonograms that resemble a cut-open snail shell.

The septations that separate the cyst components may be misinterpreted as internal structures if the probe is not optimally positioned.

Echoes can appear within a cyst due to intracystic hemorrhage or mucinous secretions (Fig. 9.**5**), at times making the cyst difficult to distinguish from a fibroadenoma. Many of these complicated cysts are noncompressible, and histological evaluation is often necessary to exclude a solid mass such as a medullary carcinoma or fibroadenoma.

The differential diagnosis of a cyst with internal echoes should include inflammation and abscess, but these conditions are usually easily diagnosed on the basis of their clinical symptoms.

As noted earlier, a small or deeply situated cyst may not display posterior enhancement, compressibility, or edge shadowing.

Fibrocystic proliferation can cause visible thickening of the cyst wall and make the cyst difficult to distinguish from a malignant tumor (Fig. 9.**6**). Similar problems of differential diagnosis arise in cysts that contain solid material, usually appearing as a wall irregularity or projecting mural mass. Histological confirmation should be obtained

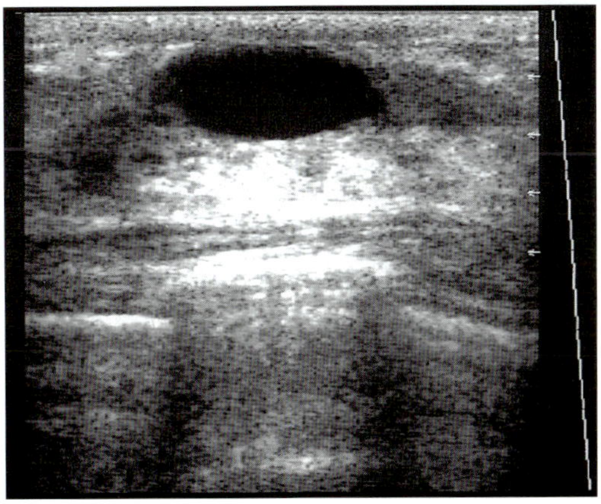
a

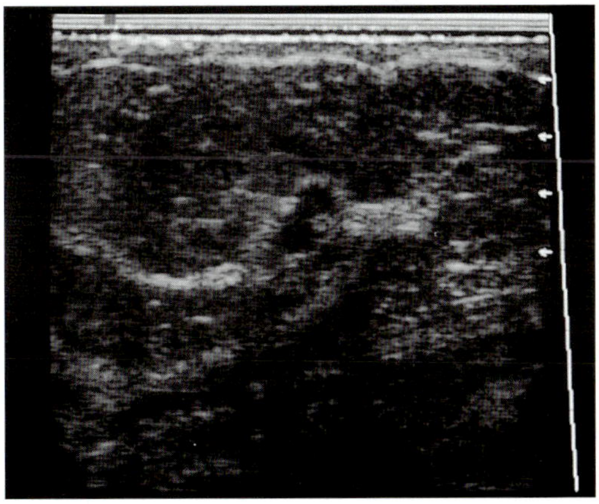
b

Fig. 9.**3a** A breast cyst about 15 mm in diameter, occurring in a relatively superficial area and showing typical posterior enhancement. **b** Small breast cysts showing no posterior enhancement.

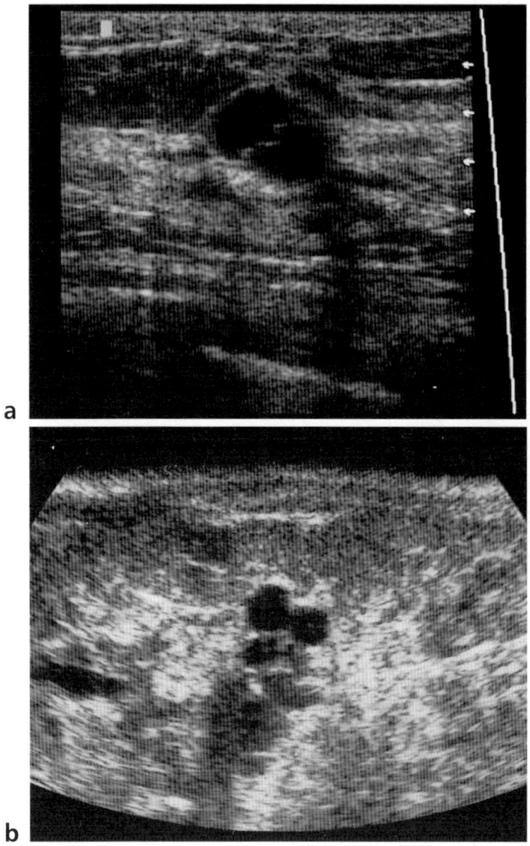

Fig. 9.**4a** A breast cyst containing a small septum. **b** Multiple adjacent breast cysts separated by thin walls.

whenever *solid intracystic structures* are detected, in order to exclude intracystic carcinoma. This procedure seems justified when one considers that 75 % of solid intracystic structures are benign (usually papillomas), 20 % are malignant, and 5 % are phyllodes tumors (Rizzatto et al. 1993).

Cyst formation may be so extensive that all of the breast parenchyma undergoes cystic transformation. In these cases it is pointless to attempt to measure the numerous cysts, since the measurements will not be reproducible. The patient may report a feeling of breast tension and other symptoms. Symptomatic cases can be managed by aspirating the cysts under ultrasound guidance and carrying out cytological analysis of the aspirated material. Aspiration

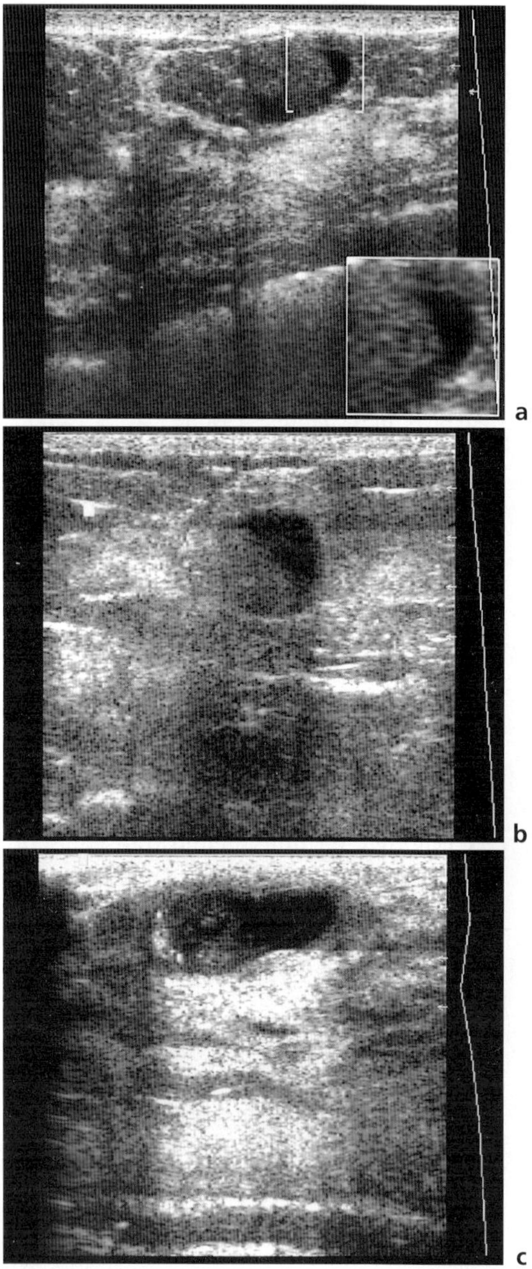

Fig. 9.**5a** A hemorrhagic breast cyst. **b** A breast cyst containing mucinous material. **c** A hemorrhagic breast cyst.

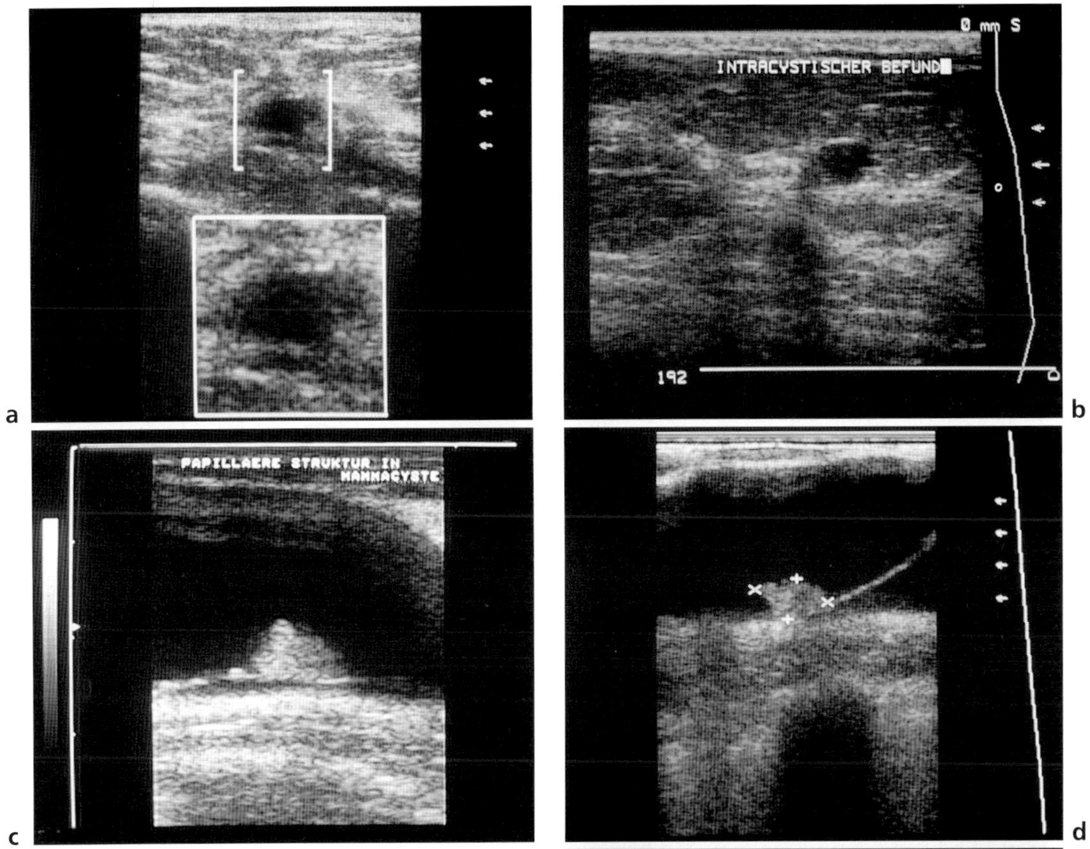

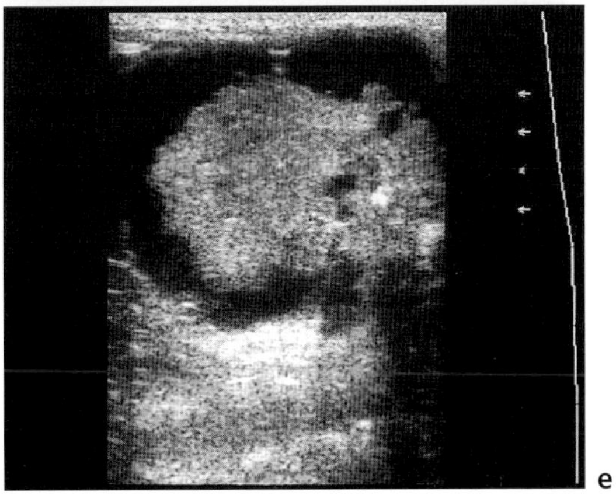

Fig. 9.**6a** A small, histologically confirmed breast cyst, the wall of which appears thickened due to fibrocystic proliferation, raising problems in the differential diagnosis. **b** A very small breast cyst showing a small, solid wall irregularity. **c** A solid intracystic papillary mass (histologically benign). **d** A solid intracystic mass (histologically benign). **e** A large intracystic carcinoma.

may also be indicated in a cystic breast so that a more useful mammogram can be obtained. In addition, pneumocystography can be performed as an adjunctive study at the time of aspiration (Fig. 9.**7**).

In summary, very large or very small cysts can pose problems in the differential diagnosis on breast ultrasonography. Large cysts can be difficult to define in their entirety and may transcend the boundaries of the

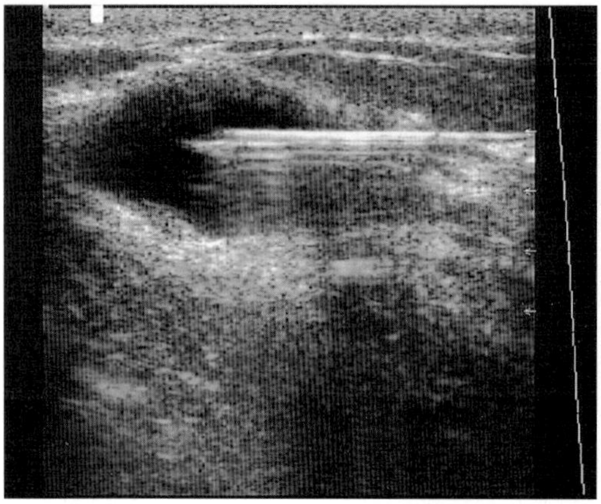

Fig. 9.7 Aspiration of a breast cyst.

acoustic window. Numerous cysts can make the intervening tissue difficult to evaluate and may give the examiner a misleading sense of reassurance ("they're just cysts!") that results in a cursory examination. Small cysts may not exhibit the sharply defined borders, lack of internal echoes, and posterior enhancement that are considered the sonographic hallmarks of simple cysts.

The following equipment-related factors should be kept in mind, as they can hamper the sonographic diagnosis of breast cysts (Fig. 9.**8**):

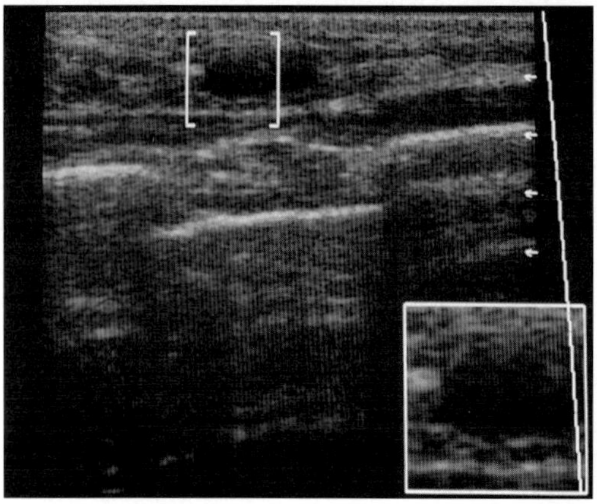

Fig. 9.**8** Section-thickness artifact causes the anterior wall of the cyst to appear indistinct, in contrast to its sharply defined posterior wall. The cyst does not appear anechoic.

- Reverberation artifacts caused by multiple reflections of the ultrasound waves inside the cyst can mimic the appearance of intracystic structures (see Fig. 2.**12**).
- Section-thickness artifact can cause unsharpness of the near wall, with apparent peripheral intracystic structures (see Fig. 2.**7**).

Fibrocystic change presents a relatively typical sonographic pattern: a mosaic of many small, hypoechoic areas (representing dilated ductal structures) against a background of very dense, hyperechoic glandular breast tissue. The tissues have a generally "unsettled" appearance. The fibrocystic breast can provide a difficult setting for the sonographic detection of true focal lesions (Fig. 9.**9**).

Nevertheless, ultrasound is more sensitive than mammography for detecting focal lesions in dense fibrocystic breasts, since mammograms usually show only a bright, radiographically dense breast that lacks clearly definable features.

Unfortunately, it is common for fibrocystic breasts to produce attenuating effects on sonograms that can mimic shadowing malignant tumors (Fig. 9.**10**). These cases warrant close-interval follow-up to watch for any changes in these acoustic effects.

Proliferative fibrocystic changes may be characterized by thickened cyst walls and by thickening and fibrosis of the interlobar stroma. The sonographic correlates of these changes are a thickened, hyperechoic supramammary fascia and the presence of hyperechoic connective tissue between the parenchymal islands and cysts.

Circumscribed areas of fibrosis appear as ill-defined hyperechoic areas that are poorly compressible and show posterior attenuation or even posterior shadowing – a pattern that is easily mistaken for carcinoma (Fig. 9.**11**).

On the whole, fibrocystic changes are very common in premenopausal women. With a prevalence as high as 80–90 %, these changes are not considered pathological unless corresponding symptoms are present.

It is typical for both the sonographic features and the symptomatology of fibrocystic change to wax and wane with the menstrual cycle. Symptoms tend to be most pronounced during the second half of the cycle. At this time more dilated ductal structures are seen at ultrasound, and cysts are larger and more numerous. Often the sonographic pattern is more heterogeneous and irregular in this phase of the menstrual cycle. In such cases, it is advisable either to repeat the examination in the first half of the cycle or to adopt the general practice of performing breast ultrasound in the early part of the menstrual cycle.

The disordered features that may be seen on ultrasound in the fibrocystic breast

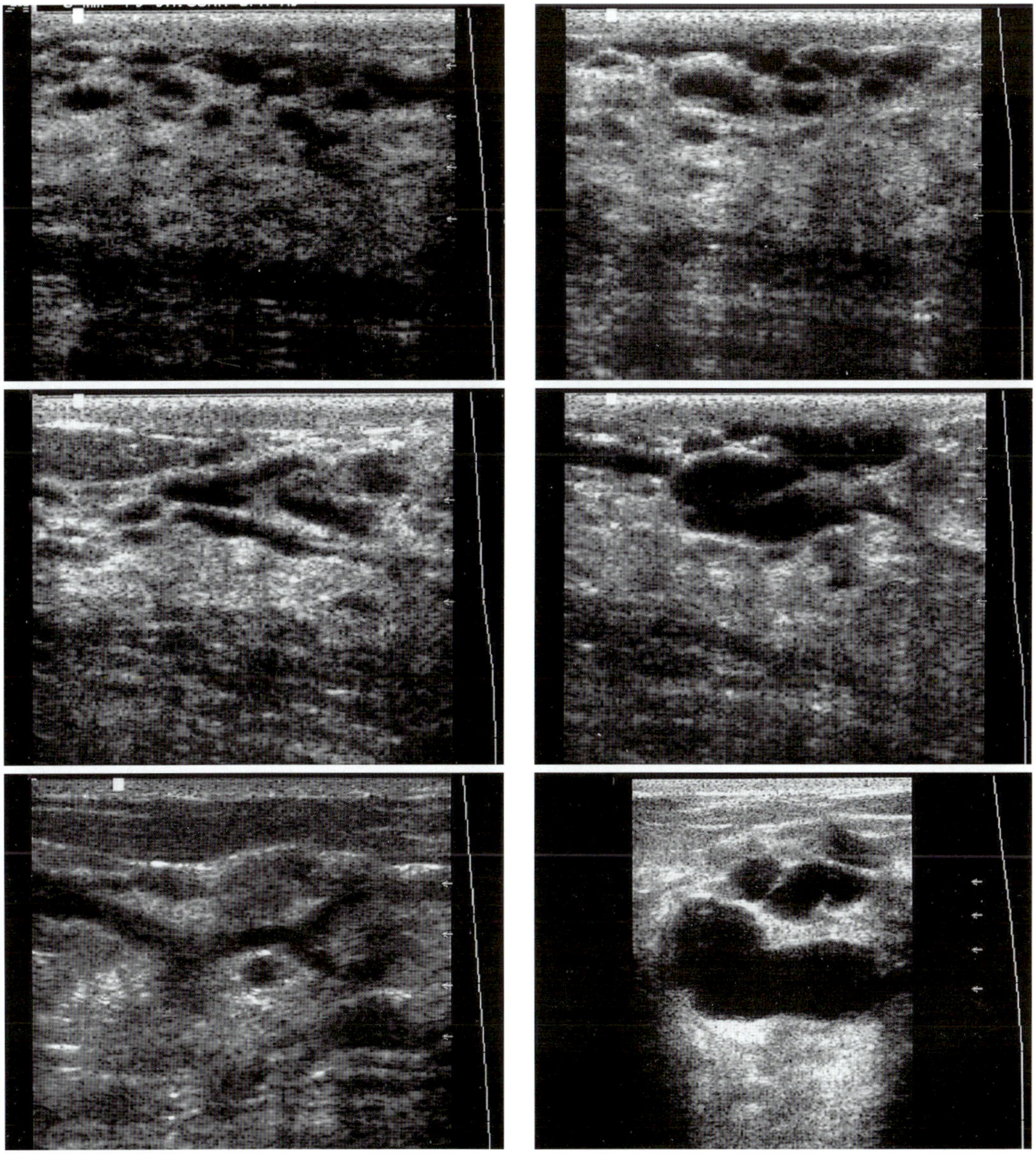

a b c d e f

Fig. 9.9 **a–g** Sonographic appearance of fibrocystic change. The parenchymal patterns can range from "honeycomb" to cystic.

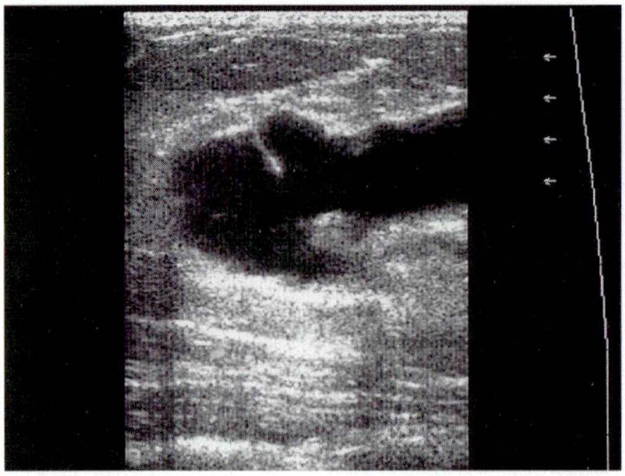

g

Fig. 9.**9** **g**.

include irregular, stellate patterns and thickened, bizarre boundaries with adjacent tissues (Fig. 9.**12**). Most of these cases defy evaluation by ultrasound or mammography, and only biopsy can provide the correct diagnosis.

Thus, the risks posed by fibrocystic change are two-fold: certain types of fibrocystic change (which cannot be differentiated by ultrasound) increase the risk of developing breast cancer, and the features of fibrocystic change can mimic the appearance of cancer. Both of these factors warrant further evaluation of the fibrocystic breast by close-interval follow-up or biopsy.

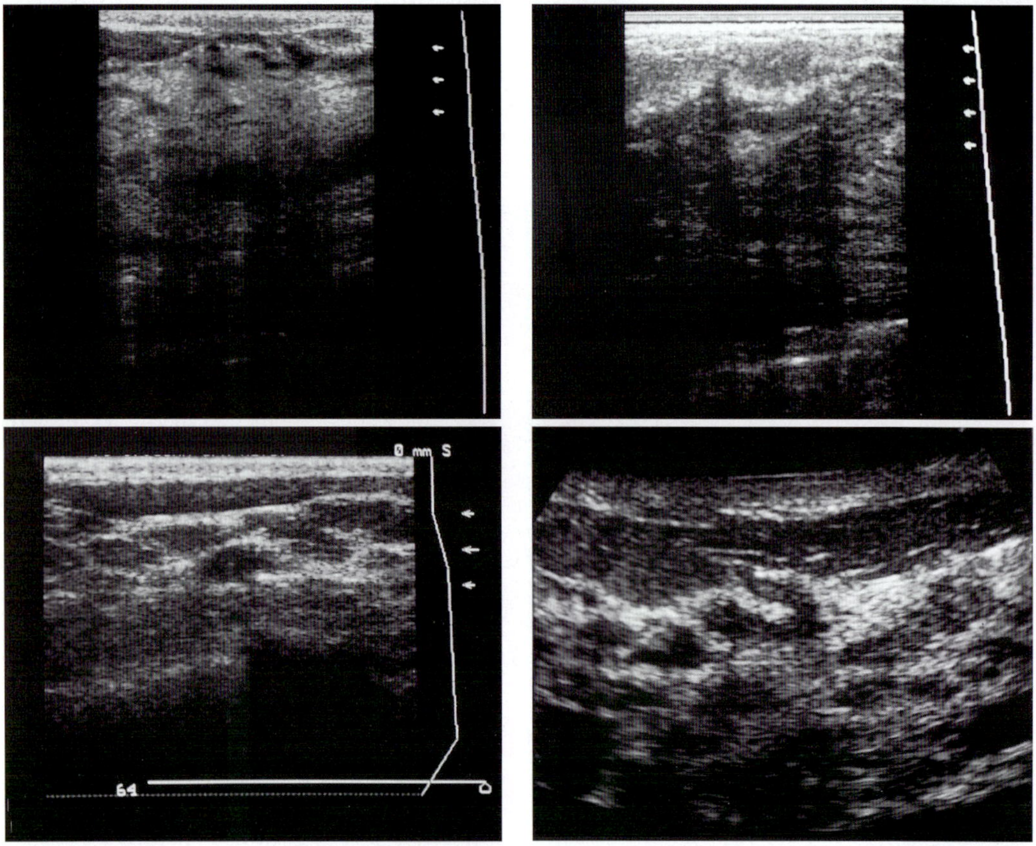

a b c d

Fig. 9.**10a** Acoustic shadows in a fibrocystic breast. **b** Shadows in a fibrocystic breast can raise problems in differential diagnosis. **c** Small fibrocystic lesions can be difficult to distinguish from malignancies. **d** The higher the transducer frequency, the more prominent the fibrocystic changes may appear.

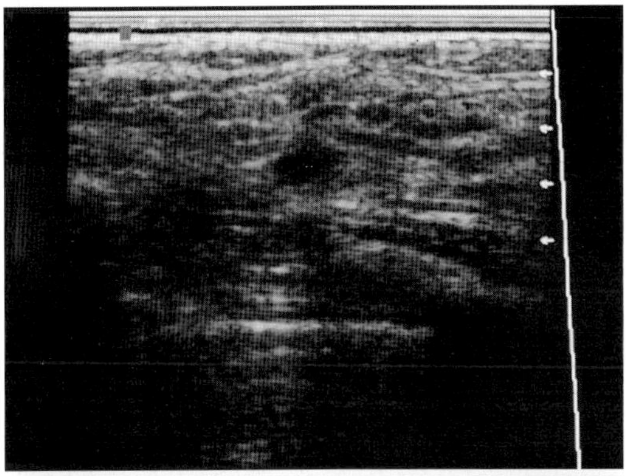
a

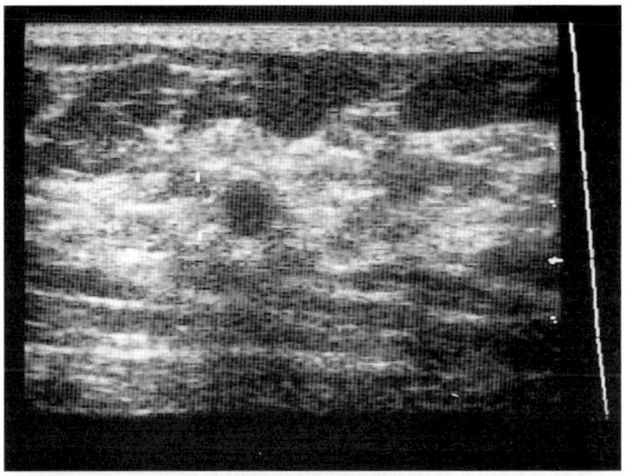
b

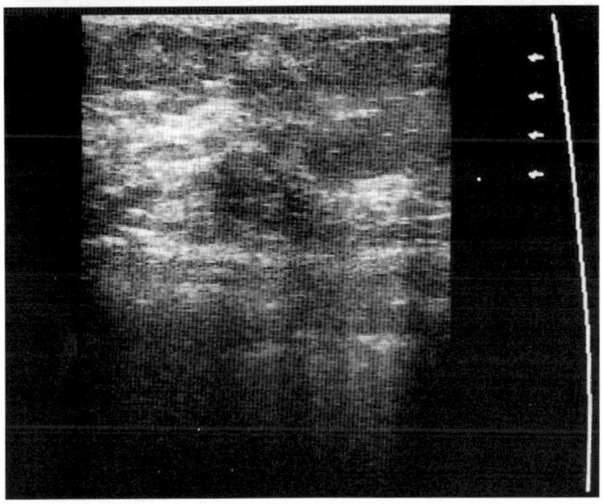
c

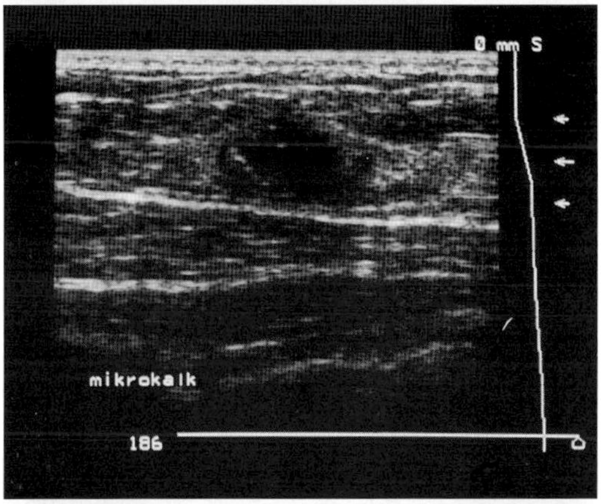

d

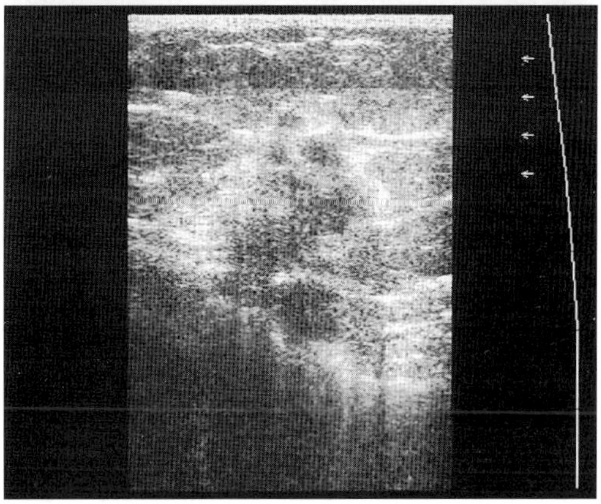
e

Fig. 9.**11a** A small lesion identified histologically as fibrocystic change. **b** The 4-mm focus in this dense breast was identified histologically as fibrocystic tissue. **c** Shadowing fibrotic tissue in a fibrocystic breast can be difficult to distinguish from carcinoma by ultrasound. **d** Microcalcifications in a fibrocystic breast. **e** The shadowing in this breast carcinoma shows marked similarities to that seen in fibrocystic lesions. **f** Macrocalcifications and microcalcifications in a fibrocystic breast. **g** Microcalcifications in a fibrocystic breast.

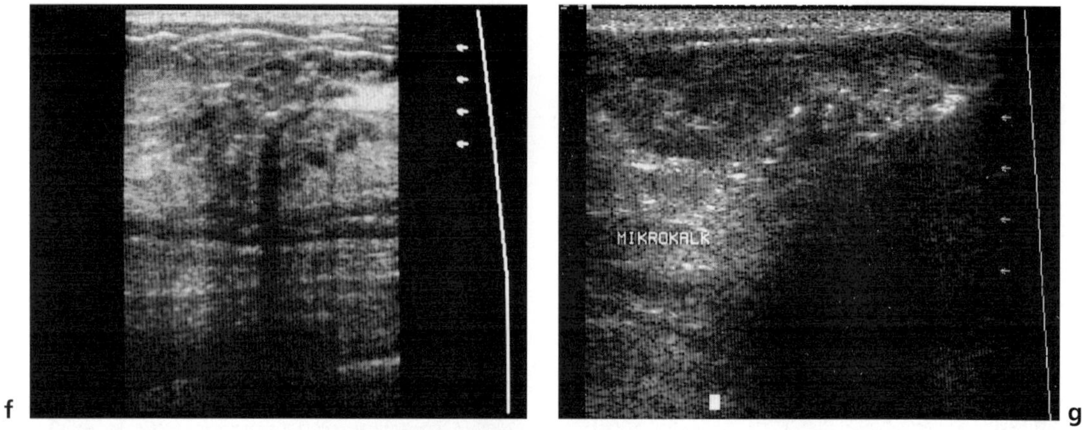

Fig. 9.**11 f, g**

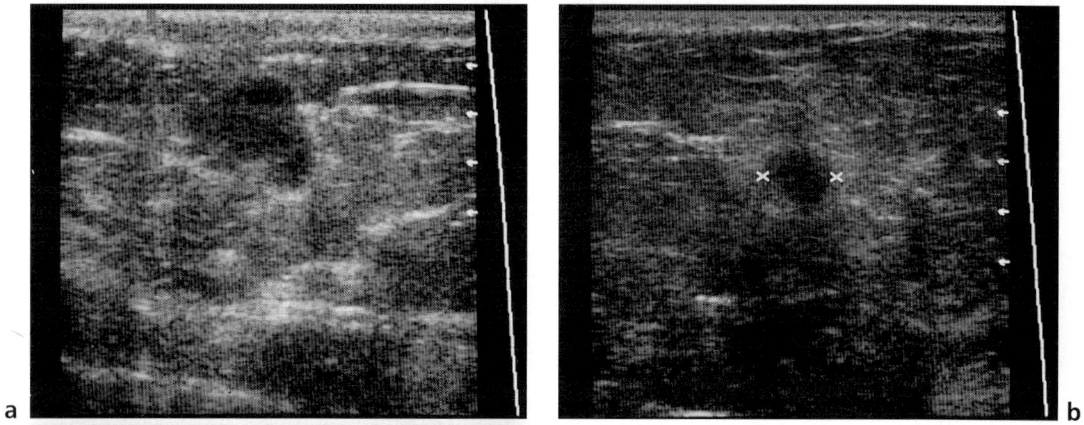

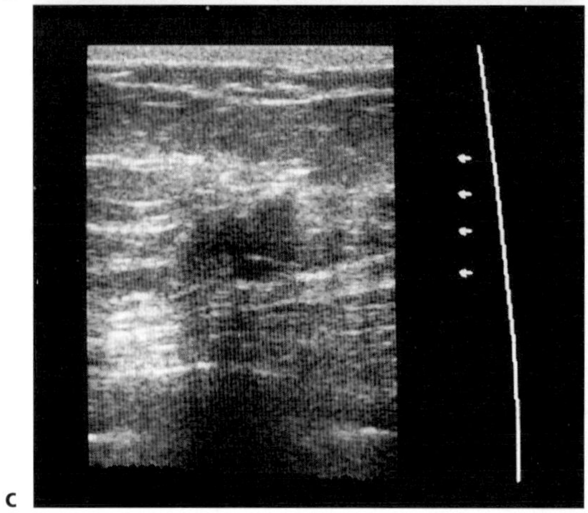

Fig. 9.**12a** A fibrocystic lesion with indistinct borders. **b** A small lesion with indistinct borders, identified histologically as fibrocystic tissue. **c** A shadowing fibrocystic lesion with indistinct borders, mimicking the sonographic appearance of a breast malignancy.

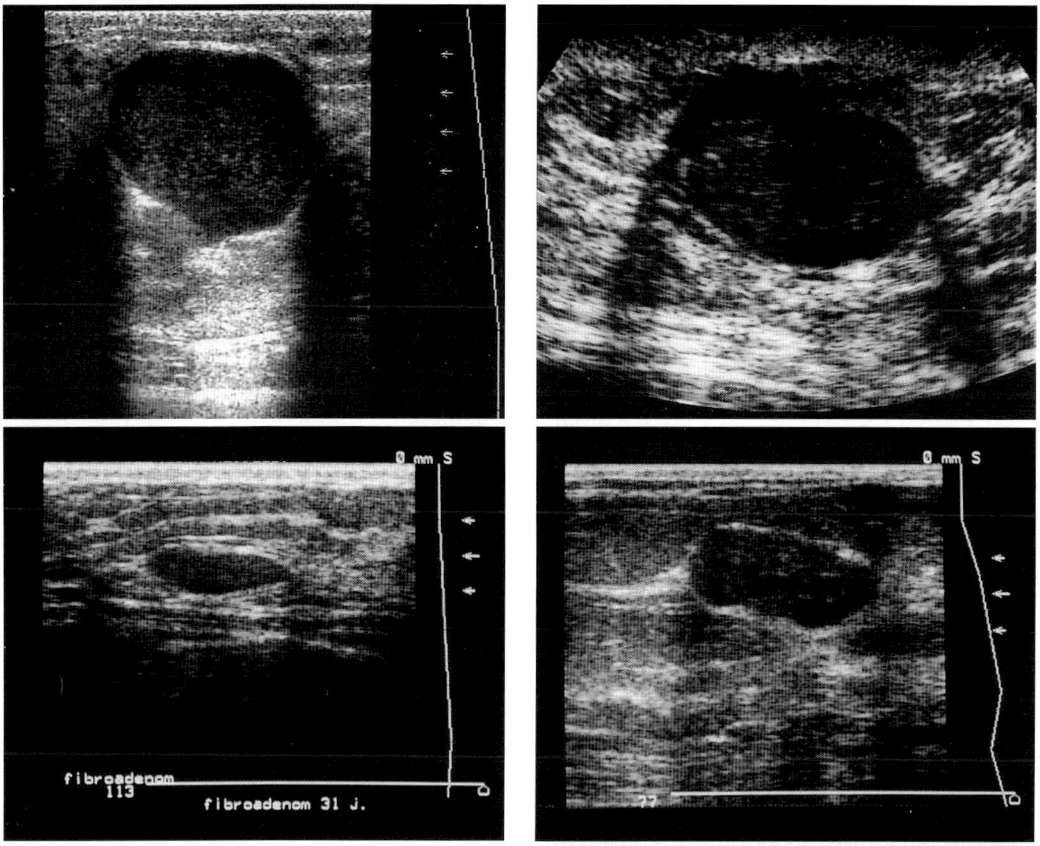

a b c d

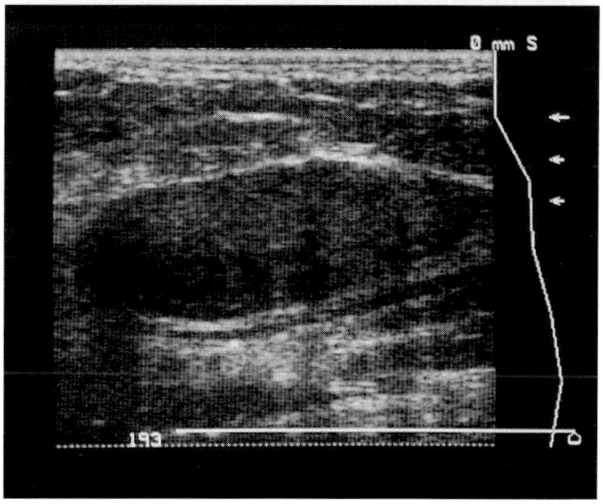

e

Fig. 9.**13a** A well-circumscribed fibroadenoma with posterior enhancement. **b** A fibroadenoma with bilateral edge shadows. **c** A fibroadenoma showing equivocal posterior acoustic effects. The transverse orientation is typical of a mass that grows by expansion. **d** A well-circumscribed fibroadenoma. **e** A large fibroadenoma showing mixed posterior enhancement and shadowing.

Fibroadenoma

Fibroadenoma is the most common benign breast tumor in premenopausal women. Though usually detected in young women and adolescents, the tumor may occur at any age. Even postmenopausal women taking hormonal therapy are subject to new occurrences of fibroadenoma. The site of predilection is the upper outer quadrant. Fibroadenomas have a very low malignant potential, with cancer developing in only about 1–2 % of cases (Bässler et al. 1989b). About 10–20 % of fibroadenomas are multiple, and few grow to more than 2–3 cm in size. Because these tumors are hormone-dependent, they usually regress at menopause.

Fibroadenoma presents clinically as a firm, rubbery, palpable mass that is frequently discovered by breast self-examination.

Sonographically, a fibroadenoma presents the typical features of a benign mass. It resembles a cyst with internal echoes and shows less shape distortion than a cyst when compressed. Most fibroadenomas exhibit sharp, smooth borders, a homogeneous internal echo texture, and moderate to high internal echogenicity. Usually there is no change in the posterior echo pattern (no enhancement or attenuation) or in the surrounding tissues, skin, or subcutaneous tissue. The sonographic appearance of fibroadenoma also depends on its composition, i.e., whether there is a preponderance of epithelial tissue or connective tissue in the tumor, and on the tissue in which the fibroadenoma is embedded (Fig. 9.**13**).

As mentioned before, fibroadenomas may appear hypoechoic to hyperechoic. Hypoechoic lesions are common in young women and signify a predominance of epithelial components. Fibroadenomas appear more echogenic within a fatty breast and may be difficult to distinguish from their surroundings (Fig. 9.**14**).

Calcification, if present, will alter the normally homogeneous appearance of a fibroadenoma.

The histological composition of a fibroadenoma also determines the posterior acoustic effects that are associated with the tumor. These can range from no effect to posterior enhancement behind predominantly epithelial tumors and posterior enhancement or shadowing behind predominantly fibrous or calcified tumors (Fig. 9.**15**).

Narrow, bilateral edge shadows are commonly seen with fibroadenomas. The expansile growth of the tumor usually causes it to assume a transverse orientation (parallel to the skin) and the lesions are "wider than tall." The tumor displaces the surrounding tissue but does not cause architectural disruption.

The list of classic sonographic features applies to most fibroadenomas (Table 9.**2**). These tumors have a spectrum of appearances, however, and lesions that do not show the typical pattern can be difficult to evaluate. The smaller the fibroadenoma, the greater the difficulty of identifying it as such with ultrasound. Small fibroadenomas are particularly difficult to distinguish from cysts. Larger fibroadenomas can resemble phyllodes tumors. Lipomas and carcinomas (particularly medullary carcinomas) can also mimic the appearance of a fibroadenoma.

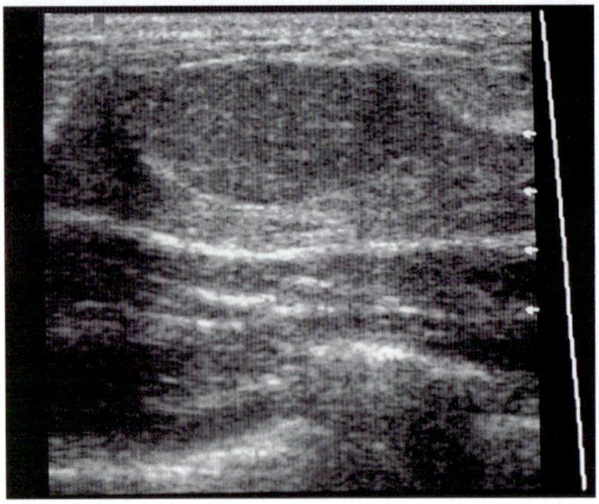

Fig. 9.**14** This fibroadenoma is isoechoic to fat, so it is poorly demarcated from the surrounding fatty tissue.

Tab. 9.**2** Typical sonographic features of fibroadenoma.

Acoustic phenomena	Description
Central echogenicity	Hypoechoic
Internal echoes	Fine, hyperechoic
Borders	Narrow, hyperechoic
Orientation of major axis	Transverse
Posterior acoustic phenomena	No effect, or homogeneous enhancement
Edge shadows	Narrow, bilateral
Compressibility	Little or none
Architectural change	None

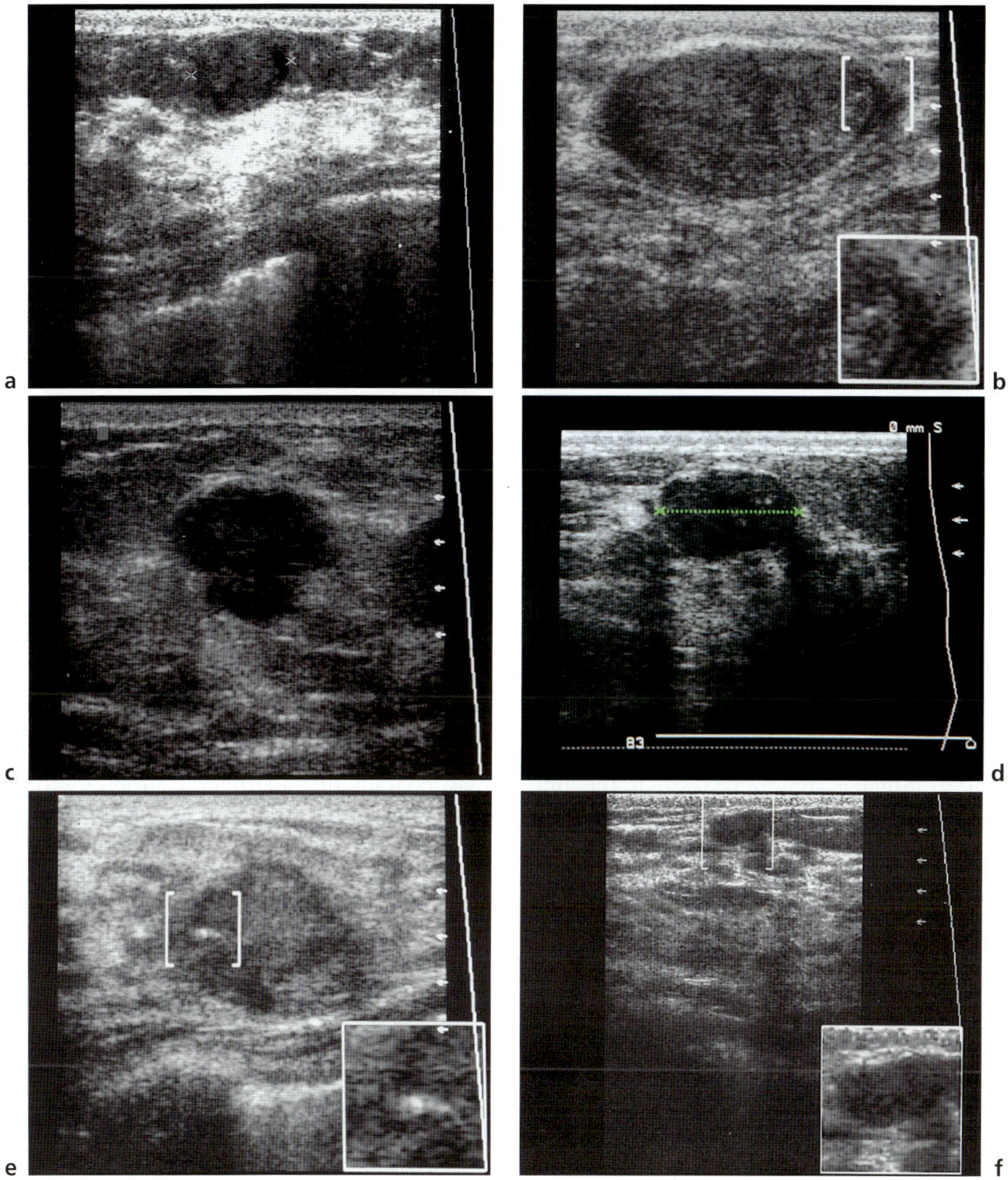

Fig. 9.**15a** A small fibroadenoma, showing a combined hypoechoic and moderately echogenic pattern. **b** This fibroadenoma is hypoechoic to surrounding tissues. **c** A hypoechoic fibroadenoma with somewhat indistinct borders. **d** A small fibroadenoma, showing indifferent posterior acoustic effects. **e** Calcifications within a small fibroadenoma.

g 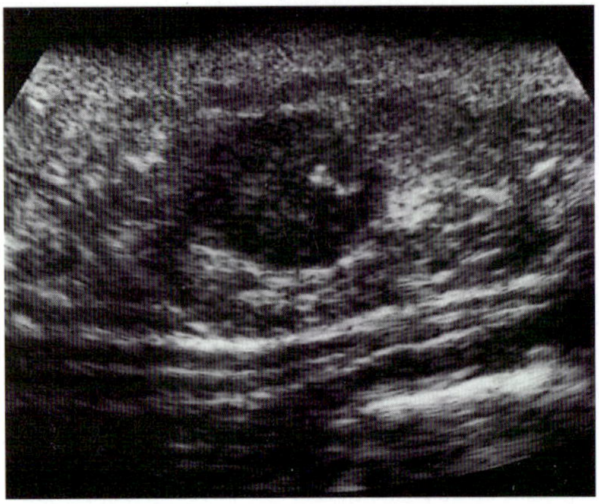

Fig. 9.**15g**

Phyllodes Tumors

The great majority of phyllodes tumors are benign, and they are sometimes referred to as "proliferative fibroadenomas" (Fig. 9.**16**). Phyllodes tumors are generally rare and are characterized by rapid growth. The peak incidence is between 50 and 60 years of age. Malignant transformation (about 10% of cases) requires a histological diagnosis. Some lesions metastasize to the lungs via the bloodstream.

Phyllodes tumors appear sonographically as predominantly hypoechoic masses, with a mixture of cystic and solid components. Ultrasound cannot differentiate between the benign and malignant variants, and sometimes it cannot distinguish phyllodes tumor from fibroadenoma.

Lipoma

Lipomas arise from fat cells and are contained within a well-defined capsule (Fig. 9.**17**). The tumor typically presents as a freely mobile palpable mass. Lipomas are usually superficial within the breast parenchyma, at the periphery of the breast, on the chest wall, or in the upper arm. They also may be embedded within the breast parenchyma.

The sonographic appearance is that of a mobile, compressible mass with thin, smooth borders. The interior of the mass is less echogenic than a fibroadenoma and is roughly isoechoic to the fatty tissue that surrounds or permeates the breast parenchyma. Because of this similarity in echogenicity, many are only identified sonographically after palpation. Some lipomas may contain fine peripheral structures of somewhat higher echogenicity representing fibrous tissue elements. Calcifications may occur within lipomas.

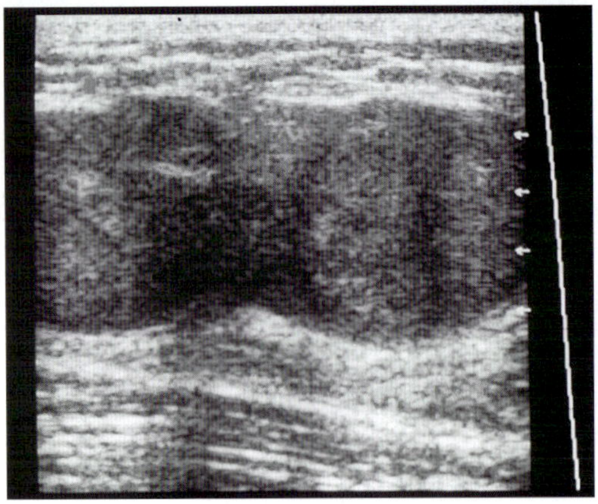

Fig. 9.**16** Phyllodes tumor.

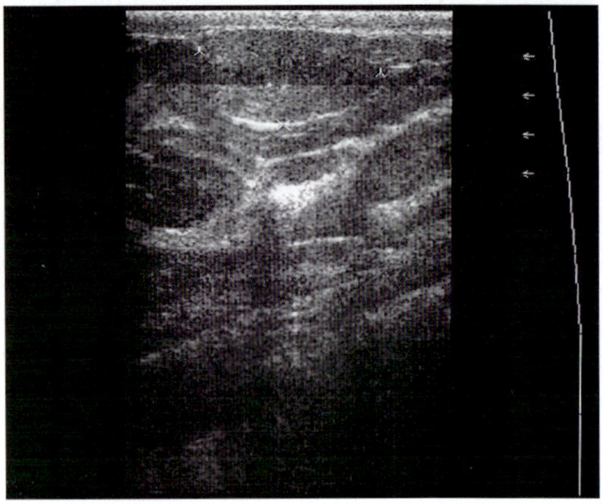

Fig. 9.**17** A lipoma that is isoechoic to surrounding fatty tissue.

Intraductal and Intracystic Papillomas

A high-resolution transducer can define intraductal papillomas as hyperechoic structures projecting into the lumina of dilated lactiferous ducts (Fig. 9.**18**). These lesions are indistinguishable by ultrasound from the early stages of papillary carcinoma. As a rule, papillomas are visible only if the duct is sufficiently dilated to permit delineation of the lesion.

Intracystic papilloma appears as a hyperechoic mural lesion that contrasts vividly with the anechoic interior of the cyst. Again, ultrasound cannot positively discriminate between benign and malignant forms. Aspiration cytology may be able to detect atypical proliferation, but a more definitive method is excisional biopsy and histological evaluation.

Fat Necrosis

Fat necrosis may be secondary to trauma or breast surgery (Fig. 9.**19**). It may present clinically as a firm, palpable mass that may even cause skin dimpling.

Fat necrosis may appear as a round, well-circumscribed lesion at ultrasound, or it may mimic the appearance of a malignant tumor. This can make it exceedingly difficult or impossible to distinguish fat necrosis from a recurrent tumor in the postoperative breast. Calcifications may occur within areas of fat necrosis.

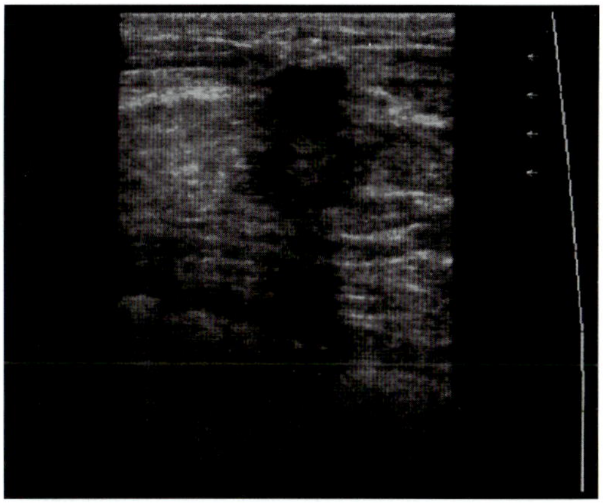

Fig. 9.**19** Fat necrosis. Ultrasound cannot positively distinguish this lesion from a carcinoma.

Galactocele

A galactocele is a benign, milk-containing cystic breast mass (Fig. 9.**20**). It is caused by obstruction of a milk-producing gland. Accordingly, galactoceles occur mainly in nursing women, and are uncommon in non-

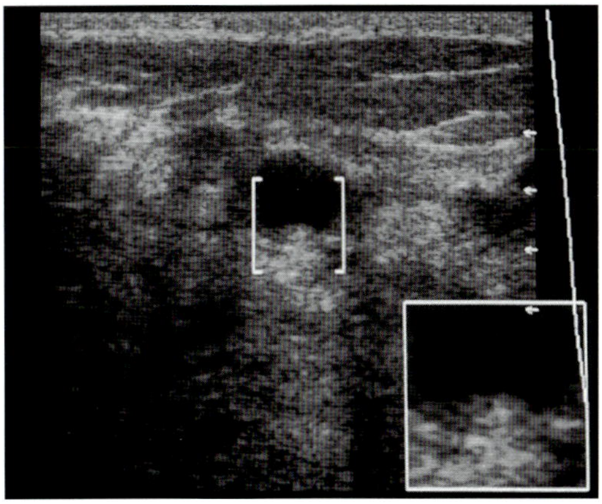

Fig. 9.**18** A small intracystic papilloma, histologically confirmed.

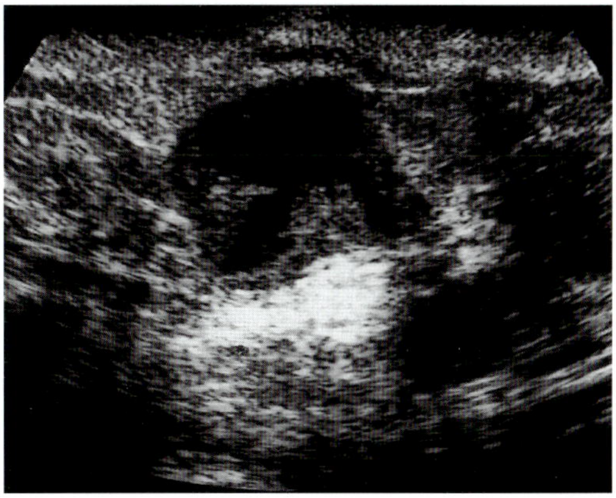

Fig. 9.**20** Galactocele.

a 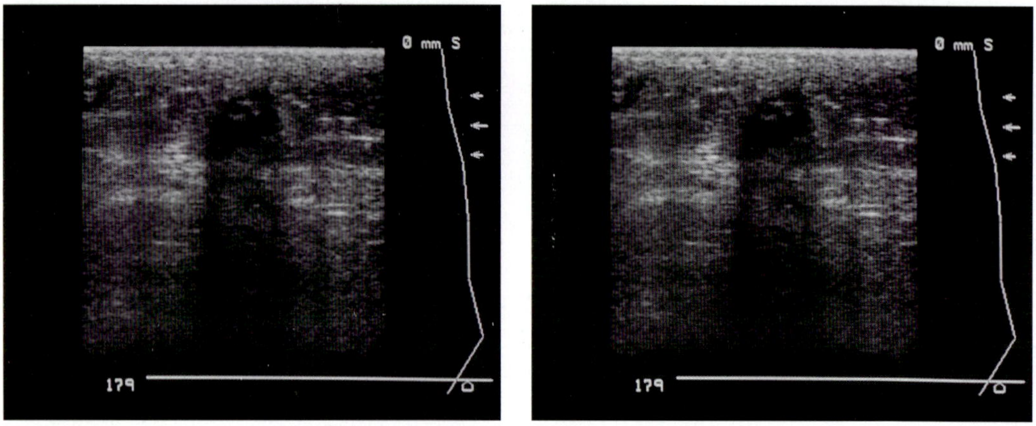 b

Fig. 9.**21a** Postoperative suture granuloma. **b** Postoperative hematoma.

lactating females and juveniles. The cysts are usually painful.

Ultrasound demonstrates a well-circumscribed cystic mass with internal echoes caused by inspissated milk. Chronic changes in a long-standing galactocele may be sonographically indistinguishable from cancer.

Postoperative Changes

Postoperative scarring has a spectrum of sonographic appearances ranging from a complete absence of echoes to marked acoustic shadowing or even a hyperechoic focal lesion. From the immediate postoperative period to about one year postoperatively, the (nonirradiated) surgical site may appear as a hypoechoic area with ill-defined contours. It borders directly on the cutaneous scar and is visible below it. The postsurgical scar may regress with time and produce no focal sonographic changes, or it may retract and draw the breast parenchyma up toward the skin, producing a visible parenchymal discontinuity.

When fibrotic scar tissue develops, it appears as a hyperechoic, shadowing area that may be indistinguishable from cancer.

The identification of recurrent tumor in a surgical scar can be difficult. But whereas scar tissue often casts an acoustic shadow without forming a distinct focal lesion, a recurrent or malignant tumor usually appears as a true focal lesion. Sensitive flow imaging techniques may help resolve the issue: recurrent tumor usually shows blood flow, scar tissue does not. Close-interval follow-up may also be useful since scar tissue, unlike tumor, usually does not change over time.

As mentioned above, fat necrosis is another possible sequela of breast surgery that can raise problems in the differential diagnosis (Fig. 9.**21**).

10 Sonography of Inflammatory Breast Diseases

Puerperal mastitis is easily diagnosed from the patient's history and clinical symptoms. Breast ultrasound is occasionally useful for assessing the response to treatment, but in the majority of cases it is unnecessary.

Nonpuerperal mastitis, on the other hand, is difficult to distinguish from inflammatory carcinoma (Barth and Prechtel 1990, Hackelöer et al. 1986, Harper 1985, Hayes et al. 1991, Pahnke et al. 1985). Acute nonpuerperal mastitis often develops in the setting of chronic mastitis for no apparent reason. Rarely, pathogenic microorganisms are identified as the cause of the inflammation, and in isolated cases it can be due to exogenous factors (drugs, trauma) (Harper 1985).

The clinical history and the inflammatory symptoms initially suggest the diagnosis of nonpuerperal mastitis. The usual workup of these patients is to proceed with mammography to exclude malignant disease. If mammographic findings are equivocal, a trial of antibiotic therapy is instituted to furnish an empirical diagnosis. Ultrasound can then be used to check for a reduction in the size of the inflammatory mass in response to antibiotic therapy (Blohmer et al. 1994).

The sonographic criteria of nonpuerperal mastitis, and particularly abscess, depend on the extent and duration of the disease (Blohmer et al. 1994, Hackelöer et al. 1986, Teubner et al. 1985) (Figs. 10.**1**–10.**3**). The criteria are as follows:

- Wide, indistinct, hyperechoic borders
- A hypoechoic center
- Attenuation behind a portion of the mass
- Limited compressibility

Pus sometimes forms a visible layer of sediment within the abscess cavity (Fig. 10.**2**). In other cases, central ductal ectasia may be the only sonographic abnormality. A circumscribed abscess collection in its early stages may not be visible with ultrasound (Fig. 10.**4a**).

Ultrasound may show subcutaneous edema developing in response to the mastitis. Along with erythema and pain, this edema is a typical manifestation of breast inflammation (Fig. 10.**4b**).

The main problem in the sonographic differential diagnosis of nonpuerperal mastitis is that the sonographic criteria may be almost identical to those of carcinoma (Chapter 8).

One way to distinguish nonpuerperal mastitis from cancer is by noting regression of the mass in response to treatment with antibiotics or bromocriptine. Doppler ultrasound can be useful for this purpose.

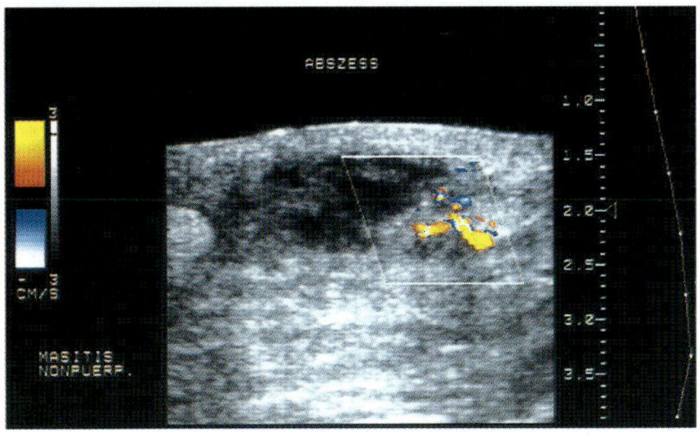

Fig. 10.**1** Sonographic appearance of an incipient breast abscess (hypoechoic septate mass) in nonpuerperal mastitis. The walls of the abscess are still indistinct. Color Doppler indicates a blood vessel at the periphery of the inflammation. A fluid offset was used due to the superficial location of the lesion.

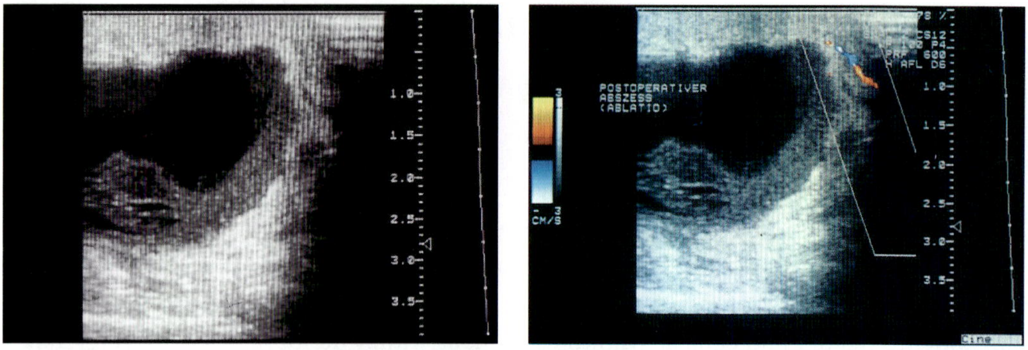

a b

Fig. 10.2**a** Sonographic appearance of a breast abscess. Purulent contents are visible within the thick, hyperechoic capsule. The overlying skin is thickened to 5 mm. **b** Color Doppler indicates blood flow in the abscess capsule.

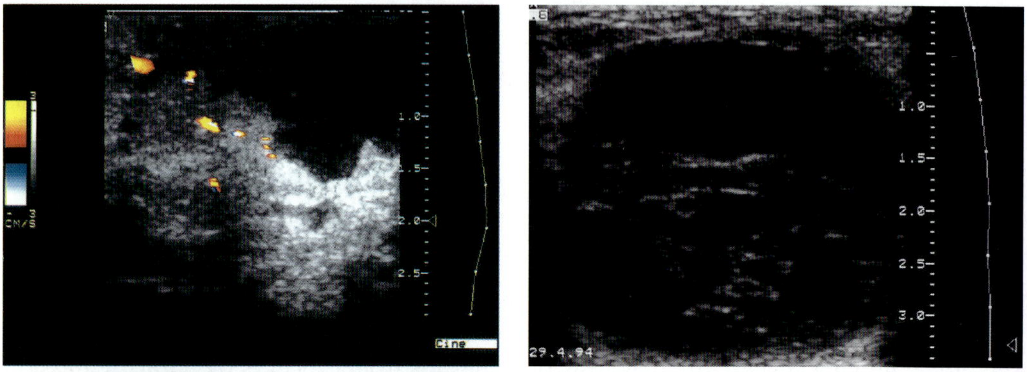

a b

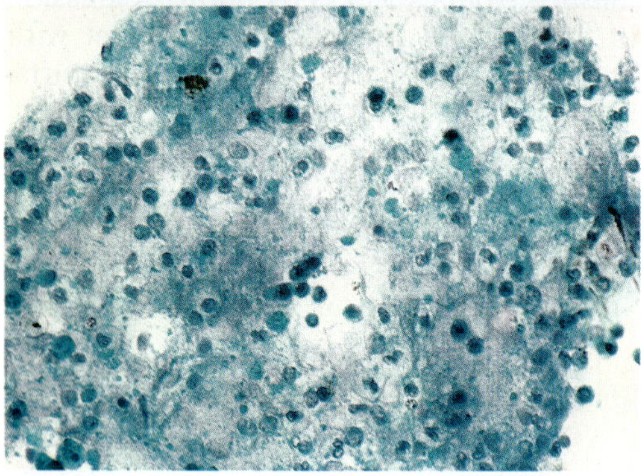

c

Fig. 10.3**a** Pulsed and color Doppler imaging after breast surgery shows pus within the wound cavity and blood flow at its periphery. **b** The pus was aspirated after unsuccessful conservative treatment. Ultrasound shows fibrin webs within the aspirated cavity. **c** Aspiration cytology (Papanicolaou stain, 100 x) shows large numbers of leukocytes, with no evidence of tumor cells.

Pulsed color Doppler (Chapter 13) can identify arterial vessels around the inflammatory process, and Doppler waveforms can be recorded from specific vessels (Figs. 10.**2**, 10.**3**).

If the absolute velocities of the Doppler indices in these vessels (Chapter 13) are measured and compared with those in the vessels of the opposite breast, the following differences will be observed:

- The peak systolic and end-diastolic velocities are higher in the "abscess vessels" than in the contralateral vessels.
- The pulsatility index (PI) and resistance index (RI) are lower in the abscess ves-

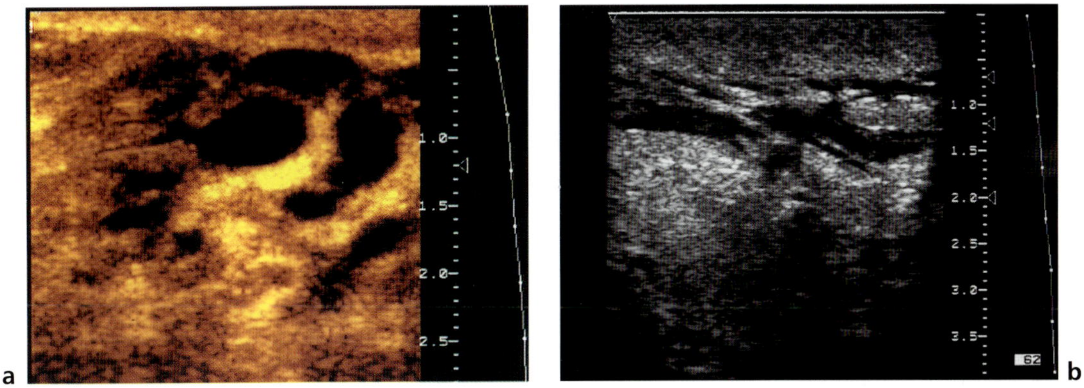

Fig. 10.4a Color B-mode image shows dilation of the central ducts in a patient with nonpuerperal mastitis. **b** Sonographic appearance of nonpuerperal mastitis in a patient who is 16 weeks pregnant. Note the thickened skin (7 mm) and the subcutaneous edema.

sels, reflecting the lower peripheral resistance in relation to the healthy contralateral breast.

The differences in the Doppler waveform parameters of the inflamed and healthy breasts can be substantial (up to 15 cm/s) (Blohmer et al. 1994).

Initial studies indicate that the Doppler waveforms and their parameters change during conservative treatment with bromocriptine or antibiotics due to suppression of the inflammation (Blohmer et al. 1994, Hayes et al. 1991). The most characteristic change is a decline in the peak systolic and end-diastolic blood flow velocities. Because the measured velocities are relatively high, and color Doppler can clearly define the course of the vessels so that optimal Doppler angles can be maintained, the absolute flow velocities in inflammatory breast diseases can be measured with sufficient accuracy.

A positive response to mastitis therapy is also associated with a rise in PI and RI, since as the inflammation subsides, the peripheral vascular resistance increases. Initial studies confirm this relationship (Blohmer et al. 1994).

If the Doppler waveform parameters, B-mode image findings (subcutaneous edema), and clinical symptoms do not show a positive response to bromocriptine or antibiotic therapy, surgical excision or incision of the breast lesion is indicated. The lesion may represent an inflammatory carcinoma or an intractable abscess.

11 Sonography of the Axilla

The ultrasound examination of both breasts should be followed routinely by axillary sonography (Fig. 11.**1**). High-frequency transducers focusing in the near field can be used in the axillary region without a standoff pad.

Axillary sonography can define the following normal anatomical structures:

- The axillary tail.
- The usual skin layers.
- Hypoechoic fat permeated by echogenic connective tissue septa.
- The axillary artery and vein, which are important landmarks located high and deep in the axilla and defining the superior limit of the examination. The artery is distinguished by its typical pulsations, the vein by its larger caliber and easy compressibility (Fig. 11.**2**).
- Muscles: the pectoralis major and minor, the latissimus dorsi, and the serratus anterior on the chest wall. Echogenic connective tissue septa are interposed between the individual muscle layers.
- Skeletal structures: the head of the humerus and the ribs.
- The thoracodorsal artery and vein, and the lateral thoracic artery and vein.
- Small lymph nodes.

As in the breast itself, a systemic scanning procedure should be followed in the axillary region. With the patient‘s arms extended upward and the hands clasped behind the head, we direct the transducer toward the axilla from the upper outer quadrant of the ipsilateral breast. As the transducer is moved along the border of the pectoralis muscle, the axillary tail is closely scrutinized for focal abnormalities. Lymph nodes are frequently detected below the pectoralis muscle. The transducer is moved upward as far as the axillary artery and vein, which define the superior limit of the axillary examination. The probe is then shifted

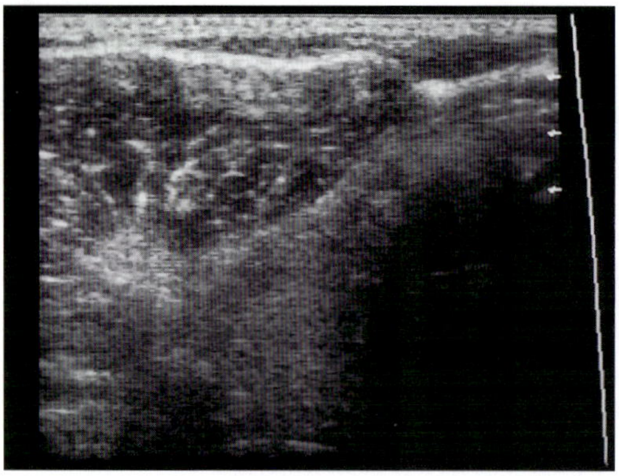

Fig. 11.**1** The pectoralis muscle, visible at upper left, is the key landmark for axillary diagnosis.

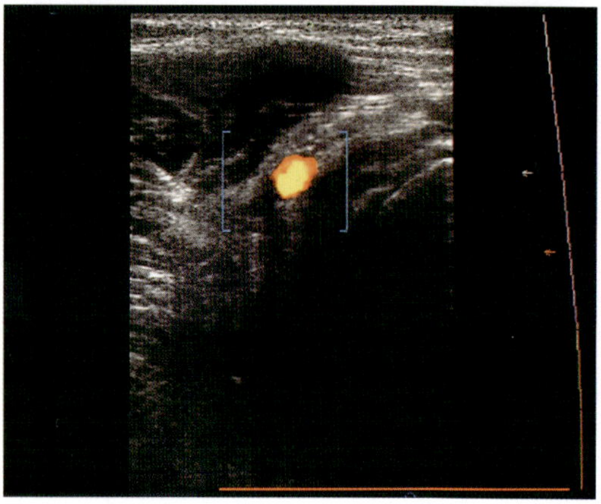

Fig. 11.**2** Color Doppler image of the axillary vein and artery.

laterally and moved downward on a line paralleling the path of the initial scan. Generally, this upward-and-downward scanning pattern is sufficient to define all of the axillary region, but scans at a more lateral site can be added if required.

Care is taken to maintain adequate probe-skin contact in the axillary region, and copious gel should be used. Sometimes the probe has to be specially angled or positioned to conform to individual anatomy; this makes it somewhat more difficult to follow a systematic protocol that will ensure complete axillary coverage.

Either a 5-MHz or 7.5-MHz transducer is suitable for most axillary examinations.

Focal lesions of the axillary tail are assessed using the same criteria as those applying to breast lesions. Particular attention is given to accessory mammary glands, which are more likely to undergo malignant transformation than orthotopic breast parenchyma.

Lymph nodes typically show a distinct structural differentiation into a hyperechoic medulla ("fatty hilum") and a hypoechoic cortex. While there are no sonographic features that are specific for an axillary node metastasis, a lymph node that lacks the normal corticomedullary differentiation is assumed to be malignant until proved otherwise. The converse is not true, however: preservation of the corticomedullary structure does not necessarily mean that the lymph node is benign. An enlarged lymph node that is mobile and not fixed to other tissues is probably benign. Fixed, matted lymph nodes are probably involved by metastatic disease.

The size of a lymph node in itself is not a useful criterion for benign/malignant differentiation (Figs. 11.**3**, 11.**4**).

The purpose of axillary sonography is to detect lymph-node metastases in a patient with known breast cancer and, more importantly, to detect tumor recurrence after surgical treatment for breast cancer. Compared with the detection of recurrent tumor, preoperative evaluation of the lymph nodes usually has little clinical significance. The diagnosis of accessory glandular

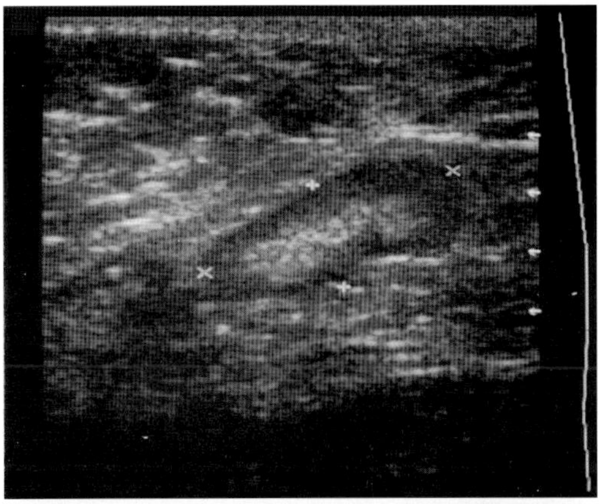
a

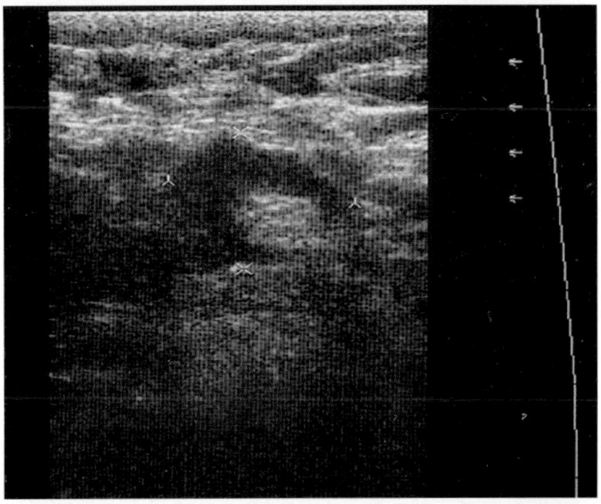
b

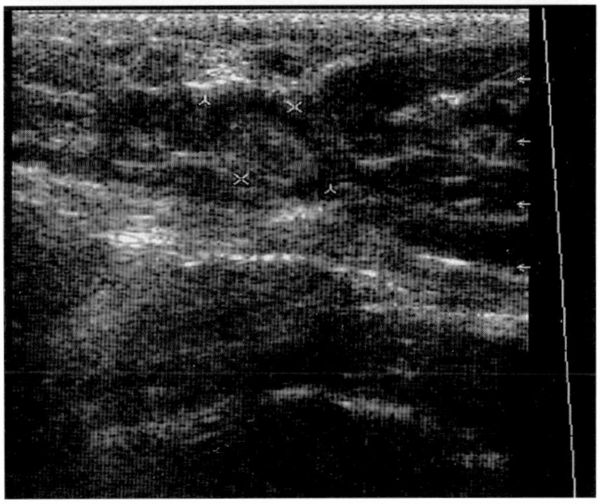
c

Fig. 11.**3a** A large lymph node showing normal corticomedullary differentiation. **b** A small lymph node with an intact corticomedullary structure. **c** A structurally intact lymph node bordering on the pectoralis muscle.

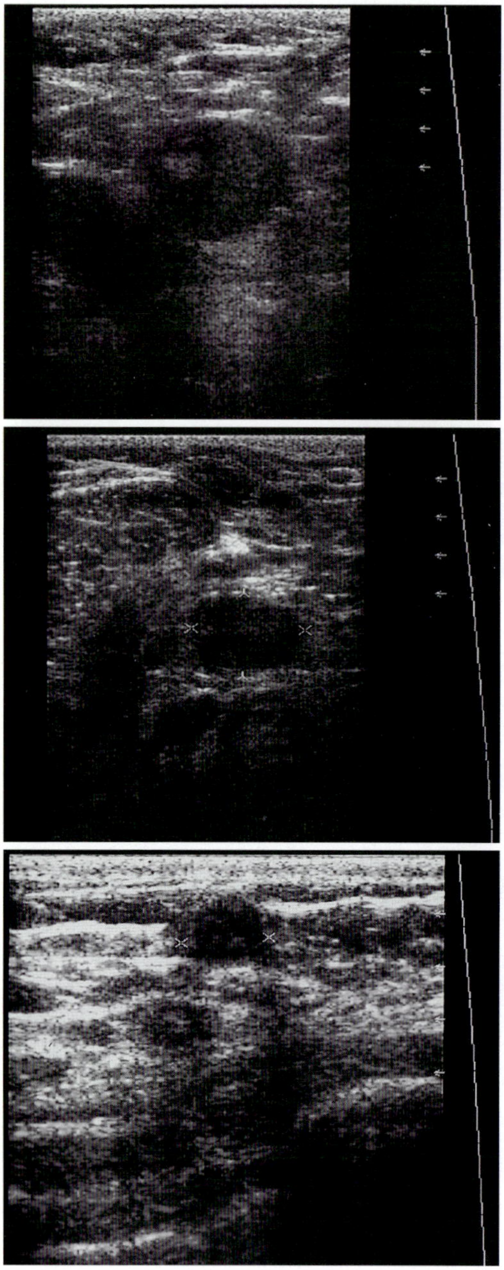

a b c

Fig. 11.4a–c Suspicious lymph nodes that lack a definite corticomedullary structure.

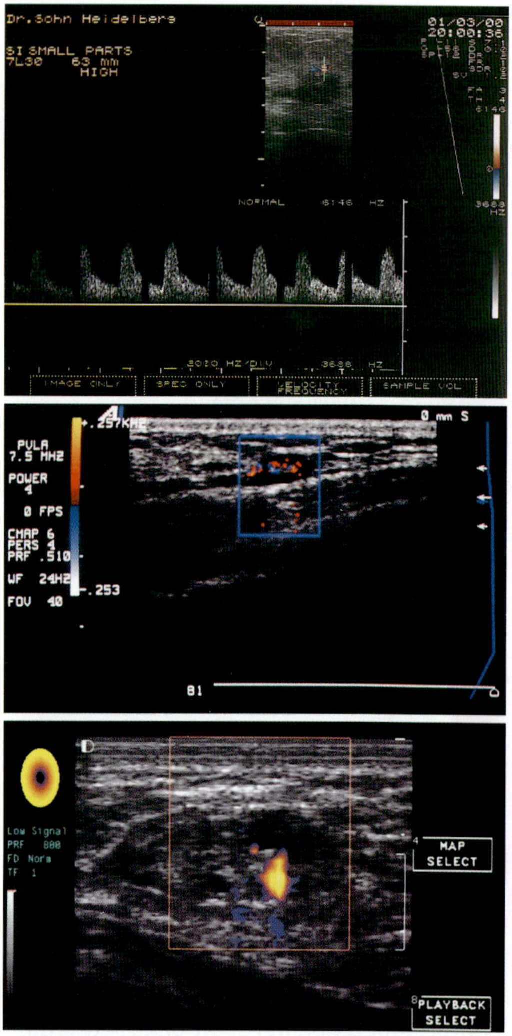

a b c

Fig. 11.5a A lymph node showing arterial blood flow (color duplex image). **b** A small lymph node with high blood flow (maximum entropy method image). **c** A lymph node with blood flow (power Doppler image).

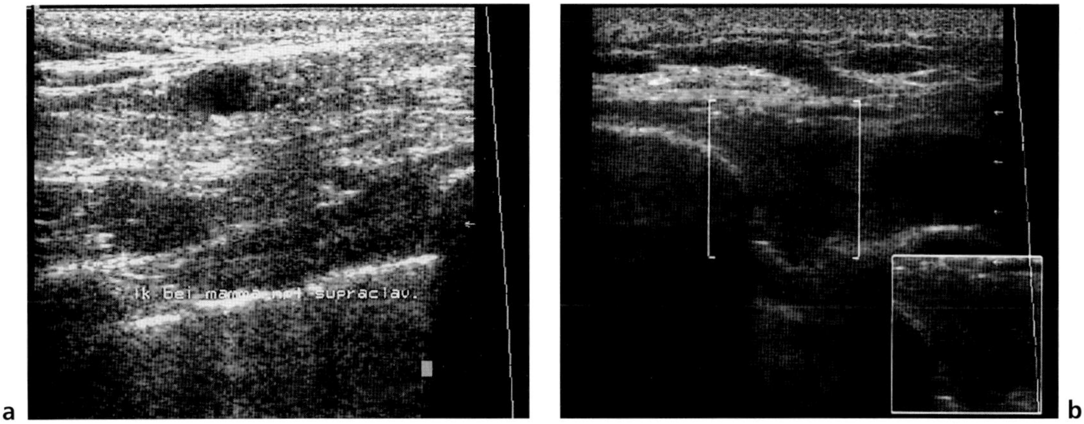

Fig. 11.6a A suspicious supraclavicular lymph node. **b** Parasternal recurrence.

tissue is very important, however, and the detection of enlarged lymph nodes accompanied by an indeterminate focal lesion in the ipsilateral breast supports the decision to carry out histological evaluation of the breast lesion.

For methodological reasons, sonography is superior to mammography in the preoperative search for lymph-node metastases. Studies have shown that sonography can correctly determine the preoperative lymph-node status in 75 % of patients (Ernst et al. 1990, Madjar et al. 1993b, Pamilo et al. 1989).

It should be noted that lymph nodes can become enlarged as a result of inflammation (especially in the arm and hand) and various systemic illnesses (malignant lymphoma, rheumatoid arthritis, dermatitis, lupus erythematosus, etc.).

Doppler ultrasound may be helpful in differentiating between benign and malignant lymph nodes. If Doppler indicates arterial blood flow in a lymph node, there is a greater likelihood of malignant nodal involvement than if the lymph node is avascular (Fig. 11.**5**). Scanning near the axillary artery can be difficult, since pulsations from that vessel are transmitted to surrounding tissues and can mask the signals from very small vessels. Blood flow may also be detected in lymph nodes that undergo reactive enlargement as a result of inflammation.

If definite metastatic involvement of the axillary nodes is found, the supraclavicular nodes and parasternal region should also be sonographically examined for staging purposes (Fig. 11.**6**).

Ultrasound can also demonstrate the chain of lymph nodes along the internal thoracic artery. This is done by slowly moving the probe downward and parallel to the sternum, using the blood vessel below the cartilaginous part of the rib as a guide which can be easily visualized and confirmed with color or pulsed Doppler ultrasound (Scatarige et al. 1989). Enlarged metastatic nodes usually appear as conspicuous masses that are easily distinguished from the small, healthy lymph nodes embedded in the fatty tissue.

12 Sonography in the Follow-Up of Breast Cancer

The performance of an adequate mammographic examination in patients who have undergone mastectomy and breast reconstruction is often hampered by serious technical obstacles. As a result, the physical findings, sonography, and magnetic resonance imaging have become the mainstays for detecting local tumor recurrence. Mammograms may also be equivocal after breast conservation in cases in which postsurgical radiation has caused increased radiographic breast density. High-resolution sonography is a logical alternative to mammography in cases of this kind.

Sonography provides a fast, simple technique for evaluating new palpable breast masses. Finding elevated tumor markers during follow-up should prompt an intensive ultrasound search for recurrent cancer at the surgical site, in the regional lymph nodes, and in the liver.

There are three stages in which ultrasound can be effectively used in the follow-up of breast cancer:

1. In the immediate postoperative period, to monitor the development and resolution of hematomas and lymphoceles.
2. During the first year after breast conservation and radiation.
3. More than one year after reconstructive or nonreconstructive mastectomy without radiation, or after breast conservation with radiation.

A frequently asked question is whether swelling in the immediate postoperative period is caused by a hematoma, edema, or lymphocele. Ultrasound can resolve the question of whether needle aspiration can and should be performed in these cases. An organizing hematoma is filled with internal echoes of varying amplitude. A fresh hematoma usually appears echo-free, as does a lymphocele. Needle aspiration can be performed safely and accurately under sonographic guidance (Fig. 12.**1**) to identify these lesions and distinguish them from an abscess.

In breast cancer patients who undergo breast conservation and percutaneous radiation therapy of the residual breast, ultrasound usually demonstrates a conspicuous edema that can be seen for up to one year after treatment. This edema hampers the detection of tumor recurrence. Because the irradiated breast is harder and less compressible, it is generally more difficult to evaluate with ultrasound. Usually the breast is permeated by hypoechoic "tracks" caused by postirradiation interstitial edema. In this setting, it can be difficult to identify focal hypoechoic lesions that signify tumor recurrence (Fig. 12.**2**).

Past the one-year mark, ultrasound can be used very successfully in the longer-term

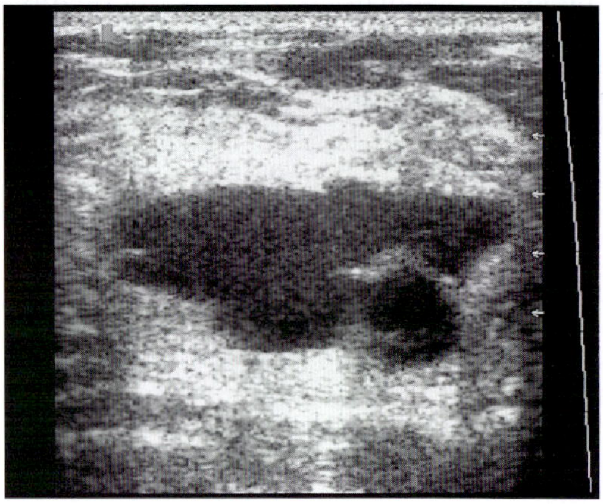

Fig. 12.1 Postoperative seroma.

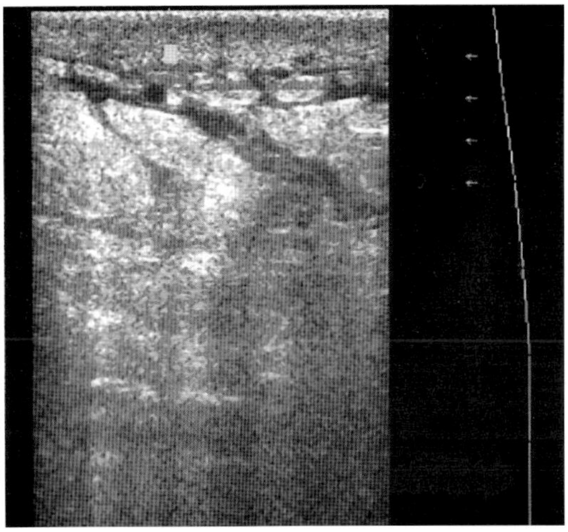

Fig. 12.**2** Typical appearance of an irradiated breast after breast-conserving therapy.

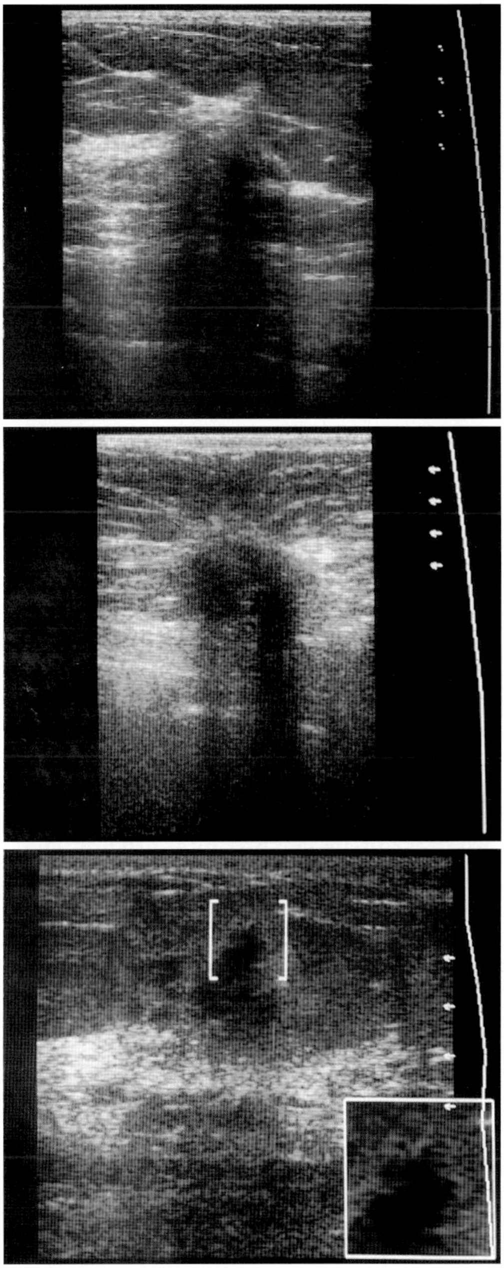

a

b

c

Fig. 12.**3a** Dense acoustic shadow cast by a postsurgical scar after breast-conserving therapy. **b** The postsurgical scar is indistinguishable from a malignant tumor. **c** Recurrence after breast-conserving therapy.

follow-up of women treated by breast conservation and radiation therapy or by mastectomy. Ultrasound can detect a recurrence with high sensitivity, though at times it is difficult or impossible to distinguish scar tissue or fat necrosis from recurrent tumor (Fig. 12.**3**).

A local recurrence of breast carcinoma can have various sonographic appearances. It may appear as a hypoechoic area within or overlying the chest wall muscle, as a metastatic lymph node, or as a primary tumor. In women who have undergone mastectomy, the recurrence usually appears as a subcutaneous, hypoechoic mass lying just beneath the skin (Fig. 12.**4**).

Basically, any change in the breast parenchyma or surgical scar should raise suspicion of a recurrence. Given the crucial importance of follow-up in these patients, it is imperative to keep accurate documentation and have the same individual perform the follow-up examinations and also document and describe the findings.

Usually, a recurrent tumor displays the same ultrasound features as the primary tumor in the same patient. Most recurrent tumors are hypoechoic.

In patients undergoing surgery for breast cancer at the University Gynecological Clinic in Heidelberg, ultrasound follow-up

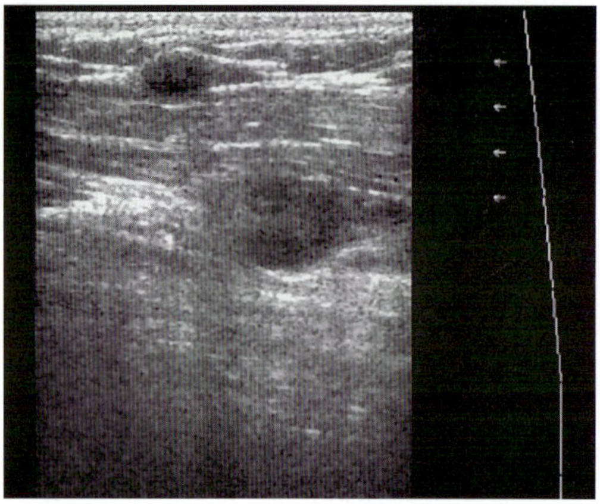

Fig. 12.**4** Recurrent tumor located superficial and deep to the pectoralis muscles.

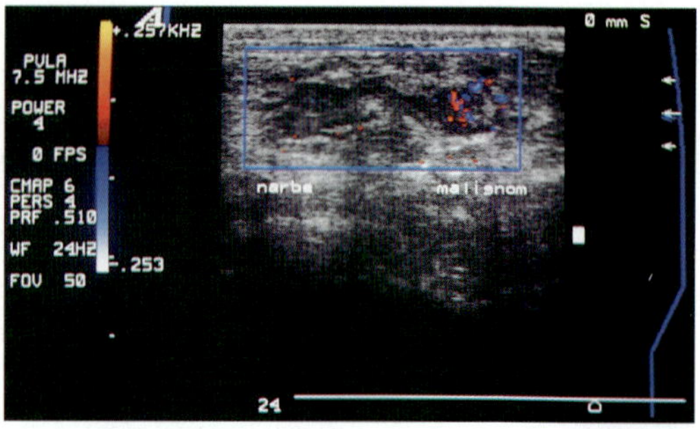

Fig. 12.**6** Recurrent tumor and scar in the same image, displaying the same B-mode characteristics. The MEM image differentiates the scar from tumor by demonstrating intratumoral blood flow.

examinations are scheduled at six-month intervals for up to five years after surgery. These relatively short-interval follow-ups enable us to detect most recurrences when they are still small and relatively well demarcated from their surroundings. The recurrence may cast an acoustic shadow, but usually this is seen only when the tumor has reached an advanced size. Differentiation from scar tissue can be quite difficult, since scars can also appear hypoechoic and cast a shadow (Fig. 12.**5**). A useful differentiating criterion is the absence of change in scar tissue on serial examinations. Color flow imaging can also be very helpful in distinguishing scar from recurrent tumor: the recurrence usually exhibits blood flow while the scar does not. This type of differentiation requires a sensitive color flow imaging system. We use the new maximum entropy method (MEM) technology exclusively for this purpose, as it can detect flow velocities as low as 0.1 mm/s, compared with 10–20 mm/s in conventional color Doppler ultrasound (Fig. 12.**6**).

a

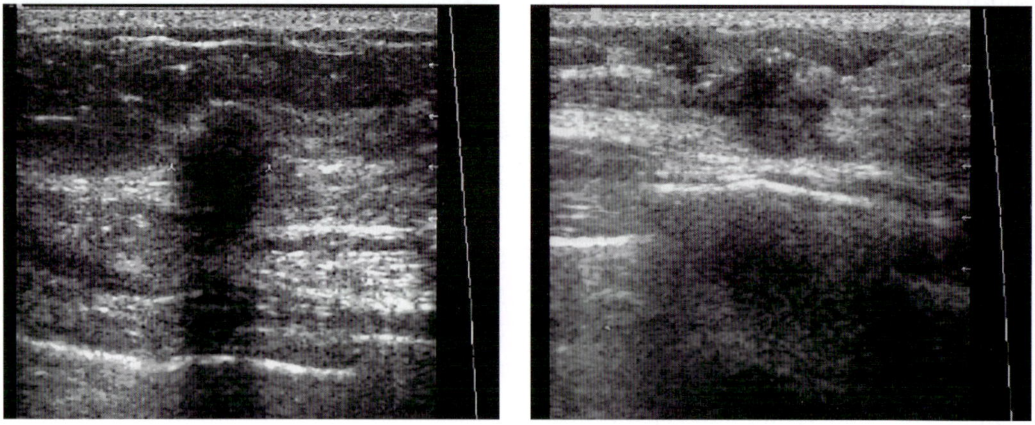

b

Fig. 12.**5a** Small recurrent carcinoma with posterior shadowing. **b** Recurrence after breast-conserving therapy.

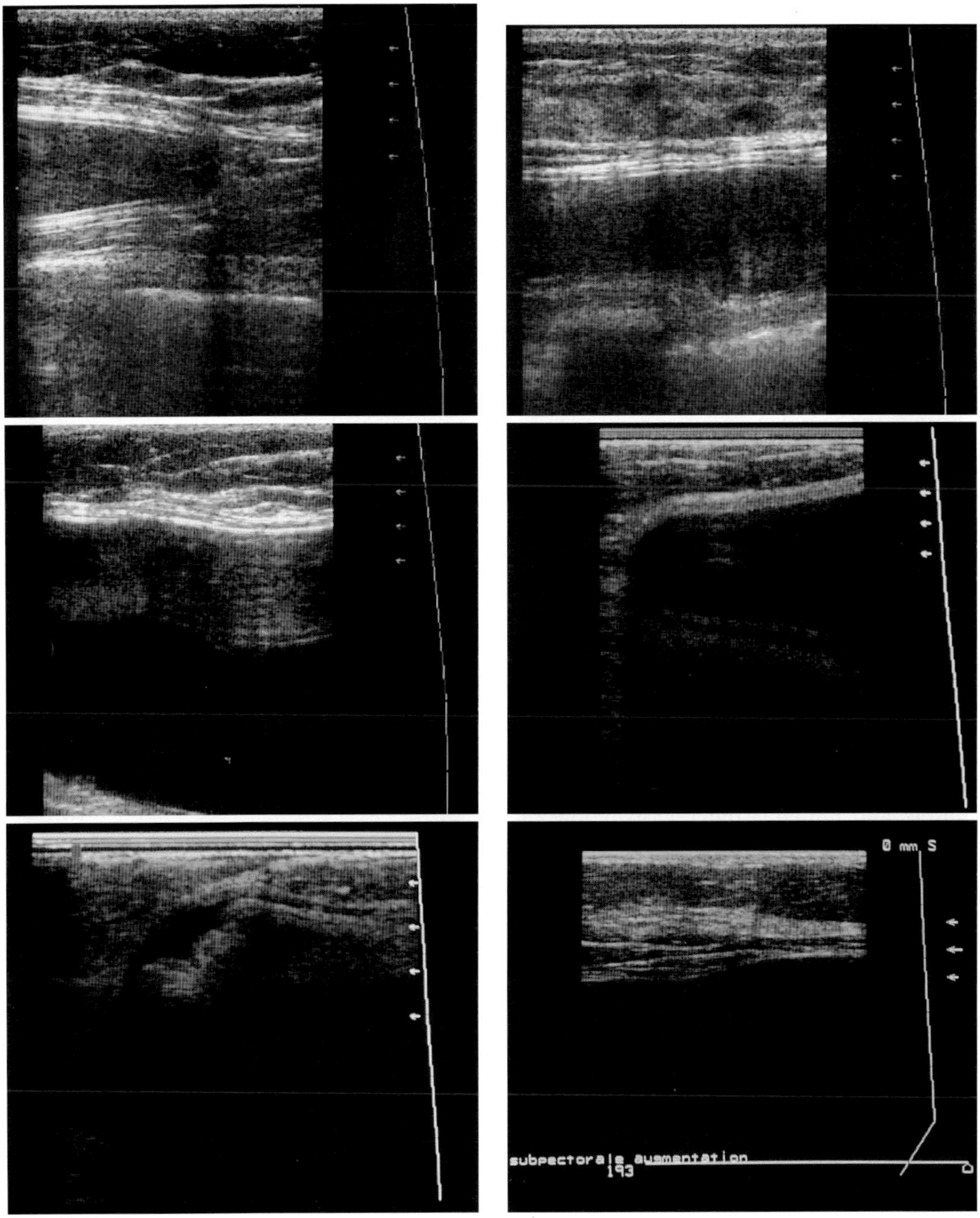

Fig. 12.7**a–c** Sequence of images showing different portions of a breast implant from the edge to the center of the implant. **d** The implant has a smooth edge. **e** It is not unusual to see a small fold at the edge of the implant and a thin peri-implant fluid layer. **f** Subpectoral implant.

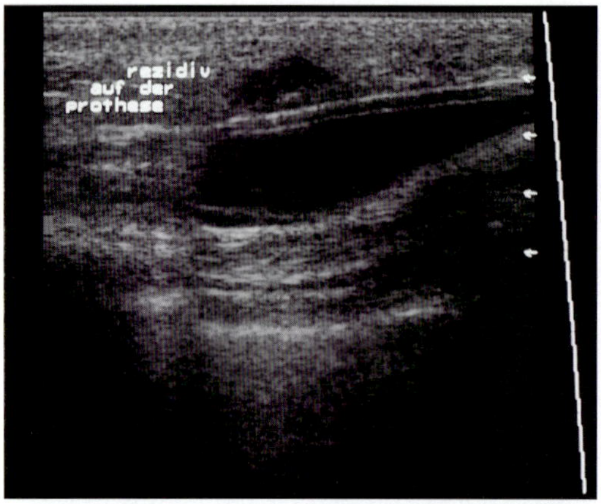

a

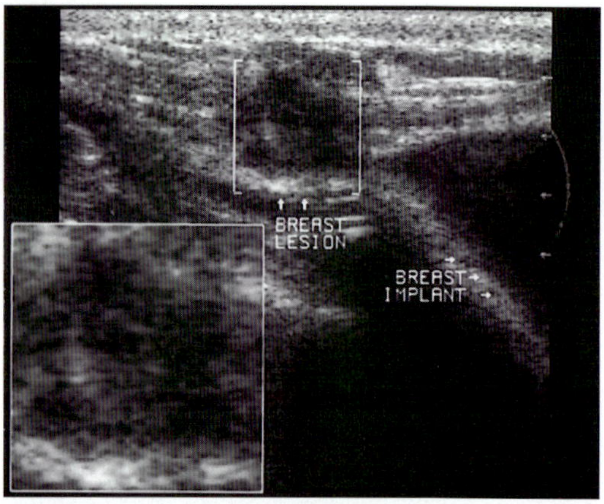

b

Fig. 12.**8a** Recurrent tumor directly overlying a breast implant. **b** Recurrent tumor adjacent to a breast implant.

Detection of Tumor Recurrence after Prosthetic Breast Augmentation

First it has to be determined whether the breast implant is superficial or deep to the pectoralis muscle, as this will direct the search for a possible recurrence. If the implant is deep to the pectoralis muscle, tumor is most likely to recur above the muscle and implant; the region below the implant is of lesser interest. We favor a meandering scan pattern like the one used in routine breast examinations (see Chapter 3) to ensure complete coverage (Figs. 12.**7**, 12.**8**).

If the implant is superficial to the pectoralis muscle and therefore lies within the region in which tumor may recur, all the tissue surrounding the implant must be examined. In these cases, the region deep to the implant is of key importance. We start by examining the border of the implant, moving the transducer in a radial pattern, always keeping the edge of the implant at the center of the image field. We then examine the tissue superficial to the implant by moving the focal zones close to the skin and using a meandering scan pattern. Finally, we use a meandering pattern to scan the region deep to the implant, with corresponding placement of the focal zones. In some cases the tissues deep to the implant are difficult or impossible to evaluate due to reverberation artifacts from the implant (Chapter 2). A more detailed discussion of the sonographic appearance of breast implants is given in Chapter 17.

Detection of Tumor Recurrence after Autologous Breast Augmentation

In cases in which autologous muscle and fat have been used to reconstruct the breast, sonography can be used in the immediate postoperative period to assess the adequacy of blood flow to the transferred tissues. Detecting tumor recurrence at a later time may prove difficult and requires a very precise examination technique, since recurrences are usually hyperechoic and therefore have the same echogenicity as fat and muscle.

13 Sonography of the Male Breast

Ultrasound evaluation of the male breast is performed so rarely that it requires special care. The normal male breast consists mostly of subcutaneous fat directly overlying the pectoralis muscle. This fat is permeated by connective tissue septa, and small amounts of glandular parenchyma may extend along the septa toward the nipple. As in females, the male breast parenchyma appears hyperechoic relative to the hypoechoic fat.

Gynecomastia is a benign hyperplasia involving all of the breast parenchyma. It may be unilateral or bilateral, and may present clinically as a painful swelling. Gynecomastia may occur without apparent cause in pubescent males, and also in the elderly. Most cases are bilateral, and the great majority resolve without treatment.

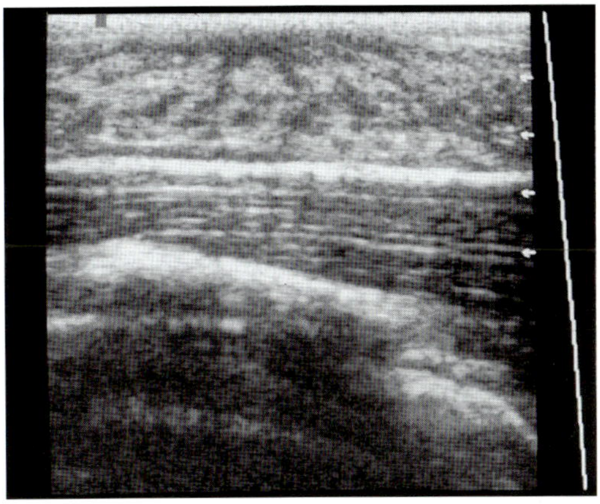

Fig. 13.**1** Ultrasound appearance of gynecomastia.

Gynecomastia in older males is probably due to falling testosterone levels.

Gynecomastia can have various internal and external causes:

Internal causes:
- Deficient androgen levels (e.g., due to trauma, Klinefelter's syndrome, or castration)
- Elevated estrogen levels (e.g., due to testicular tumors or adrenal disease);
- Estrogen-androgen imbalance (e.g., due to hepatic cirrhosis or renal disease).

External causes:
- Drugs with estrogenic activity (e.g., digoxin)
- Drugs with antiandrogenic activity (e.g., spironolactone)
- Certain drugs with unexplained mechanisms of action (e.g., diazepam, penicillins, heroin, etc.).

In one-third of cases, the etiology remains unknown.

Sonographically, the breast in gynecomastia appears structurally normal. The ductal system opens into the nipple below the areola, and the glandular tissue resembles that in the female breast (Fig. 13.**1**).

Since the male breast is subject to (although generally less susceptible to) any and all of the disorders that can also affect the female breast, including benign and malignant tumors, every focal sonographic lesion found in the male breast warrants cytological, or preferably histological, evaluation. The same criteria used in the female breast are applied to the analysis of focal lesions.

14 Sonographic Evaluation of Blood Flow in Breast Masses

The sonographic assessment of blood flow in the breast and in breast masses is still highly controversial. It would therefore be wrong to characterize it as a reliable, established procedure. Currently, the ultrasound evaluation of blood flow offers no advantage over other imaging studies in its ability to differentiate between benign and malignant breast disease.

This chapter deals with the biological principles of the sonographic evaluation of blood flow, the various technical methods that are available for sonographic flow imaging, clinical experience with these methods, and future developments.

Biological Principles of Sonographic Blood Flow Imaging

The biological principles of ultrasound flow imaging are based on tumor angiogenesis. Most malignant tumors have a copious blood supply. The formation of new blood vessels is vital for the rapid growth of solid malignant tumors (Folkman 1971). Tumors with a volume of 1–2 mm^3 or more have to acquire a vascular supply in order to grow. Folkman (1992) distinguishes between a prevascular and a vascular phase of tumor growth. A tumor in the prevascular phase grows slowly and rarely metastasizes. A tumor in the vascular phase acquires a blood supply, grows rapidly, and is more likely to metastasize. Because tumor angiogenesis determines the metastatic potential of a carcinoma, measurement of the vascularity of the primary tumor could provide an extremely useful means of predicting subsequent metastasis (Weidner et al. 1991, Horak et al. 1992).

New vessels tend to develop around the advancing edge of a malignant tumor. The tumor-associated vessels show irregular patterns of proliferation, which can include corkscrew tortuosity and marked variations in caliber. Tumor vascularity is also characterized by high-velocity arteriovenous shunts (Bouck 1994) and by an abundance of new vessels entering the tumor itself.

Sonographic blood flow evaluation in breast tumors is based on the hypothesis that the increased number of (irregularly shaped) vessels, the decreased peripheral resistance in the vascular bed of the breast malignancy, and the elevated flow velocities caused by arteriovenous shunting all create a distinctive pattern that can be quantitatively analyzed with ultrasound. In addition to the high-velocity arteriovenous shunts, there are numerous peripheral tumor-feeding vessels that are perfused by very low-velocity flow.

Modern technical capabilities such as high image resolution and sensitivity to low flow velocities have made it possible to apply Doppler ultrasound techniques in the differential diagnosis of breast masses. While the results published to date have been contradictory (Adler et al. 1990, Birdwell et al. 1997, Blohmer 1995, Britton and Coulden 1990, Cosgrove et al. 1990, Dock 1993, Halliwell 1993, Harper 1985, Konishi 1992, Kubek et al. 1996, Madjar et al. 1986, 1990, 1992, Raza and Baum 1997, Sohn 1992, 1993), it is very difficult to compare different studies due to differences in the equipment used and areas of interest (arteriovenous shunts, feeding vessels, newly formed tumor vessels) and due to a lack of established reference values. In addition, blood flow in a normal breast is strongly influenced by the patient's age, hormone status (replacement), peripheral arterial blood pressure, and by atherosclerotic processes (Blohmer et al. 1995).

Thermography is based on similar biological principles but is not widely used in the differential diagnosis of breast masses because of its low sensitivity and specificity (Barth and Prechtel 1990).

Techniques of Blood Flow Imaging

Doppler Sonography

In Doppler sonography, the sound waves reflected from a moving medium undergo a frequency shift (the Doppler effect), which is used to image red blood cells moving within tumor vessels and measure their velocity. The magnitude of the frequency shift depends on the frequency of the emitted sound waves and the velocity of the blood flow. When Doppler ultrasound is used to evaluate blood flow in breast masses, the velocities to be measured are often in the millimeter per second range and do not exceed several centimeters per second. Only high-frequency Doppler probes can register flows of such low velocity. Madjar et al. (1989) tested various transducer frequencies and documented the advantage of higher frequencies in continuous-wave Doppler investigations of tumor blood flow.

The Doppler system records the magnitude of the frequency shift of the reflected sound waves and can convert it directly into an audible output (in Hz) or into a visible waveform expressing the velocity of the red blood cells (in cm/s).

Continuous-Wave Doppler

In a continuous-wave (CW) Doppler system, sound waves are continuously transmitted and received by the transducer. The Doppler shift can generate an audible output or can be displayed on the monitor as a Doppler waveform (Fig. 14.**1**). The transducer consists of a small, pencil-shaped probe. The CW Doppler probe cannot generate a simultaneous B-mode image. Nor can it selectively record signals from a specified depth; the Doppler interrogation is "blind," covering the entire breast and recording all detectable flow signals encountered by the beam. In this type of examination, the total blood flow in the breast is measured by the summation of all moving reflectors and is compared with the healthy contralateral breast. The advantage of CW Doppler is its high sensitivity in detecting blood vessels owing to the high Doppler frequency (10 MHz) that is used.

An examiner evaluating nonpalpable breast masses with CW Doppler must have

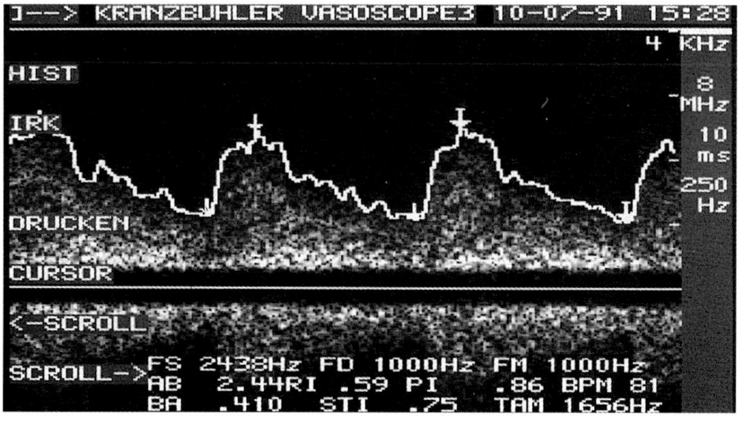

Fig. 14.**1** CW Doppler trace of blood flow in a breast tumor.

extensive experience with the method. Tumor-associated vessels cannot be selectively examined. This accounts for the low acceptance of CW Doppler among clinicians.

The results achieved with CW Doppler in comparing healthy and tumorous breasts laid the groundwork for the development of pulsed and color-coded Doppler imaging techniques. CW Doppler was the first modality to reveal subtle changes in mammary blood flow relating to the menstrual cycle and to demonstrate the bilateral symmetry of mammary blood flow in most women. Also, researchers working with CW Doppler introduced quantitative analysis of breast perfusion based on the analysis of Doppler waveform parameters (Madjar et al. 1992, Schild and Fendel 1991, Schild et al. 1993, Sohn et al. 1993).

Duplex Sonography

Duplex sonography combines pulsed Doppler signal acquisition with B-mode imaging. The sound waves are transmitted and received at designated intervals. The length of these intervals can be modified to select a specific tissue depth from which Doppler signals are acquired. This depth is selected by positioning the sample volume at the desired location in the B-mode image (Fig. 14.**2**). Pulsed Doppler can selectively interrogate a focal breast abnormality. Because the blood vessels of interest are not defined in the B-mode image, however, it can be very tedious to locate blood vessels using this technique. Also, it is uncertain whether all vessels have been interrogated and whether some vessels have been sampled more than once.

The following *Doppler waveform parameters* can be analyzed when CW or duplex sonography is used:

- Peak systolic velocity (max v sys): A
- Minimum end-diastolic velocity (min v dias): B
- Resistance index (RI): RI = A–B/A
- Pulsatility index (PI): PI = A–B/Q
- A/B ratio: Q = A/B.

Pulsed Color Doppler Sonography

Pulsed color Doppler ultrasound is the method most commonly used to study the blood flow in focal breast lesions. For this reason, it will be described here in somewhat greater detail.

In color Doppler sonography, the Doppler signals received from flowing blood are

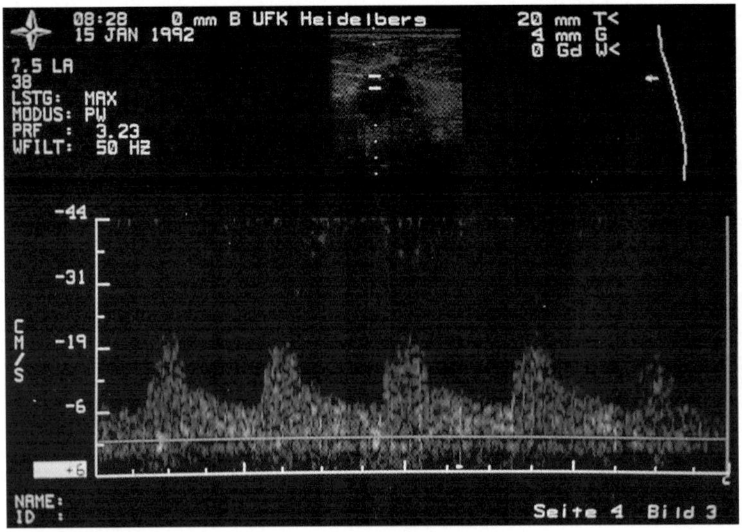

Fig. 14.**2** Duplex display (B-mode image plus Doppler spectrum) of blood flow in a breast tumor.

processed and color-encoded. The blood flow velocities are displayed in various colors and brightness levels. The direction of the blood flow is immaterial in this type of examination. The presence of color Doppler signals can identify blood vessels too small to be resolved in the B-mode image, and the color signals themselves provide a source of additional information. In a color duplex system, moreover, Doppler waveform analysis can be performed by positioning the sample volume within the vessel that is generating color signals.

The following equipment features are needed in a system for duplex imaging:

- A Doppler frequency of 5 MHz or higher
- Simultaneous display of the B-mode image and Doppler waveform
- Variable sample volume size
- Variable Doppler angle (to adapt the scan to the course of a specific vessel)
- Angle correction capability
- Selection of a low range of detectable frequencies (1 cm/s or lower)
- Good separation of equipment noise or artifacts (respiration) from the flow image
- System software for displaying the Doppler waveform and analyzing key Doppler parameters (peak systolic velocity, minimum end-diastolic velocity, A/B ratio, PI, RI)
- A lightweight transducer that is easy to handle (the probe must be held stationary for longer periods of time during Doppler signal acquisition)

A wall filter or high-pass filter is used to eliminate intrinsic movements of the vessel walls that would interfere with signal acquisition from moving red cells. Because this can also filter out signals from low-velocity flow components, the cut-off frequency of the high-pass filter used in breast ultrasound must be set low enough to detect low-velocity flow within the breast lesion. The Doppler instruments used for breast examinations are so sensitive that they can even register respiratory effects on the blood flow velocities in veins.

Examination technique: The first step in carrying out a pulsed color Doppler breast examination is to locate the tumor in the B-mode image. Any color Doppler signals appearing in the image field will indicate the presence of blood flow. Then, while maintaining a shallow beam-vessel angle, the sample volume of the pulsed-wave (PW) Doppler system is positioned within the vessel of interest. The Doppler waveform is displayed on the monitor and can then be evaluated. If a Doppler signal is not acquired with a shallow beam-vessel angle, systems with angle correction can factor the beam-vessel angle into the velocity calculation to correct for a more vertical angle.

Because image generation in the triplex mode (B-mode + color flow + Doppler waveform display) is a slow process, we recommend displaying only the Doppler waveform while other display options are held in freeze-frame.

Non-Doppler Techniques

These techniques either do not use the Doppler effect at all or use it in a highly modified form to detect extremely low blood flow velocities. Because color flow imaging with these techniques is more sensitive than waveform imaging with duplex systems, the non-Doppler techniques are essentially qualitative studies and often do not yield a Doppler waveform that can be quantitatively analyzed.

The two most important and innovative techniques at present are MEM imaging and power Doppler imaging.

Maximum Entropy Method (MEM) (Fig. 14.**3**)

Compared with conventional Doppler ultrasound, which can detect blood flow velocities no lower than about 1–3 cm/s, MEM technology can produce high-quality color images of flow velocities as low as 0.1 mm/s.

The algorithm for this type of imaging was developed by the United States Navy for sonar applications. The algorithms were

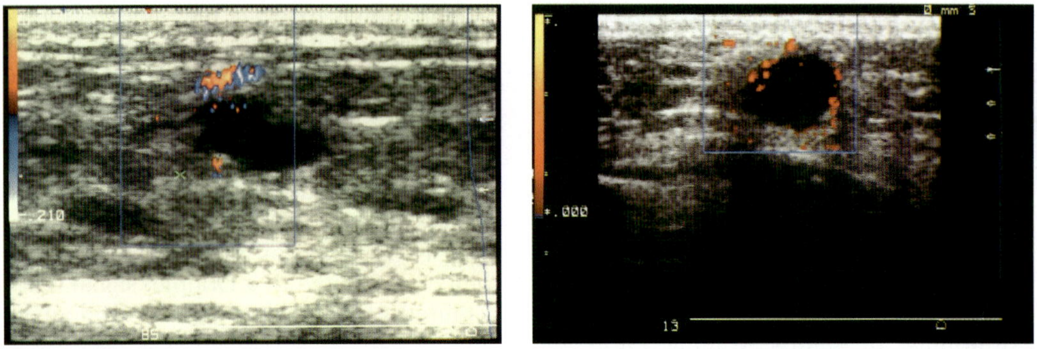
a b

Fig. 14.3 MEM technique. **a** Image showing high blood flow at the periphery of a very small breast carcinoma. **b** Blood flow in a small breast carcinoma.

later modified to improve spectral resolution and noise detection. MEM solves the problem of noise masking the useful signal by providing optimum separation of flow information from unwanted noise.

MEM, a nonlinear method of spectral analysis, was first described by Burg in 1967. It is based on selecting for analysis the spectrum in which the time series happens to fall outside the observed patterns. By maximizing the entropy of the unknown spectra, this method allows an unbiased evaluation of the subthreshold spectrum.

MEM defines the distribution of noise for the useful information contained in an ultrasound volume. By accurately modeling the noise, MEM optimizes the separation of useful flow information from noise. MEM algorithms are so powerful and effective in an acoustic environment that they can even detect signals fainter than the background noise level.

Traditional color Doppler algorithms and MEM can be compared on the basis of eight key criteria: sensitivity, penetration, resolution, frame rate, accuracy, velocity ranges, velocity resolution, and the visualization of flow that cannot be seen in the B-mode image.

Studies to date have shown that MEM:

- can depict extremely low-velocity flows by minimizing all noise sources;
- can extract Doppler shift information from a minimum of reflected ultrasound energy and thus can optimize the frame rate without loss of resolution or sample volume size;
- provides a markedly enhanced signal-to-noise ratio in the extracted Doppler information, with an improved depth of penetration;
- can record Doppler spectra with greater sensitivity despite a high noise content;
- shows excellent robustness in the presence of noise, even with Doppler signals of extremely low intensity;
- can register flow not displayed in the B-mode image and can better differentiate Doppler signals from other signals.

These properties underscore the potential clinical usefulness of MEM imaging, particularly in the visualization of slow blood flow such as that occurring in tumors and organs. One drawback of this method is that it does not yield quantitative flow data. Pulsed Doppler in a duplex system can quantitate blood flow, but it cannot analyze the extremely slow flows that are characteristic of malignant tumors.

Power Doppler (Fig. 14.4)

Power Doppler imaging, known also as "ultrasound angiography," is similar to conventional color Doppler in that it superimposes color-encoded flow information onto the B-mode image in real time. It differs

a
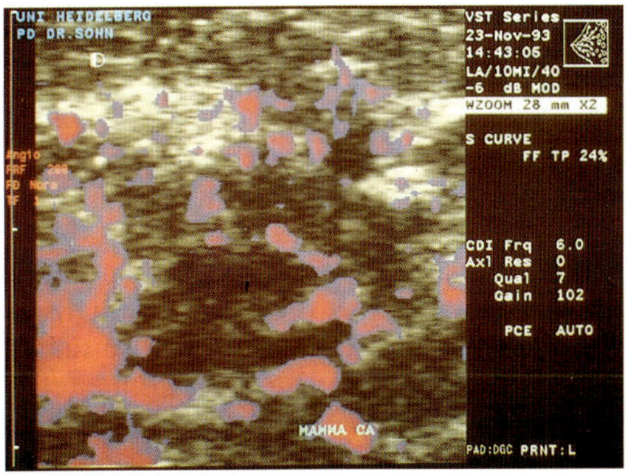

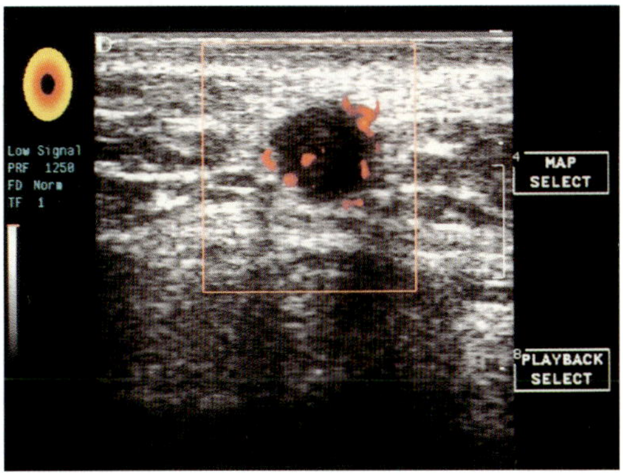

b

Fig. 14.4 Power Doppler images. **a** High blood flow in and around a small breast carcinoma, appearing as a combination of single color pixels and color areas. **b** Blood flow in a small breast carcinoma.

from color Doppler, however, by using a fundamentally different physical parameter of the reflected ultrasound to generate a color image: power Doppler analyzes the amplitude, rather than the frequency shift, of the reflected signals. The amplitude is determined by the quantity or density of the blood cell aggregates that are detected within the sample volume of the ultrasound beam; hence it is unaffected by the angle between the direction of blood flow and the interrogating beam (the frequency shift in color Doppler is determined by the velocity of the reflectors).

Amplitude is a less "noisy" parameter than frequency shift. This is particularly true in broad-band signals, which represent the sum of many frequencies of comparable intensity. The amplitude results from the summation of these various frequency components, whereas the frequency shift is a mean value. Since there is less noise in the amplitude signals, power Doppler can use higher gain settings than color Doppler, yielding a more sensitive and more continuous vascular image.

In power Doppler, signals of higher amplitude are encoded in yellow, and signals of lower amplitude are encoded in dark blue. Noise occurs stochastically throughout the frequency band but has a uniformly low amplitude. Thus, while noise in color Doppler produces a mosaic-like color pattern, noise in power Doppler is assigned a specific color value: dark blue. This color can be electronically "wiped" from the image, leaving only signals whose intensity is greater than that of noise.

A high persistence setting is currently used in power Doppler studies to further improve the signal-to-noise ratio. This technique of signal averaging is much more effective in power Doppler than in color Doppler. This is because power Doppler is less velocity-dependent than color Doppler, and because amplitudes are less pulsatile than velocities, resulting in less variation of signal amplitudes from one image to the next.

Another key element of the power Doppler system is the tissue discriminator, which tags the returning ultrasound signals as originating from solid tissue or from flowing blood. These signals are separated for further processing, tissue signals being processed to generate the B-mode image and blood signals to generate the "angiographic" flow image. Ideally, this technique offers considerably higher sensitivity than color Doppler. Other advantages of power Doppler over color Doppler are that it is relatively angle-independent and is not subject to aliasing (Cosgrove et al. 1990; Rubin et al. 1994). Disadvantages of the technique include the extreme motion sensitivity and lack of flow velocity or directional information.

Clinical Experience with Blood Flow Imaging in Breast Tumors

There is still no consensus regarding the interpretation of sonographic blood flow images (Sohn et al. 1992, 1993, Madjar et al. 1989a, b, 1990a, 1991b, Jellins 1988, Cosgrove et al. 1990, Rubin et al. 1994). Presented below is an attempt to review all the interpretative aspects of color flow imaging and determine which are the most useful.

The following features can be studied and evaluated:

- The number of blood vessels
- Calculated Doppler waveform parameters (resistance index, A/B ratio, pulsatility index)
- Comparison of blood flow in the healthy and diseased breasts of the same patient
- The size and number of tumor-associated color pixels or color areas
- The appearance and characteristics of the Doppler waveform

Determining the number of blood vessels is fraught with difficulties. The number of vessels in a color flow image can be determined only by analyzing the pattern of individual or contiguous color pixels, and this will depend on how many vessels—or how many times one vessel—may intersect the image plane. With CW or pulsed Doppler, the number of blood vessels can be determined only by counting the vascular signals that are found, and this depends largely on how systematically the examination is conducted. In many cases, only isolated color pixels can be found in and around a tumor, and these cannot be unequivocally assigned to a particular vessel. Another problem is the potential for counting a vascular segment more than once when calculating the number of vessels.

The standard Doppler parameters (resistance index, A/B ratio, pulsatility index) appear to be the most reproducible parameters for Doppler waveform analysis. Although these parameters cover only certain properties of the waveform (i.e., the peak systolic and end-diastolic velocities), they are the most objective tools available for characterizing a Doppler waveform.

The main parameter for waveform analysis is the resistance index. Ranging in value from 0 to 1, this ratio can express the vascular resistance as a percentage.

When characterizing a breast lesion, most examiners use only the lowest resistance index that can be recorded in a tumor or its immediate surroundings. The rationale for this approach is that the difference between benign and malignant tumors is most pronounced at the capillary level, where neovascularization occurs and very low vascular resistances prevail. It is easier to detect the low-resistance vascular bed created by the numerous tumor-associated capillaries than to identify the higher blood flow that occurs in large feeding vessels. This explains why the lowest measured resistance index is used for tumor blood flow characterization, and clinical experience justifies this practice.

The first studies on color Doppler breast imaging applied a simple criterion for differential diagnosis: if color Doppler signals were detected in a focal breast lesion, the lesion was probably cancerous; otherwise, the lesion was probably benign (Britton and Coulden 1990).

Adler et al. (1990), however, were unable to detect color Doppler signals in 18 % of malignant breast lesions. Using the same method, they detected blood vessels in the breast tissue of 97 % of all patients who did not have a focal breast lesion. Thus, the simple qualitative visualization of intratumoral vessels is no longer considered an adequate basis for differential diagnosis.

As a result, increased attention has been focused on the quantitative analysis of the Doppler parameters that are recorded from tumor vessels (see above) (Blohmer 1995, Dock 1993, Konishi 1992, Madjar et al. 1991, Sohn et al. 1992, 1993). Quantitative measurements of blood flow velocities can be obtained from the Doppler waveforms. The velocity determination depends, however, on the angle of the incident sound beam (Sohn et al. 1992, 1993).

As it is virtually impossible to maintain a constant beam–vessel angle for all measurements, attention turned to the largely angle-independent Doppler indices of PI and RI. Sohn et al. (1992, 1993) found that side-to-side disparities of RI were useful in the differentiation of benign from malignant breast lesions. Medl et al. (1994) and Peters-Engl et al. (1995) (the same group of authors) claim that an RI less than 0.7 is an excellent criterion for differentiation between benign and malignant focal breast lesions using Doppler ultrasound. In their studies, Doppler ultrasound showed a sensitivity of 84 %, a specificity of 80 %, a positive predictive value of 71 %, and a negative predictive value of 90 % in the evaluation of breast lesions. However, given the various types of carcinomas, their varying grades of differentiation and patterns of vascularization, the diversity of benign lesions affecting the female breast, age-associated changes in blood flow, and many other variables, there seems little point in using an absolute value as the cut-off level for benign-malignant differentiation. The authors did not consider the possibility of blood flow changes due to hormone replacement, or the dependence of findings on the size of the focal lesion.

As for the disadvantages of pulsed color Doppler in breast tumor diagnosis, the slow flows that typically occur in intratumoral vessels (neovascularization) cannot be reliably depicted or measured with conventional Doppler technology, which is not sensitive enough and is subject to heavy interference from equipment noise in this range of velocities (see above) (Sohn 1995). Conventional Doppler is best for evaluating the flow in tumor-feeding arteries. Given the high demand of malignant tumors for blood supply, these feeding vessels carry a high-velocity flow which, in theory, may be accompanied by a low vascular resistance.

Another disadvantage of conventional Doppler ultrasound is the lack of reference values. For example, what does it mean to characterize a breast tumor as "hypervascular" by Doppler ultrasound? Can the values measured in postmenopausal women (velocities, indices) be compared with those in premenopausal women? And what are the effects of hormone replacement, vascular status, and other factors?

Comparing the blood flow in the healthy and diseased breasts can be accomplished by comparing the Doppler waveform parameters with those of an artery in the matching quadrant of the contralateral breast. The results of one study (Blohmer et al. 1995) are shown in Table 14.**1.**

Significant differences in maximum systolic velocity, minimum end-diastolic velocity, and median velocity were found between the tumor-feeding vessels in the diseased breast and the vessels in the matching quadrant of the contralateral breast. Higher flow velocities were measured in the tumor vessel than in the control vessel of the opposite breast. The magnitude of this disparity was significantly greater than that associated with benign focal lesions.

The large range of variation in the data in Table 14.**1** indicates, however, that this method may fail in individual cases.

The data for PI and RI show no significant difference between the carcinoma ves-

Table 14.**1** Differences and statistical significance of absolute flow velocities and Doppler indices determined in the vessels of a focal sonographic lesion (tumor breast, T) and a vessel in the matching quadrant of the contralateral breast (control or comparison breast, C).

Parameter	Malignant tumors	Benign tumors	Significance
δ v max T/C (cm/s)	10.8 ±14.6	2.1 ±8.6	$p<0.001$
δ v min T/C (cm/s)	2.7 ± 4.7	0.2 ±3.8	$p<0.01$
δ v mean T/C (cm/s)	5.6 ± 8.4	0.8 ±5.5	$p<0.001$
δ PIT/C	0.2 ± 2.4	0.06±0.6	n.s.
δ RIT/C	0.03± 0.17	0.02±0.1	n.s.

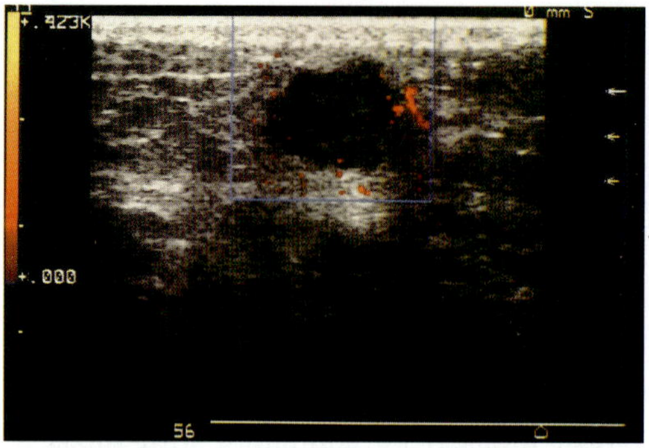

Fig. 14.5 Color Doppler image of a dense breast with invasive lobular carcinoma. The usual criteria for benign-malignant differentiation are of little value in this image. A blood vessel in the wall of the focal lesion may signify a malignant tumor.

sel and control vessel, a finding that has been confirmed by other authors (Konishi 1992, Madjar et al. 1992). Explanations offered for the unexpectedly high velocities in the (feeding) vessels are as follows: new vessels tend to develop at the advancing edge of a malignant tumor. The tumor-associated vessels show bizarre shapes and arrangements (corkscrew tortuosity, caliber variations), resulting in turbulence and elevated flow velocities (Kurjak et al. 1992). Arteriovenous shunts are also common in tumor vessels and are associated with high-velocity flow (Bouck 1994).

The new color flow techniques described above may one day enable radiologists to analyze the low-velocity tumor blood flow at the capillary level, which may portray most clearly the hemodynamic hallmarks of malignancy.

Examples. The first features of breast carcinoma noticed in the color Doppler image are the bizarre vascularization pattern and the concentration of blood vessels at the tumor periphery (Figs. 14.**5**–14.**7**). The Doppler waveform provides more definitive evidence of malignancy, revealing flow patterns that strongly support the diagnosis of carcinoma when compared with the contralateral breast (Figs. 14.**6**–14.**8**).

None of the investigated Doppler waveform parameters showed a significant difference between the arterial vessels in benign lesions and corresponding vessels in the opposite, healthy breast (Table 14.**1**).

Examples. Figure 14.**9** shows the color Doppler image of an arterial vessel at the periphery of a cyst. A Doppler waveform can also be recorded from fibrotic areas in the breast (Fig. 14.**10**).

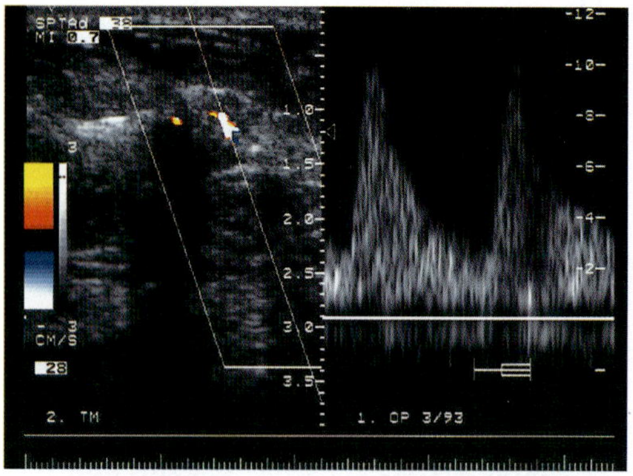

Fig. 14.**6** Pulsed and color Doppler examination of a recurrent breast carcinoma. In the B-mode image, the focal lesion is difficult to identify within the dense glandular tissue. The presence of blood vessels at the periphery of the lesion (proved by the Doppler waveform) yields additional information.

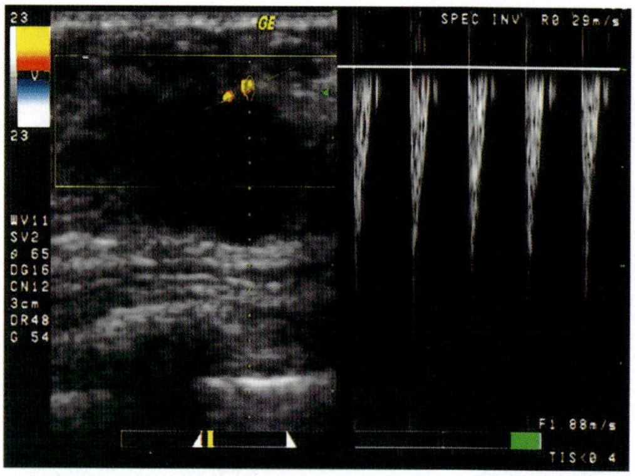

Fig. 14.**7** Color Doppler image of a blood vessel at the periphery of a carcinoma. Angle correction is used to determine the absolute flow velocities in the tumor vessels.

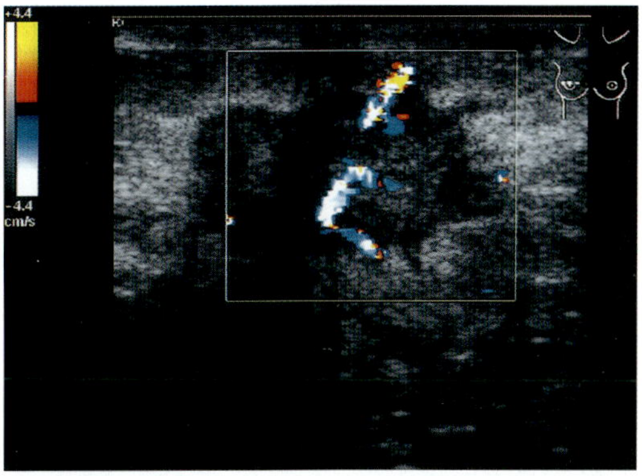

a

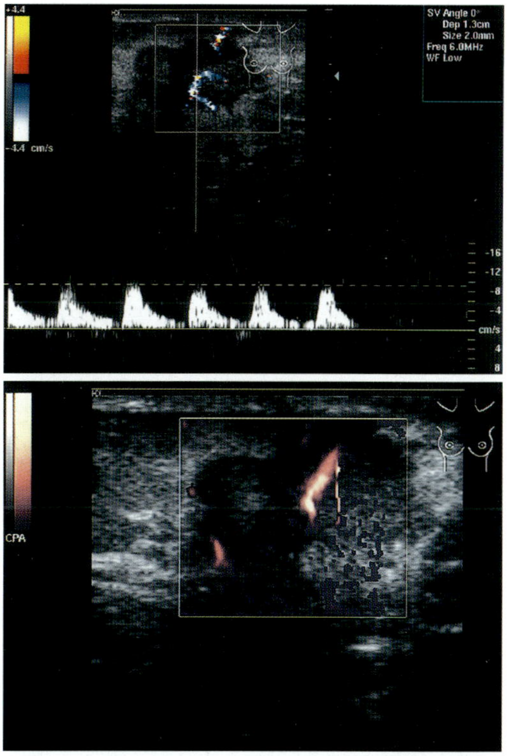

b

c

Fig. 14.**8a** Color Doppler image of high-velocity, turbulent flow in an arterial vessel (see Fig. 6.**10**). **b** A Doppler spectrum was recorded from this vessel at an acute angle, and the absolute flow velocities and RI were determined from the waveform. **c** Additional slow flow visualized by color power angiography (CPA).

Figure 14.**11** shows the color Doppler image and corresponding waveform recorded from a blood vessel in a fibroadenoma.

While the new color flow techniques can depict intratumoral blood flow with very high sensitivity, they do not, at present, yield quantitative flow information. The strongest criterion for malignancy is the presence of numerous color pixels within a lesion.

The presence of typical waveform characteristics signifying high or low vascular resistance is an important aspect of tumor blood flow studies. Early diastolic notching of the Doppler waveform indicates a high vascular resistance. This feature is typical of waveforms acquired from vessels with a muscular wall and therefore characterizes the normal blood flow in a healthy breast.

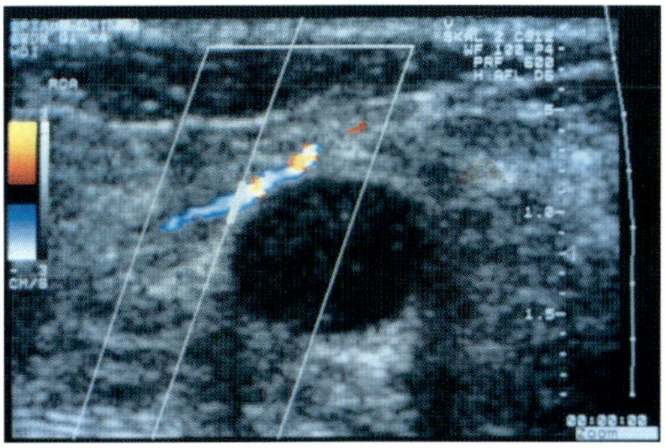

Fig. 14.**9** Color Doppler image of an arterial vessel at the periphery of a breast cyst.

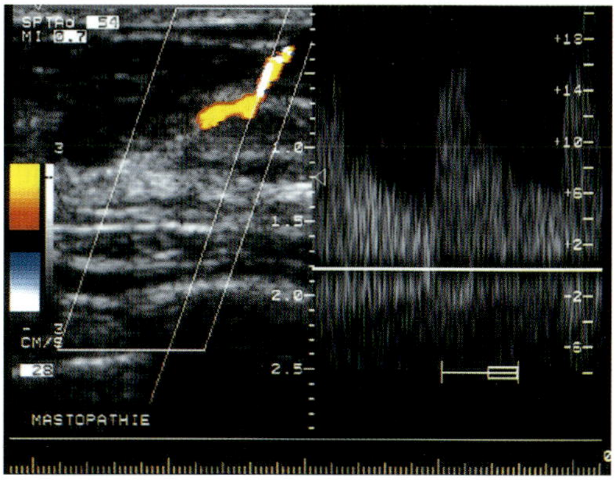

Fig. 14.**10** Color Doppler image of a blood vessel in fibrocystic tissue, and the corresponding Doppler waveform.

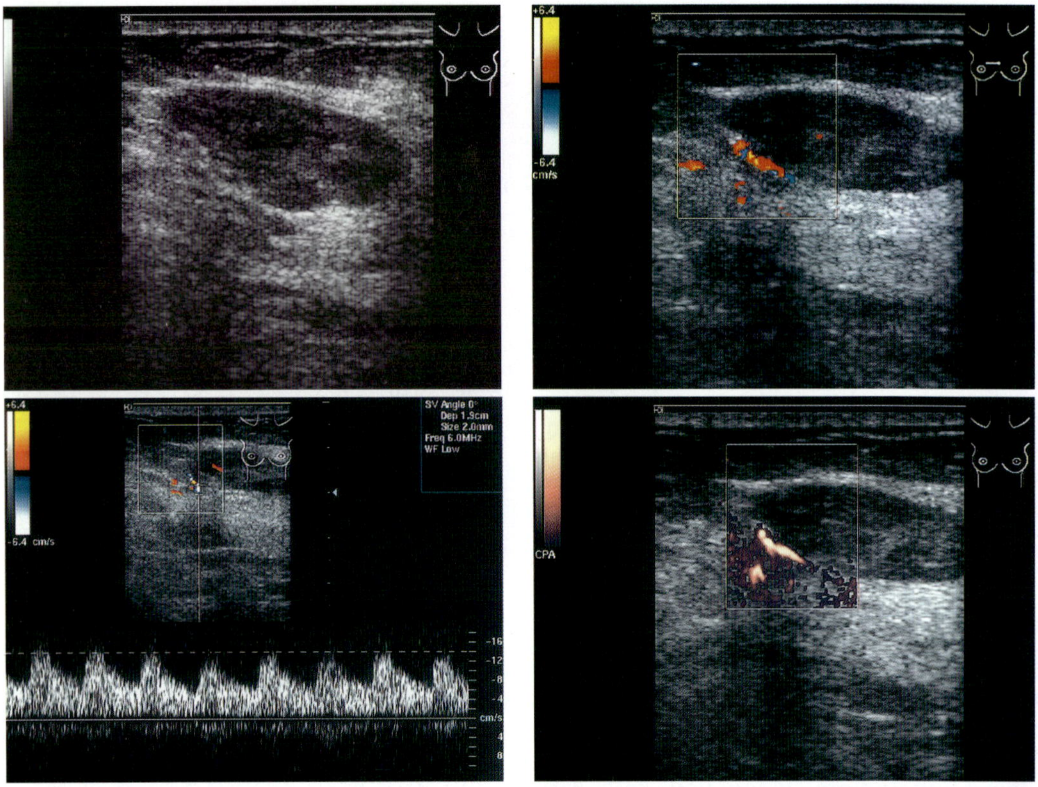

Fig. 14.**11a** Typical B-mode appearance of a fibroadenoma. **b** Color Doppler image of an arterial vessel at the tumor periphery. **c** Corresponding Doppler waveform indicating absolute flow velocities and RI. **d** When CPA is activated, no additional vessels are seen.

Ideally, this pattern is also seen in benign tumors. When there is a preponderance of vessels that lack a muscular coat, as in malignant tumors, the early diastolic notch does not appear, indicating a very low vascular resistance. It should be noted, however, that minute capillaries without a muscular coat occur in normal tissues and in benign and malignant tumors, and that different types of pathology vary only in the number of low-resistance vessels that are carrying low-velocity flow. Thus, the absence of notching is not pathognomonic for malignant lesions and serves merely as a suggestive sign that may be helpful to an experienced examiner (Figs. 14.**12,** 14.**13**).

Another difficulty is that notching in some vessels may be so subtle that different examiners will draw different conclusions about whether or not the sign is present. To some extent, then, notching is a subjective parameter.

One problem with using a slow-flow-sensitive color technique is that integrated pulsed Doppler cannot be used to quantitate the individual color pixels. The only alternative is to attempt a direct, albeit imperfect and incomplete, quantification by analyzing the color area and the intensity of the color pixels. This can be done by determining the quantitative ratio of the color areas to the rest of the image area, or by combining this measurement with an assessment of color intensities. This analysis sounds simple, but it can be difficult to accomplish by computer, since not all systems allow a specific color signal to be selected from an image and transferred to a computer for analysis (Figs. 14.**14,** 14.**15**).

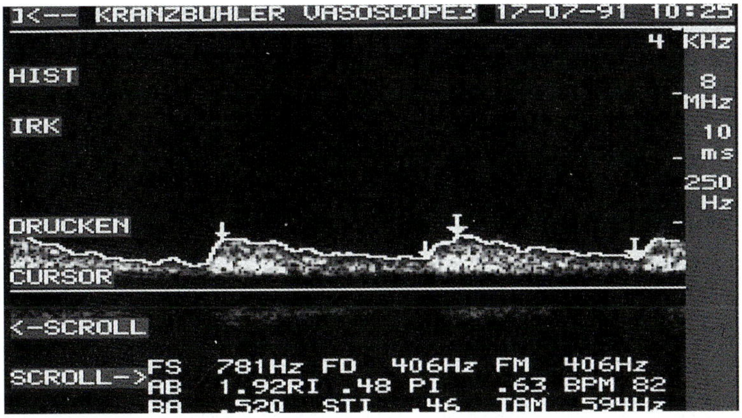

Fig. 14.**12** Doppler trace from a malignant breast tumor. The relatively low systolic peak and high end-diastolic velocities signify a very low vascular resistance. The flat waveform with a smooth, gradual downslope from systole to end-diastole is a pattern commonly seen with malignant tumors.

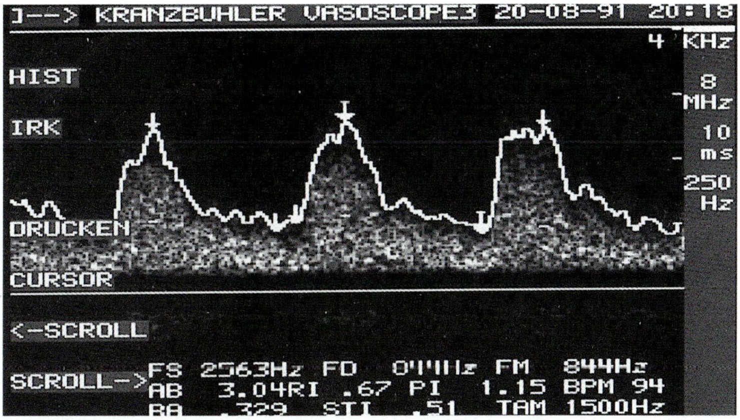

Fig. 14.**13** This Doppler trace from a benign breast tumor shows a typical high-resistance pattern marked by a high systolic peak and very low end-diastolic frequency. Systole and diastole are clearly differentiated, and the trace shows an abrupt rather than smooth progression from systole to end-diastole. This pattern is commonly seen with benign tumors.

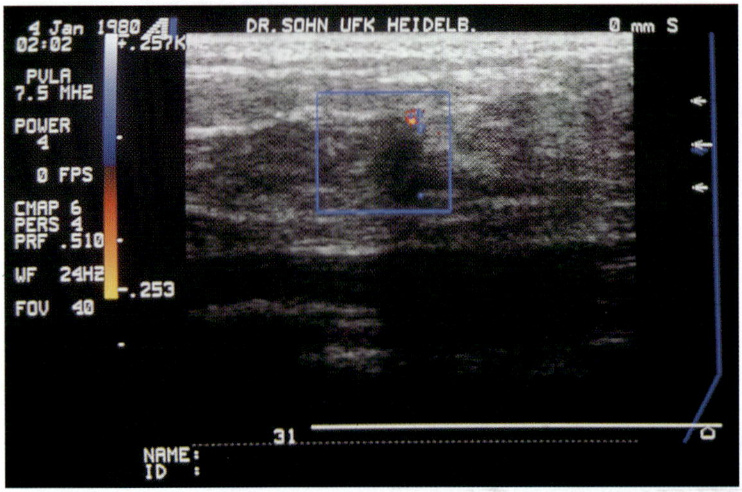

Fig. 14.**14** Scant blood flow in a small breast carcinoma produces an isolated color signal in this MEM image. The disadvantage of "non-Doppler" color flow techniques is that often the color pixels cannot be analyzed by pulsed Doppler, and blood flow must be assessed subjectively based on the number and size of the visible color areas.

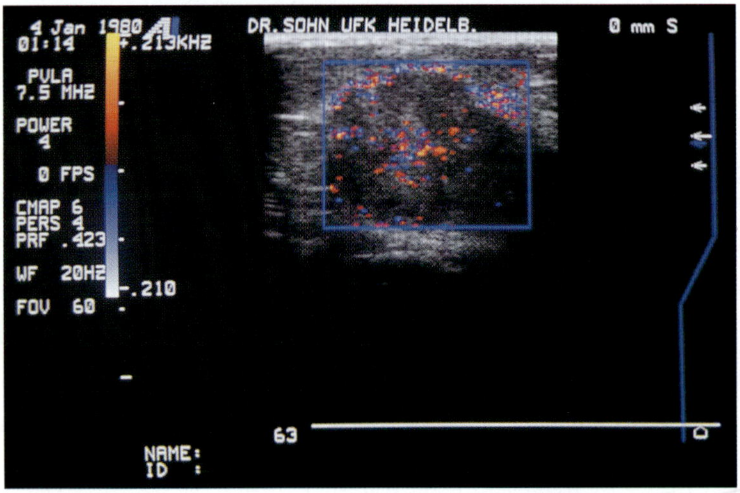

Fig. 14.**15** Clusters of color pixels signifying high blood flow in a relatively large breast carcinoma.

How Reliable are Conventional and Color Flow Ultrasound Imaging in the Evaluation of Breast Masses?

To answer this question, we present here a study that was designed to investigate whether modern color flow techniques could improve the differentiation between benign and malignant breast masses. In the study, 192 women with a palpable breast mass or a mammographically suspicious breast lesion were examined using conventional B-mode sonography and MEM color flow imaging the day before surgery. The B-mode and MEM findings were classified as benign or malignant, and the results of the preoperative sonographic diagnosis were compared with the subsequent histologic findings.

Equipment

The examinations were performed with a prototype MEM color flow imaging system (Acoustic Imaging, Tempe, Arizona) using a high-resolution 7.5-MHz transducer.

Compared with conventional Doppler, which can detect minimum flow velocities of about 1–3 cm/s, MEM can detect extremely slow flows (0.1 mm/s) and produce flow images of exceptionally high quality. The main drawback of MEM imaging is its qualitative nature, i.e., its inability to quantitate flow. While pulsed Doppler in an integrated duplex system can quantitate flow, it cannot analyze the extremely slow flow velocities that are common in malignant tumors.

In this study conducted at the University Gynecology Clinic in Heidelberg, we evaluated the color signal directly, based on the visual impression of the examiner. The results were based on the subjective assessment by an experienced examiner rather than the less sensitive pulsed Doppler method. Cosgrove et al. (1990) were successful in similar studies of flow characterization.

Patient Population

The patients consisted of 192 women with a palpable or mammographically detected unilateral breast mass who were examined on the day before surgery. Patients who did not have a sonographically detectable lesion were excluded from the study.

Examination Procedure

The ultrasound examination was always performed by the same examiner, who was blinded to the findings of mammography and other clinical findings. After taking a brief history and palpating the breast, the examiner proceeded to locate the mass in the high-resolution B-mode image and classify the lesion as malignant or benign.

Subsequently, a separate assessment was performed on the basis of the color flow image, disregarding the B-mode diagnosis. The sample volume extended past the lesion by 5 mm on all sides. Flow registration was set to maximum sensitivity and detected only the slowest blood flows (pulse repetition frequency 210 Hz).

Interpretation of Color Flow Images

The number of color pixels was used to determine whether a large or small amount of blood flow was detectable in a mass. This type of classification, though subjective, is the results of years of experience indicating that benign tumors imaged at maximum sensitivity tend to show a small number of isolated color pixels, while malignant tumors show greater numbers of pixels and especially "color areas" formed by contiguous pixels. The human eye can readily distinguish between isolated and contiguous color pixels.

The classification criteria used in this study were as follows: a focal lesion showing fewer than five color pixels, indicating little or no blood flow, was classified as benign. A lesion showing more than five color pixels or complex color areas, indicat-

Table 14.**2** Differentiation between benign and malignant breast tumors using B-mode imaging, MEM color flow imaging, and a combination of the two techniques.

Sonographic technique	Number of tumors correctly diagnosed	
	Malignant tumors (n=121)	Benign tumors (n = 71)
B-mode imaging alone	83.47 % (n = 101)	76.06 % (n = 54)
Color flow imaging alone	89.26 % (n = 108)	76.06 % (n = 54)
Combination of B-mode and color flow imaging	95.87 % (n = 116)	90.14 % (n = 64)

Table 14.**3** Malignant breast tumors correctly classified by the combined use of B-mode and color flow imaging.

Correctly classified as malignant by both techniques	76.86 % (n = 93)
Equivocal B-mode appearance with high blood flow	10.74 % (n = 13)
Benign B-mode appearance with high blood flow	1.65 % (n = 2)
Malignant B-mode appearance with scant blood flow	6.61 % (n = 8)
Total	95.87 % (n = 116)

Table 14.**4** Benign breast tumors correctly classified by the combined use of B-mode and color flow imaging.

Correctly classified as benign by both techniques	63.38 % (n = 45)
Equivocal B-mode appearance, without detectable blood flow	11.27 % (n = 8)
Malignant B-mode appearance, without detectable blood flow	2.82 % (n = 2)
Benign B-mode appearance, with high blood flow	12.68 % (n = 9)
Total	90.14 % (n = 64)

ing markedly increased flow, was classified as malignant. It was found that this assessment was highly reproducible.

The lesions were thus classified preoperatively as benign or malignant by evaluating the B-mode image and the color flow image. If there was a discrepancy between the B-mode and color flow findings, the examiner took the less equivocal finding as definitive. On completion of the examination, the sonographic results were immediately documented in writing. The study outcome was evaluated by comparing the sonographic diagnosis with the subsequent histologic diagnosis.

The total study population (n = 192) was divided into a malignant tumor group (n = 121) and a benign tumor group (n = 71), based on the histopathologic diagnosis. The overall results of the study are summarized in Tables 14.**2**–14.**4.**

Group 1: Malignant Tumors (Table 14.**3**)

Breast carcinoma was histologically confirmed in 121 of the patients. In 116 of these patients, the sonographic assessment (based on the B-mode or color flow image, or both) agreed with the histologic diagnosis. An evaluation based solely on the B-mode image correctly identified 101 of the tumors as malignant, and an assessment based solely on color flow correctly identified 108 of the malignant tumors.

Accordingly, the conventional B-mode image had a sensitivity of 83.5 % (101 of 121) in detecting malignancy, and the color flow image had a somewhat higher sensitivity of 89.3 % (108 of 121). The combination of B-mode and color flow increased the sensitivity to 95.9 %, correctly identifying 116 of the 121 tumors as malignant. This means that in 116 cases, the lesion was correctly diagnosed as malignant based on the findings of one or both of the sonographic techniques.

Agreement between the two methods, with both the B-mode and color flow images indicating a malignant tumor, was noted in 76.9 % of the cases (n = 93). In 23 of the cancer patients, the two methods did not agree. These cases require closer scrutiny.

In 13 cases (10.6 %), the B-mode assessment was equivocal because the lesion showed predominantly benign criteria such as sharp borders and narrow, bilateral acoustic shadows, while other criteria were suggestive of malignancy. But the color images demonstrated high blood flow in all of these cases, showing more than five color pixels or color areas, as described above, and supporting a diagnosis of malignancy.

In another 1.7 % of the cases (n = 2), the B-mode appearance of the lesion initially suggested a benign process, but the color images showed increased blood flow consistent with a malignant tumor.

Low blood flow, uncharacteristic of malignancy, was found in eight women with breast cancer (6.6 %), but the B-mode image showed definite malignant criteria that suggested the correct diagnosis.

A total of five women in group 1 (4.1 %) had a false-negative preoperative ultrasound diagnosis, i.e., both the B-mode and color flow image findings were classified as benign despite the presence of a malignant tumor.

Group 2: Benign Tumors (Table 14.4)

Seventy-one patients had a histologically confirmed benign breast lesion.

As noted earlier, an examiner faced with discrepant B-mode and color findings took the less equivocal finding as definitive. In 64 of the 71 benign cases, this procedure correctly identified the lesion as benign, i.e., a correct, benign preoperative sonographic diagnosis was made in 64 women. The lesion was correctly diagnosed as benign in 54 patients by B-mode findings alone, and in an equal number by color flow findings alone. Thus, B-mode alone and color flow alone were found to have equal specificities of 76.1 % in the diagnosis of benign breast disease. When the two techniques were combined, the specificity increased to 90.1 % (64:71).

In 45 of the 64 patients correctly diagnosed with benign breast disease by ultrasound (63.4 %), both techniques agreed in classifying the lesion as benign. The remaining 19 cases in which only one of the methods indicated a benign lesion are briefly reviewed below.

In 11.3 % of these cases (n = 8), the color flow image was crucial in making the correct diagnosis, the absence of slow blood flow in the color image identifying the equivocal B-mode lesion as benign. The reasons for the failure of the B-mode assessment included:

- Normal architecture of the glandular breast tissue with an equivocal focal lesion
- Scar tissue casting an acoustic shadow
- Equivocal echogenicity of the focal breast lesion

In another two cases (2.8 %) the B-mode image showed a malignant-appearing lesion, but the color image did not show increased blood flow, and the lesion was therefore assumed to be benign.

Although increased flow was visible in 12.7 % of the cases (n = 9), the tumor had to be classified as benign because of obvious benign criteria in the B-mode image.

In seven cases (9.9 %), the tumor was incorrectly classified as malignant by both sonographic methods. Histologically, these tumors consisted of fibrocystic lesions and one foreign body granuloma.

These results show that MEM color flow imaging adds significant diagnostic information to the conventional B-mode examination. B-mode imaging alone has a sensitivity of 83.5 %, and color flow imaging alone has a sensitivity of 89.3 %. Combining the two methods increases the sensitivity to an impressive 95.9 %. Combined B-mode and color flow imaging had a specificity of 90.1 % in this study.

Discussion of the Study

These results, consistent with those of many other authors in recent years, show that color-coded sonographic studies provide improved accuracy in the differential diagnosis of breast lesions.

The addition of color flow imaging in this study increased the accuracy of benign-malignant differentiation by 12.4 % for malignant breast tumors and by 14.8 % for benign lesions compared with B-mode imaging alone. B-mode and color flow imaging were found to have equal specificities for benign lesions – 70.1 % – when each method was used alone. Combining the two methods increased the specificity to 90.1 %.

Thus, B-mode and color flow imaging are complementary rather than alternative techniques, providing greater than 90 % specificity when combined. Similarly, a sensitivity of almost 96 % in the detection of malignant tumors could be achieved only when B-mode criteria were evaluated in conjunction with the color flow image. While MEM imaging is a powerful new technique, the separate evaluations described above prove that it complements rather than replaces the conventional B-mode image: eight malignant tumors and nine benign lesions were misinterpreted by evaluation of the flow image alone. These errors can be explained by noting that both fibrocystic lesions and foreign body granulomas (composed of organizing inflammatory tissue) are associated with a local, physiological increase in blood flow.

In one case in this series, the sonographic findings were suspicious for fibrocystic change, but histological examination revealed invasive ductal carcinoma with a predominantly intraductal component. Presumably, the lesion was misdiagnosed as benign at ultrasound because the largest invasive focus was only 3 mm in diameter.

With 21 focal lesions (13 malignant, eight benign), it was not possible to differentiate between benign and malignant lesions using the B-mode findings, and MEM imaging was essential for accurate characterization of the lesion.

In four cases (two malignant, two benign), the unequivocal color flow findings overruled the result of the B-mode examination, i.e., lesions that appeared malignant in the B-mode image were correctly reclassified as benign, and benign-appearing lesions were reclassified as malignant.

These results correlate well with those of other authors, indicating that an accuracy rate of 90–94 % can be achieved in differentiating between benign and malignant breast lesions using various Doppler techniques. Differences in technical methods must be taken into account, however, when the results of different authors are compared. The basic advantage of the prototype MEM imaging system used in this study is that it can demonstrate extremely low flow velocities. Its main drawback is its inability to quantitate flow. The development of an objective, automated method of signal registration and analysis is urgently needed.

When Doppler techniques are used, different authors use completely different parameters for interpreting the blood flow measurements. Given the variable nature of these parameters, the similarity of the results is remarkable.

Madjar et al. (1993) suggested using the peak systolic flow velocity, mean tumor blood flow, and the sum of the flow velocities as quantitative flow parameters for tumor differentiation by color Doppler sonography. In the search for uniform examination standards, Madjar believes that the mere display of color pixels is not a very useful criterion. We do not share this opinion. In our experience, the combination of conventional B-mode imaging and low-velocity color flow imaging by a non-Doppler technique provides the greatest diagnostic accuracy, despite the basically subjective nature of both techniques. The new color-coded techniques for imaging extremely low flow velocities place us on the threshold of being able to detect and visualize tumor angiogenesis.

Even in examinations using the latest duplex systems or CW Doppler, there is no clear consensus on the selection of analytic parameters. Schild et al. (1993) pointed to high diastolic flow as a conspicuous feature of malignant lesions. Burns et al. showed that the difference in maximum systolic frequency relative to the contralateral breast was a very useful criterion for differentiating between benign and malignant lesions.

Other useful criteria are increased frequency shifts (Madjar et al.) and comparing the number of blood vessels between the healthy and affected sides (Madjar et al., Heilenkötter and Jagella 1993). In our view, the number of blood vessels cannot be accurately determined due to the possibility of counting the same vessels more than once. Two recent reports by Raza and Baum (1997) and Birdwell et al. (1997) evaluating the use of power Doppler ultrasound for solid breast lesions show conflicting results. While Raza and Baum considered power Doppler ultrasound to be a useful and potentially important tool to predict malignancy, the study by Birdwell et al. (1997) did not come to the same conclusion. Their experience with power Doppler imaging suggested that both benign and malignant lesions could be avascular, and that the presence of color within a solid breast mass was a nonspecific finding and therefore of limited value in the diagnostic evaluation of solid breast masses.

In summary, color Doppler and the latest non-Doppler techniques have significantly improved the blood flow analysis of breast masses and the ability to distinguish between benign and malignant lesions. These techniques enable us to investigate blood flow in vessels that are below the resolution limit of ultrasound. Techniques based on the Doppler principle (duplex scanning, CW Doppler) are unable to detect the very low flow velocities that occur in malignant tumors.

Despite the substantial diagnostic gain achieved with Doppler and non-Doppler techniques, we still cannot differentiate benign and malignant breast tumors with 100 % accuracy (Figs. 14.**19**–14.**31**). Noninvasive sonographic blood flow studies have a particularly important role in patients with equivocal B-mode image findings, shadowing scar tissue, mammographically dense breasts, and follow-up after breast conservation. Given the profound implications of a diagnosis of breast cancer, however, it would be wrong to deprive any patient of histological confirmation. Not even the most modern imaging procedures can furnish an absolutely reliable preoperative diagnosis in patients with a breast mass.

Consequently, it may be desirable to move the emphasis of investigations in another direction. It has been possible to show that the level of blood flow to a malignant tumor correlates with its biological behavior. This implies that color flow imaging may be useful for the prognostic evaluation of malignant breast tumors, i.e., ultrasound may be able to differentiate between higher-grade malignancies and less aggressive lesions. Further studies are needed to resolve this question.

Future Developments in Sonographic Blood Flow Investigations of Breast Masses

Color Flow Imaging: a New Prognostic Factor?

While sonographic blood flow studies have advanced the benign-malignant differentiation of breast lesions as described above, they have not removed the need for histological confirmation. As a result, attention has increasingly turned to the potential of ultrasound as a prognostic indicator. In their studies of malignant breast tumors, Sohn et al. have observed a basic distinction between breast cancers with high blood flow and breast tumors with low blood flow. This distinction appears to relate to the known prognostic factors for breast carcinoma. A special study was conducted to determine whether these observations could be objectively confirmed. In the study, 119 women with breast cancer were examined sonographically on the day before their primary operation, and the result was compared with postoperative findings.

The goal of the study was to learn whether the biological behavior of a malignant breast tumor could be inferred from its color flow imaging characteristics.

Equipment

The examinations were performed with a prototype MEM color flow imaging system (maximum entropy method; Acoustic Imaging, Tempe, Arizona).

Patients

The criterion for inclusion in the study was the presence of a sonographically detectable breast mass. Sonographic flow imaging was carried out on the day before surgery. On the day of the operation, all patients with benign lesions were excluded from the study based on the frozen section result (later confirmed by the definitive histological diagnosis), yielding a group of 131 patients with histologically confirmed breast cancer. From that population, 119 patients with invasive ductal carcinoma were selected to form a homogeneous group with a uniform histology. In these 119 patients, the sonographic result and the result of several prognostic factors – tumor size, lymph-node status, receptor status, ploidy, and S phase – were recorded and correlated.

Due to a data collection error, receptor status and ploidy are available for only 60 of the patients.

Since subdivision into the minimum number of subgroups was desired for the 119 patients, lymph-node status was simply assessed concerning the presence or absence of metastatic lymph-node involvement. The number of involved lymph nodes and the presence or absence of capsular penetration were to be analyzed and correlated with blood flow classes (see below) in a larger patient population.

For the same reason, tumor size was classified either as T1 or as a stage higher than T1.

The patients ranged in age from 27 to 82 years, with an average age of 55.7 years.

The sonographic examinations were always performed by the same examiner. Initially, the breast tumor was located in the B-mode image. Then the size of the sample volume was adjusted so that it encompassed the tumor and extended 5 mm past it on all sizes. In all cases, blood flow registration was set to maximum sensitivity so that the very slowest blood flows could be detected (pulse repetition frequency 253 Hz). Most flows imaged by this technique are too slow for quantitation by pulsed Doppler (unsuccessful attempts were made to record a Doppler signal in the first 69 patients). It was therefore necessary to evaluate the color signal directly, instead of analyzing a Doppler waveform.

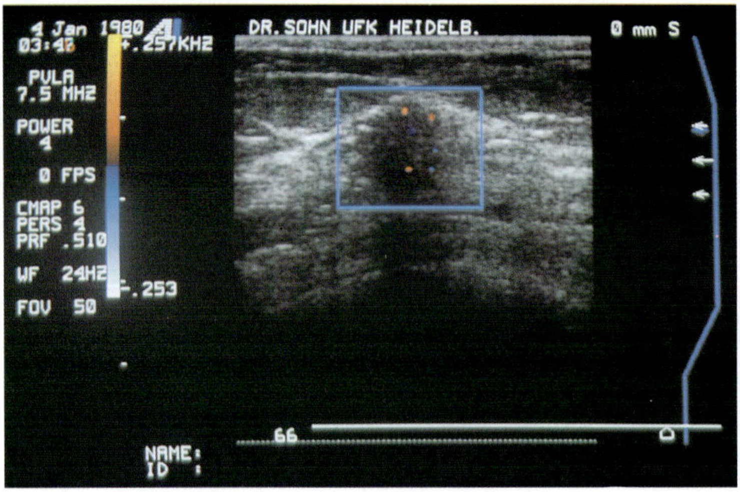

Fig. 14.16 Example of class I blood flow in a breast carcinoma based on subjective classification.

The intensity of the blood flow was expressed in terms of the number and characteristics of the color pixels – a method that proved to be reproducible. Given the current lack of an objective, automated recording system, the tumors were visually analyzed by the examiner and assigned to one of three classes:

- Class I: a lesion showing only isolated, noncontiguous color pixels (i.e., no color area) (Fig. 14.**16**)
- Class II: a lesion associated with one visible color area (Fig. 14.**17**)
- Class III: a lesion associated with more than one color area (Fig. 14.**18**)

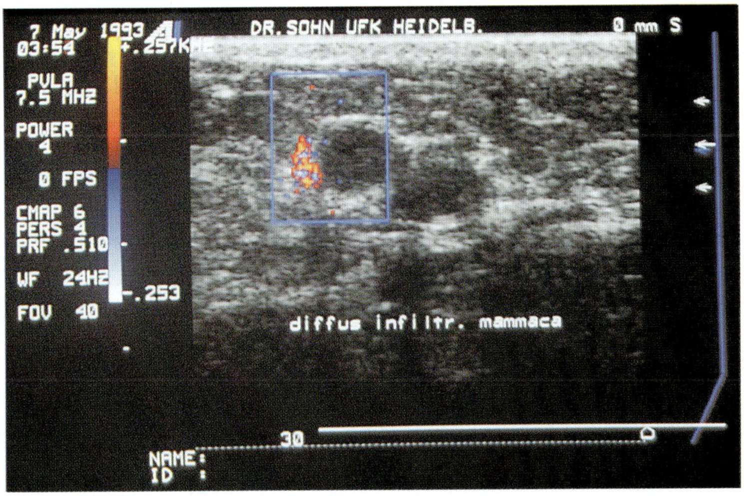

Fig. 14.**17** Example of class II blood flow in a breast carcinoma based on subjective classification.

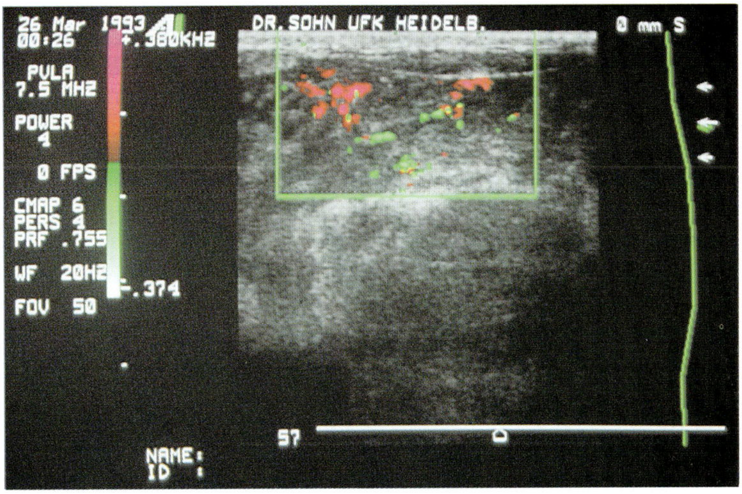

Fig. 14.**18** Example of class III blood flow in a breast carcinoma based on subjective classification.

While this classification is subjective and involves some uncertainty, it is based on a straightforward visual task that is practical and reproducible.

In order to prove this assumption, we had two physicians read five sample images from each of the three classes before the study began. In their independent readings of the images, both physicians agreed in their classification of all 15 images, confirming the excellent interobserver reproducibility of this method.

Tumor Classifications in the Study

Roughly equal numbers of tumors were assigned to blood flow classes I and II, and fewer tumors were assigned to class III:

- Class I: 46 patients (38.7 %)
- Class II: 42 patients (35.3 %)
- Class III: 31 patients (26 %)

Tumor Size

To minimize the number of patient subgroups, we simply differentiated T1 lesions from larger tumors. Twenty-two patients in Class I (48 %), 21 patients in Class II (50 %), and seven patients in Class III (23 %) were diagnosed as having a T1 lesion.

Lymph-Node Status

A minimum of 17 and a maximum of 24 axillary lymph nodes were removed in all patients. Thus, on average more than 20 lymph nodes from each patient were available for histological evaluation.

Most of the patients in Class I (slight flow, n = 46) had no detectable lymph-node involvement: 41 (89 %) of the Class I patients had no lymph-node metastases, and only five (11 %) of the patients had positive nodes.

A very different picture emerged in the Class II patients (moderate flow, n = 42): 28 (67 %) of these patients had lymph-node metastases, and only 14 (33 %) had negative lymph nodes.

Most of the patients in Class III (high flow, n = 31) were found to have lymph-node metastases: 25 (81 %) had positive axillary nodes, while only six (19 %) had negative nodes.

Receptor Status

Information about the receptor status was available for only 60 of the patients.

Estrogen and progesterone receptors were positive (> 20 fmol/mg) in 15 patients assigned to class I, in 10 patients assigned to Class II, and in six patients assigned to Class III.

Other patients were either estrogen-receptor-positive or progesterone-receptor-positive, but not both: four patients in Class I, five patients in Class II, and four patients in Class III.

Three patients each in Class I and II and 10 patients in Class III were negative for both estrogen receptors and progesterone receptors.

Ploidy

Information on ploidy was available for only 60 patients. Aneuploid cells were found in seven patients from Class I, nine patients from Class II, and 17 patients from Class III. Diploid cells were found in 15 patients from Class I, nine from Class II, and three from Class III.

S Phase

To correlate the S phase with blood flow classes, the patients were subdivided into a group with a low S phase (< 5.0 %) and a group with a high S phase (> 5.0 %).

Fifty-seven patients had an S phase less than 5.0 %, and 62 patients had an S phase greater than 5.0 %. Forty of the patients in the low S phase group were in blood flow Class I, 14 were in Class II, and three were

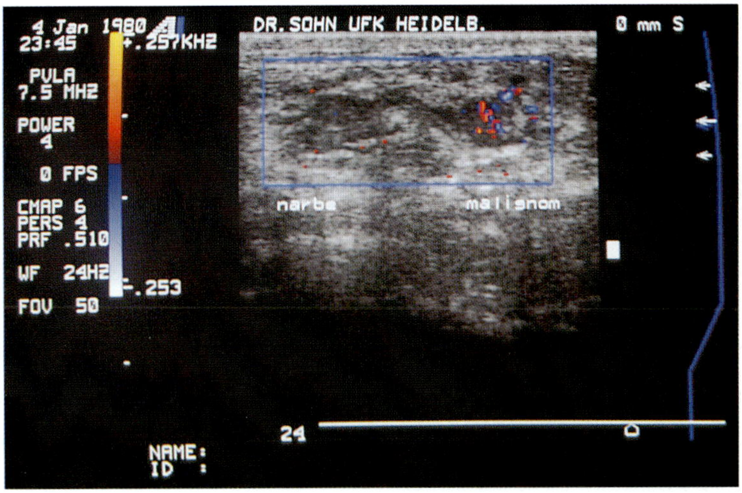

Fig. 14.**19** On the right side of the image is a small recurrent breast carcinoma; on the left side is scar tissue following breast-conserving cancer surgery done years earlier. Blood flow is not detected in the scar tissue, but conspicuous flow signals are recorded in the recurrent tumor.

in Class III. By contrast, a high S phase (> 5.0 %) tended to correlate with higher blood flow classes: only nine of the high-S-phase patients were in Class I, 23 were in Class II, and 30 were in Class III.

Discussion of the Study

As described above, in our experience color flow imaging can increase the confidence of conventional sonography in differentiating between benign and malignant breast lesions. The fact that malignant breast tumors often have a higher blood flow than benign lesions can be used for diagnostic purposes. This difference is based on the neovascularization of malignant neoplasms. There has been a notable lack of consensus, however, as to whether high or low flow velocities should be investigated. However, setting aside the question of what flow ve-

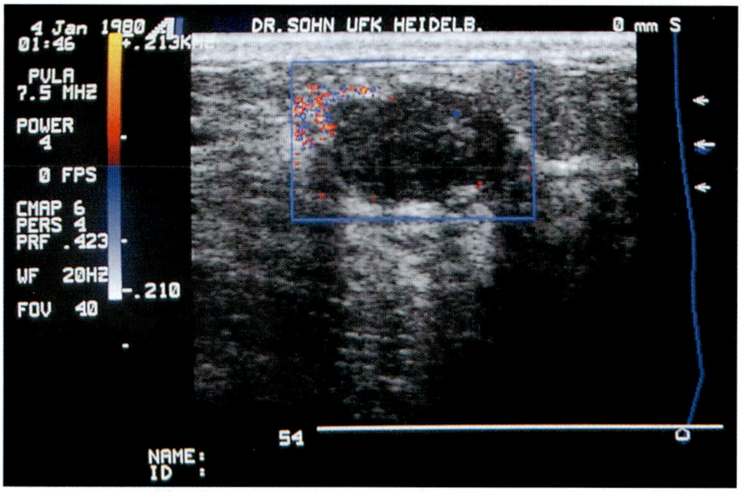

Fig. 14.**20** Blood flow is detectable only at the periphery of this fibroadenoma.

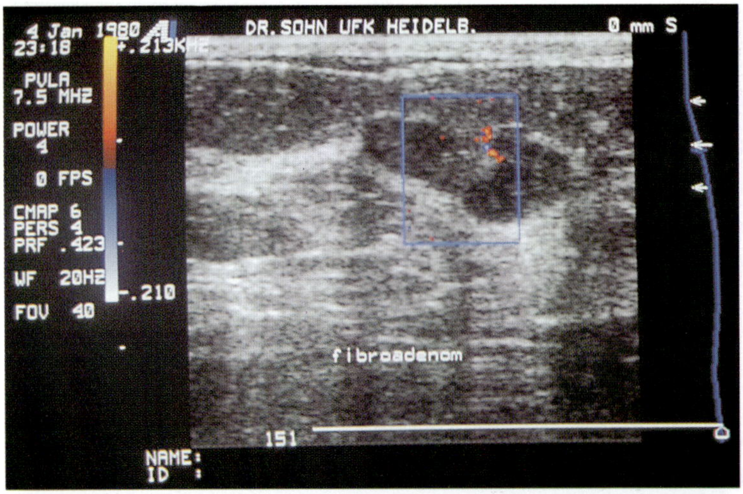

Fig. 14.**21** Intratumoral blood flow in a fibroadenoma. It is common for benign tumors to show a relatively "ordered" vascular pattern in which segmental vascular morphology can be appreciated. This is not characteristic of malignant tumors.

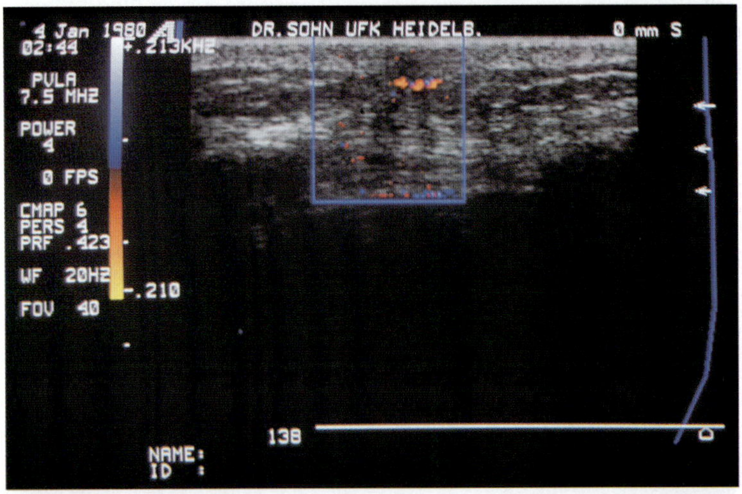

Fig. 14.**22** Color Doppler image showing relatively high blood flow in a very small breast carcinoma.

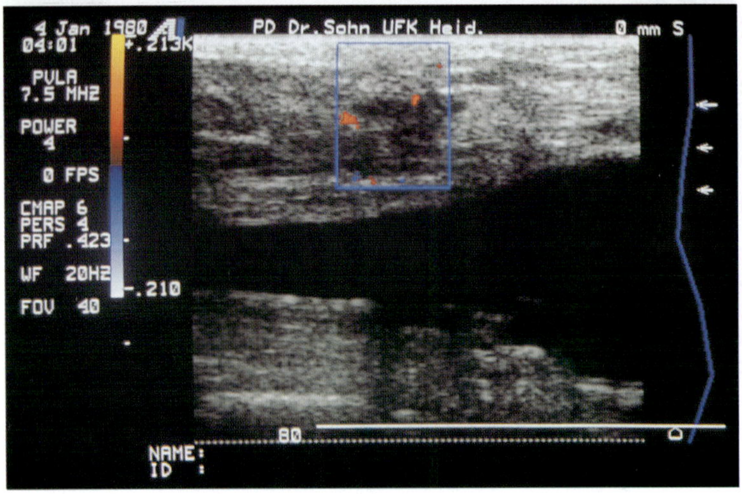

Fig. 14.**23** Blood flow in a recurrent breast carcinoma overlying a breast implant in place for five years. This case illustrates the potential value of color flow imaging in the follow-up of breast cancer.

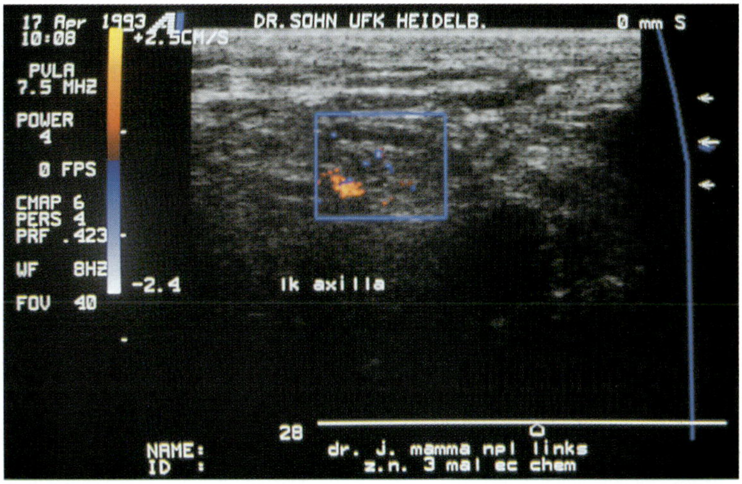

Fig. 14.**24** Blood flow around an axillary lymph node in a patient whose breast cancer was treated by preoperative neoadjuvant chemotherapy. Metastatic and inflamed lymph nodes are indistinguishable using color flow imaging, as both may be associated with increased blood flow.

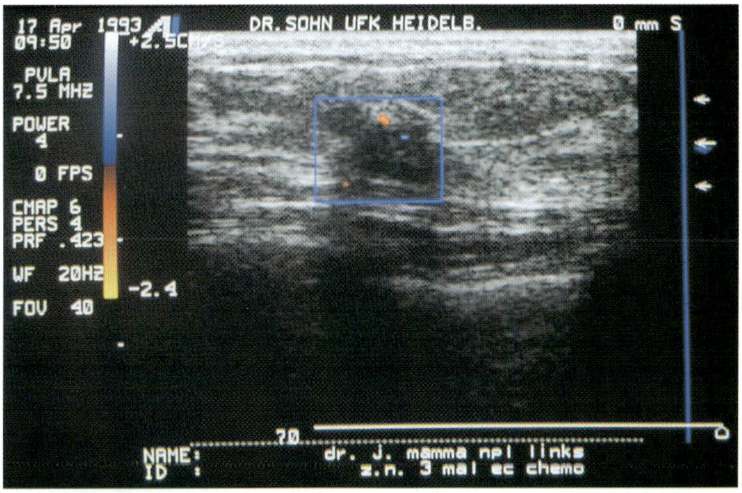

Fig. 14.**25** Scant blood flow in a breast carcinoma treated by neoadjuvant chemotherapy. This therapy reduced the tumor size from 4.8 cm to 1.1 cm, with a corresponding decrease in blood flow.

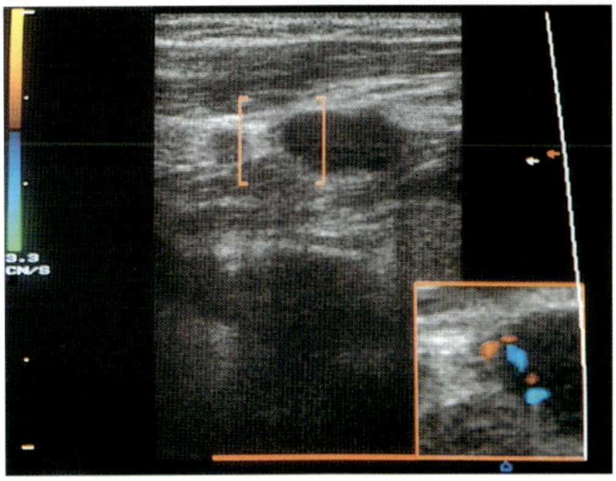

Fig. 14.**26** High blood flow at the periphery of this fibroadenoma demonstrates that even benign tumors may have a copious blood supply.

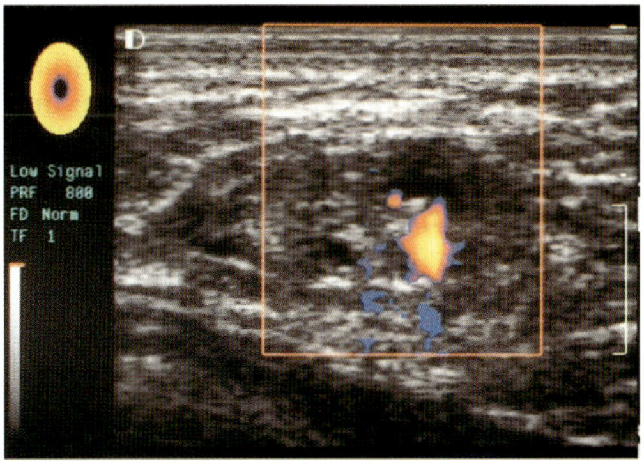

Fig. 14.**27** Blood flow in an area of fibrocystic change.

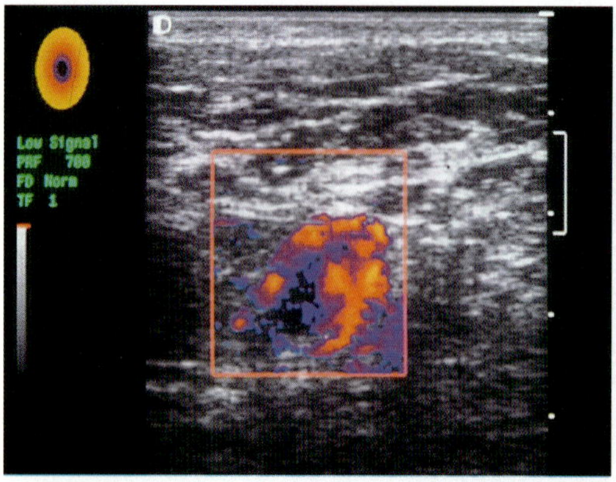

Fig. 14.**28** Small carcinoma with marked blood flow. The area of blood flow visualized by power Doppler completely covers the B-mode image of the focal lesion.

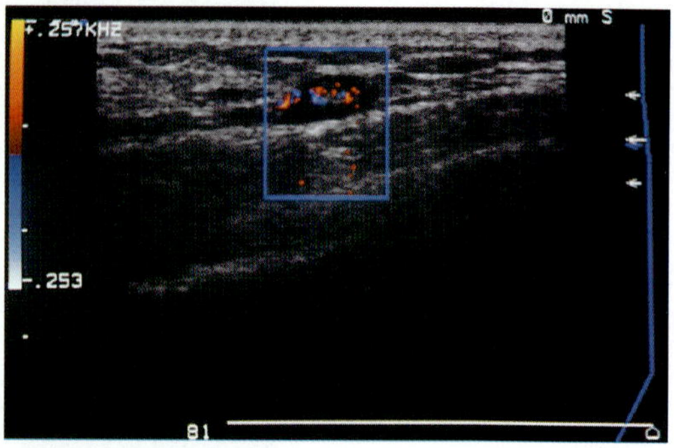

Fig. 14.**29** Blood flow in a small axillary lymph node.

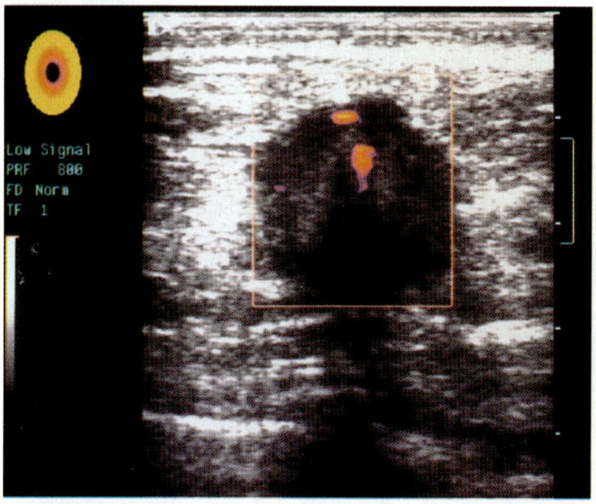

Fig. 14.**30** Carcinoma with relatively minimal blood flow.

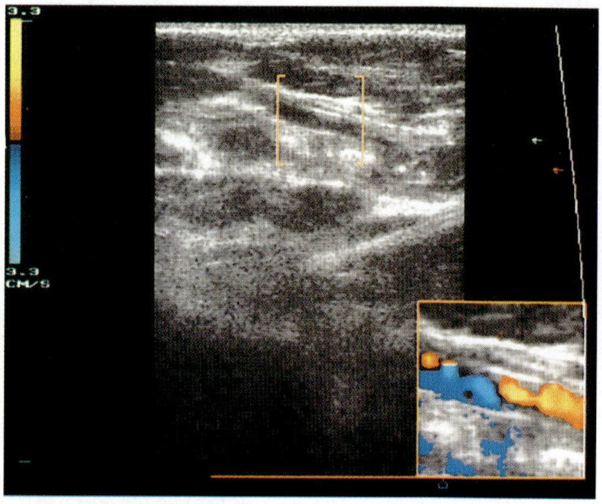

Fig. 14.**31** The color flow image clearly differentiates the blood vessel from mammary ducts.

locities should be used to differentiate between benign and malignant lesions, one fact remains clear: imaging studies cannot determine with absolute confidence whether a tumor is malignant or benign (Figs. 14.**119**–14.**31**). Consequently, the primary task of color flow imaging is in our view different from distinguishing between benign and malignant disease.

In the course of studying the problems of differentiating between benign and malignant breast masses, we noticed that malignant tumors showed marked differences in their levels of blood flow and degrees of vascularity. These observations prompted the present study correlating the various classes of tumor blood flow with the known prognostic factors for breast cancer. A sonographic technique capable of detecting and imaging very slow flow velocities was used. Initially, an attempt was made to define the differences in malignant tumor blood flows using conventional Doppler ultrasound, but this was unsuccessful. Since previous work had already shown considerable success with the use of MEM technology to image slow flows in distinguishing between benign and malignant lesions, it was decided to use this technique. The advantages and disadvantages of the method are described above. As it was not possible to quantitate MEM flow data, it was necessary to devise a three-level scheme for the visual classification of tumor flow patterns. Repeated studies of the same lesions confirmed the excellent reproducibility of this classification method. The human eye can readily differentiate between isolated color pixels, single color areas, and multiple color areas as a criterion for assigning lesions to specific blood flow classes.

In the initial study presented above, the sonographic findings were compared with the postoperative findings characterizing the biological behavior of breast carcinomas. Although this research is still preliminary, a remarkably high correlation was observed between minimal blood flow detected at ultrasound (Class I pattern) and the absence of axillary lymph-node metastases. By contrast, the majority of patients with a Class III type of blood flow had positive axillary nodes. Even in patients with moderate flow (Class II), metastatic lymph-node involvement was present in two-thirds of the cases. It appears that a definite relationship exists between the level of blood flow in a malignant tumor and the presence of lymph-node metastases.

Roughly equal numbers of patients were assigned to Classes I and II, and fewer patients were assigned to Class III. The size of the tumor probably had no effect on assignments to Class I and II, but it may well have affected Class III, as these patients had relatively few T1 lesions.

Patients with a low S phase were mainly represented in Class I, while a high S phase usually correlated with high blood flow. Aneuploid tumor cells tended to correlate with high tumor blood flow, while diploid tumor cells were frequently associated with low tumor blood flow. Patients having tumor cells with estrogen and progesterone receptors were mainly assigned to Class I or II, while patients with negative receptors were mostly assigned to Class III.

These results indicate a relatively uniform trend in which low tumor blood flow correlates with favorable prognostic factors, while high blood flow correlates with a less favorable prognosis. These results are preliminary and require confirmation in long-term studies with larger case numbers.

The study substantiates the argument above that only vessels carrying slow blood flow should be evaluated, as they form the basis for the results presented.

It should be emphasized again that color flow imaging does not significantly improve the ability to distinguish between benign and malignant tumors, since it is less than 100% accurate and B-mode imaging already yields very good results in this area. However, the potential of color flow imaging in evaluating the biological behavior of malignant breast tumors is encouraging. It can be hoped that, in the future, there may be less concern among researchers with the question of differentiating between benign and malignant disease and greater attention to the issue of prognostic assessment. As mentioned earlier, suitable equipment and technology are necessary for this type of investigation, although this is not yet uniformly available.

Contrast Agents in Breast Ultrasound

F. Geka and C. Sohn

Introduction

For several years now, blood flow imaging using power Doppler ultrasound has been available in addition to the traditional sonographic criteria for differentiating between malignant and benign breast lesions. The method involves superimposing a color-coded flow image over the standard B-mode image in real time. Power Doppler is a technique in which the amplitude of the echo is analyzed to determine the number of blood cells that are encountered by the ultrasound beam. The results of this technique are not affected by the incidence angle of the beam relative to the perfused vessel. The main advantage of power Doppler over conventional color Doppler, which relies on the frequency shift caused by moving blood cells, in that power Doppler is approximately 40 times more sensitive than color Doppler and can therefore detect and evaluate very low flow velocities such as those that occur in the capillary beds of tumors. The slowest flow velocity detectable by power Doppler is 0.4 mm/s (Sohn et al. 1996).

Clinical Significance of Blood Flow Assessment in Breast Masses

When a malignant breast tumor grows beyond several millimeters in size, it triggers the release of angiogenesis factors in order to meet its nutritive requirements, which can no longer be met by diffusion alone (Folkmann et al. 1972). Similar observations have been made in fast-growing benign lesions (Folkman et al. 1973). These tumor vessels show an irregular growth pattern and an atypical wall structure that lacks a muscular coat, so that the vessel wall is unable to dilate or contract to regulate flow. A variety of features, often coexisting, have been found to characterize these vessels, such as the presence of shunt vessels carrying high-velocity flow, vascular loops with caliber variations leading to heterogeneous flow patterns, and tumor-associated capillaries with low vascular resistance and low flow velocities (Kurjak et al. 1992, Bouck 1994, Horak et al. 1992). The analysis of primary tumor vascularization could be of value in predicting future metastasis, since the metastatic potential of a tumor has been found to correlate with the number and density of the tumor-associated vessels (Weidner et al. 1991).

Since even some benign processes – such as inflammatory and proliferative breast lesions and pregnancy-related and lactation-related breast changes – lead to increased blood flow, it is clear that differentiating between benign and malignant lesions using noninvasive diagnostic methods is of key importance (Madjar et al. 1997, 1998, Leucht and Madjar 1995).

Advantages of Ultrasound Contrast Agents

Echo-enhancing contrast agents are often helpful in assessing the degree of vascularization of a focal lesion. An intravenous contrast agent with the brand name Levovist has now been available for some time. The agent consists of granules of a galactose-based material that are mixed with a specified amount of solvent before use. The mixture is shaken, forming microbubbles that adhere to the surface of the granules. These microbubbles increase the echogenicity of the blood by creating an interface that has a high acoustic impedance. A special property of this contrast agent is the transpulmonary stability of the galactose suspension, achieved by adding 1 mg of palmitic acid to the D-galactose.

Use, Effects, and Side Effects of Levovist

The use of Levovist in more than 1200 patients has shown a significant improvement in vascular definition, increasing the intensity of echo signals by 10–20 dB (Schlief 1991). Rare cases of side effects have been reported, such as transient headache and heat or cold sensation (Schlief 1993, Madjar et al. 1997, 1998). The only recognized drug-related contraindication to the use of Levovist is hereditary galactosemia.

Various concentrations of the contrast agent, controlled by the amount of water added to the injection solution, can be used in Doppler ultrasound examinations. For example, a concentration of 200 mg/ml of contrast agent is sufficient to enhance Doppler signals that are detectable but not clearly demonstrated in noncontrast imaging. A concentration of 300 mg/ml or 400 mg/ml is preferred in cases in which noncontrast signals are weak or absent. The agent is administered as a peripheral intravenous bolus injected at 1–2 ml/s to ensure uniform Doppler signal enhancement. Initial enhancement occurs 15 seconds after contrast administration. The enhanced signals appear mostly in the periphery of the tumor during the inflow phase. Intratumoral vessels show enhancement following a plateau phase of variable duration, and the signal intensities fade during the washout phase (Duda et al. 1995). This triphasic pattern of signal enhancement could provide an important clue to the growth dynamics of the tumor.

Technique of Blood Flow Measurement

Before an ultrasound contrast agent is administered, a high-frequency B-mode examination is performed at frequencies of 10–13 MHz. The axial resolution in this frequency range is 0.15–0.12 mm.

As a reference for evaluating blood flow in the suspicious area, power Doppler imaging is first performed in normal breast parenchyma. The intensity of the color pixels in the reference scan can be lowered to a minimum level at which only scattered signals are recorded. The same setting is then used to evaluate the suspicious area and compare it with the reference scan. This evaluation is based on vessel count, signal intensity, and blood flow changes such as decreased, increased, or absent blood flow. The color intensity within the suspicious area can again be lowered to help differentiate the effect of the contrast agent from the precontrast findings.

Results Published to Date

Most invasive carcinomas show an increase of blood flow in the power Doppler image, the diameter of the tumor correlating with the increase in flow. But hypervascularization is also found in about 30 % of benign breast lesions, most notably fibroadenomas, inflammatory processes, and fibrocystic changes. Conversely, in situ carcinomas and some early invasive cancers (T1a) show blood flow patterns similar to those of benign lesions, with little or no detectable increase in flow.

In pulsed Doppler studies as well, authors have been unable to define a useful cutoff value to distinguish between benign and malignant tissue. Findings indicate that the maximum systolic velocity in feeding vessels is different in benign and malignant lesions, but practical limitations of angle correction make it impossible to conduct a precise velocity analysis. It has been shown that stage T1 and T2 breast carcinomas have a significantly lower maximum systolic velocity and higher resistance index (RI) than stage T3 and T4 tumors. But these parameters are of limited use for differentiating between benign and malignant lesions, as they are very similar in stage T1 and T2 carcinomas and benign breast lesions (Milz et al. 1997). Madjar et al. (1997, 1998) also found that resistance indices and flow velocity measurements are inadequate for differentiating breast malignancies from benign focal lesions.

This uncertainty factor that is inherent in blood flow measurements alone, using either power Doppler or pulsed Doppler, underscores the importance of combining the flow image with high-frequency B-mode ultrasound. Milz et al. (1997) achieved a sensitivity of 87 % and a specificity of 82.5 % with this combined approach.

Madjar et al. (1997, 1998) noted differences in the enhancement characteristics of benign and malignant breast lesions after the administration of a contrast agent. Images obtained after the administration of Levovist demonstrated vessels in malignant tumors that had not been shown by power Doppler imaging without the contrast agent.

Further studies and larger case numbers are needed in which flow indices, perfusion patterns, and flow velocities are accurately documented and correlated with the histological findings so that we can differentiate more accurately between benign and malignant tissue and improve the prognostic assessment for various lesions. Greater importance should be attached to effects specific to the contrast agent, with the goal of improving the interpretation of focal lesions (Duda et al. 1993).

Sohn et al. (1997) have described a method for the quantitative evaluation of tumor perfusion. They used the latest instrument technologies (VST Synergy from Diasonics/Sonotron) to plot graphic displays of blood flow changes in breast tumors while the systemic blood pressure was temporarily raised by exertion. In future studies, an ultrasound contrast agent will be administered by peripheral injection so that the increase in blood flow can be visualized.

Other Contrast Agents and Indications for Use

The use of contrast agents in the investigation of breast lesions is familiar from the field of magnetic resonance imaging (MRI). The rise in signal intensity per unit of time is used to evaluate dynamic processes in areas in which neovascularization has occurred (Duda et al. 1995).

Ductography (galactography) is a classic method for diagnosing ductectasia or intraductal lesions. A radiopaque contrast medium (aqueous or iodinated) is injected by catheter into the lactiferous ducts to visualize the ductal structures of the breast.

Use of Contrast Agents for Investigating Tumor Blood Flow

Initial studies indicate that an intravenously administered transpulmonary ultrasound contrast agent traditionally used in echo cardiography can enhance the Doppler signals recorded from tumors. When injected intravenously, this contrast agent can improve the imaging of breast lesions by increasing the signal intensities. This can improve the diagnostic results in some circumstances, particularly when less sensitive equipment is being used. Contrast agents in color Doppler, for example, can provide a clearer depiction of blood flow.

These contrast agents may have the same range of applications as in magnetic resonance imaging, in which contrast enhancement is commonly used to study the dynamics of tumor blood flow. Further research in this area is needed. Contrast enhancement should, however, never be used to compensate for deficient equipment.

Given the controversy surrounding published results and the technological constraints noted above, it is clear that there is no standard methodology for the time being that can be applied to the differential diagnosis of breast lesions by ultrasound flow imaging. A uniform standard is yet to be defined. Nevertheless, we believe that color flow imaging shows promise not only for differentiating between benign and malignant breast masses but also for the prognostic evaluation of malignant disease.

15 Ultrasound-Guided Interventional Procedures in the Differential Diagnosis of Breast Lesions

H. Junkermann and U.M. Hamper

Aspiration Cytology

With the increasing use of mammography and sonography for early cancer detection, it is common to discover breast lesions that require further investigation. While this can be accomplished by imaging studies (special mammographic views, ultrasonography, magnetic resonance imaging), fine-needle aspiration biopsy (FNAB) is an important procedure that is performed in some countries (Sweden, for example) routinely before every open biopsy and therapeutic breast operation. FNAB can reduce the rate of biopsies of benign lesions and assist in surgical planning, reducing the need for multiple surgical interventions in the same breast. Although FNAB has been successfully performed by some, it has not been widely embraced as a technique, due to several drawbacks. These include the need for a skilled and highly trained breast pathologist, persistent problems with insufficient tissue acquisition, and a high false-negative rate (Dowlatshaki et al. 1989, Ciatto et al. 1990). Consequently, histology is preferable to cytology for most pathologists and has led to the introduction of the "modern" core biopsy era, which began with the introduction of larger automated core biopsy "guns." Ultrasound is an excellent modality for monitoring and guiding needle insertions for aspiration cytology or core biopsies.

Technique

FNAB should be performed with a 20–40-gauge needle. Most authors carry out a negative-pressure aspiration with syringe suction. FNAB without suction will provide equally good cell yields from malignant tumors, but will collect less cellular material from benign tumors (Ciatto et al. 1991). A Cameco or similar type of hand grip is recommended. With the transducer positioned on the breast, the needle is inserted in a direction roughly parallel to the transducer face to allow optimum monitoring of the insertion (Fig. 15.**1**). The needle can deviate up to 30° from the long axis of the transducer and still be well visualized; steeper angles will limit or prevent adequate monitoring. Under sonographic guidance, the needle is advanced to a point just short of the target lesion. The plunger of the syringe is now retracted to produce suction, while the needle tip is moved back and forth in the lesion under constant ultrasound vision. Before the needle is withdrawn from the tissue, suction is discontinued so that material

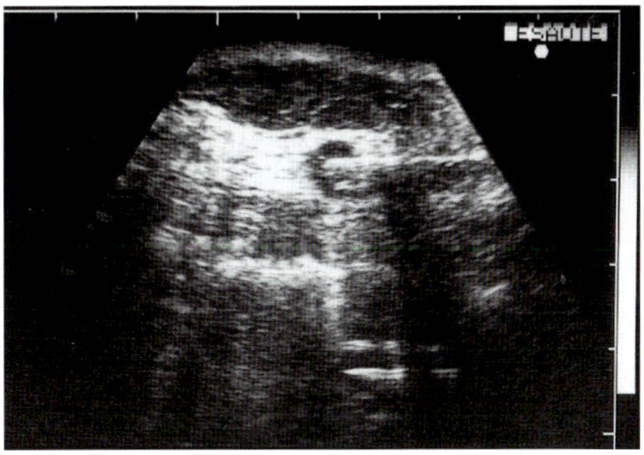

Fig. 15.**1** Ultrasound-guided aspiration of a 7-mm solid breast mass. Cytology yielded atypical cells, and histology identified the lesion as invasive ductal carcinoma. The needle is entering the image from the right side. It is directed parallel to the transducer face, and its path is clearly displayed on the monitor.

is not drawn into the barrel of the syringe, where it would be difficult to retrieve. The material collected in the needle is ejected onto a glass slide and spread into an even smear. Depending on the stain preference of the cytologist, the specimen may be air-dried (for May-Giemsa-Grünwald staining) or fixed in a solvent (for Papanicolaou staining).

Evaluation and Results

It should first be determined whether adequate cellular material has been collected from the lesion (Fig. 15.**2**). In 20–30 % of cases, insufficient material has been sampled for a definitive diagnosis (Löfgren et al. 1988, Ciatto et al. 1990). Further management of these cases depends on the nature of the mammographically or sonographically detected lesion. If there was definite mammographic or sonographic evidence of malignancy, or if the lesion had a typical "carcinoma feel" during the needle insertion (Svane et al. 1993), surgical excision should be performed regardless of the cytological result. Otherwise, depending on the result of the imaging studies, the patient can be followed up on an outpatient basis, aspiration cytology can be repeated, or histological confirmation can be obtained.

Fine-needle aspiration cytology can significantly improve the accuracy of the preoperative diagnosis. While imaging studies alone have a predictive accuracy of about 25 % for breast carcinoma, FNAB can usually increase this rate to more than 50 % (Fig. 15.**3**) (Svane et al. 1993). Experienced examiners can achieve accuracy rates of 75 % or even 87 % (Azavedo and Svane 1991). For FNAB to be used to its full potential in breast diagnosis, close cooperation is needed between the breast diagnostician and the cytologist. These specialists should confer on the details of the aspiration technique and specimen preparation, and ideally they should jointly discuss every case, since there are many cases in which cytology alone cannot furnish a confident diagnosis. The best results are achieved when cytology is used as part of an integrated breast workup that includes clinical findings, mammograms, and ultrasound.

Reservations about cytology in Germany and the United States are due partly to the lack or unavailability of trained, experienced breast cytologists on site and partly to a lack of the interdisciplinary cooperation described above. As a result, there are relatively few examiners who can combine the various methods and achieve good results.

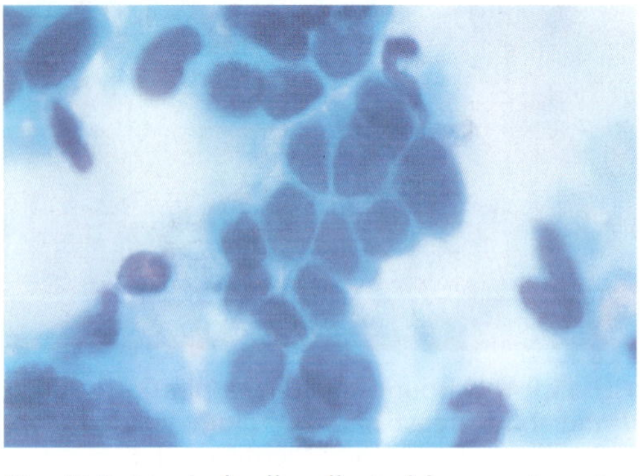

Fig. 15.**2** Atypical cells collected from an invasive ductal carcinoma (courtesy of Dr. Melsheimer, Department of Gynecological Morphology, University of Heidelberg).

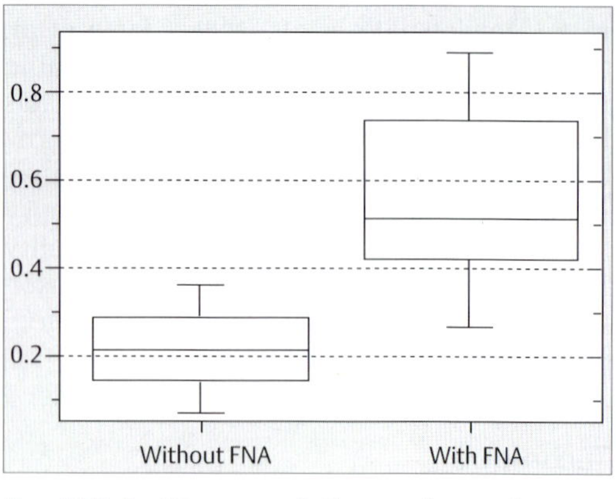

Fig. 15.**3** Positive predictive value of open biopsy performed without (left) and with (right) prior fine-needle aspiration (FNA) (after Svane et al. 1993).

Core Biopsy

High-speed automated large-core biopsy is a new technique that is rapidly gaining widespread use. Because it is less traumatizing and easier to perform, automated core biopsy has completely replaced manual core biopsies at most centers (Junkermann et al. 1993, Parker et al. 1991, 1994, 1995a, 1995b, Parker and Burbank 1996, Liberman et al. 1994). For lesions that can be localized with ultrasound, we always perform the core biopsy under sonographic guidance, as this is simpler and more comfortable for both the patient and the physician than stereotactic guidance. In patients with a palpable breast mass, we routinely check the needle placement with ultrasound, since the central tumor mass itself is often considerably smaller than the palpable mass caused by the perifocal reaction, which contains few or no tumor cells at its periphery. A core biopsy of the breast may be technically more demanding and traumatic than FNAB. Its advantage is that it yields a histological specimen that the pathologist can evaluate for histopathological criteria; unlike cytological material, the histological specimen can demonstrate the invasiveness of the tumor.

Technique

Automated core biopsy of the breast is usually performed with a 14-gauge (2.1-mm) core needle. The biopsy gun should have an excursion of 20–22 mm (Parker et al. 1993). After the lesion has been located in the ultrasound image and the puncture site has been selected (it should allow needle insertion parallel to the transducer), local anesthesia is administered at the puncture site, infiltrating the area from the skin surface down to the tumor. It is unnecessary to infiltrate all of the area surrounding the tumor. Before the needle is introduced, either a small stab incision (2–3 mm) is made in the skin, or a 13-gauge trocar is inserted (Fig. 15.**4**). Some prefer the trocar, as it allows multiple cores to be obtained

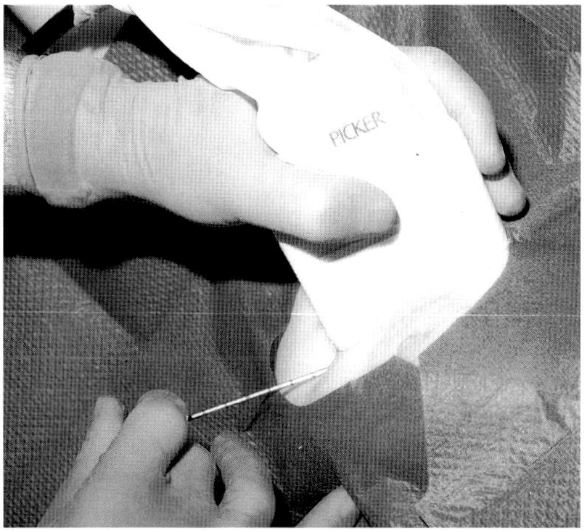

Fig. 15.**4** Insertion of the 13-gauge trocar. The puncture site is chosen so that the needle can be inserted roughly parallel to the transducer face.

from a single puncture and reduces the risk of hematoma formation and seeding of tumor cells along the needle track (Harter et al. 1992). The cocked needle is advanced to the tumor under ultrasound guidance, and the needle is fired (Fig. 15.**5**). The needle is then withdrawn, and the tissue core is removed from the notch in the needle shaft (Fig. 15.**6**). Most radiologists recommend that several cores be obtained – a minimum of five from circumscribed

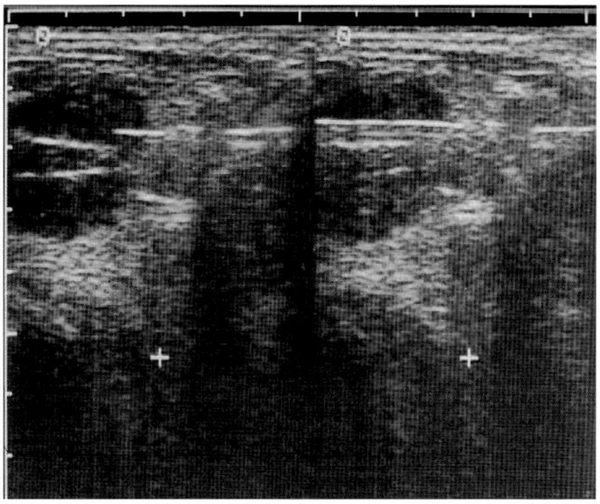

Fig. 15.**5** Insertion of the needle: prefire (left) and postfire views (right). The tracks from two previous needle insertions appear as linear echoes.

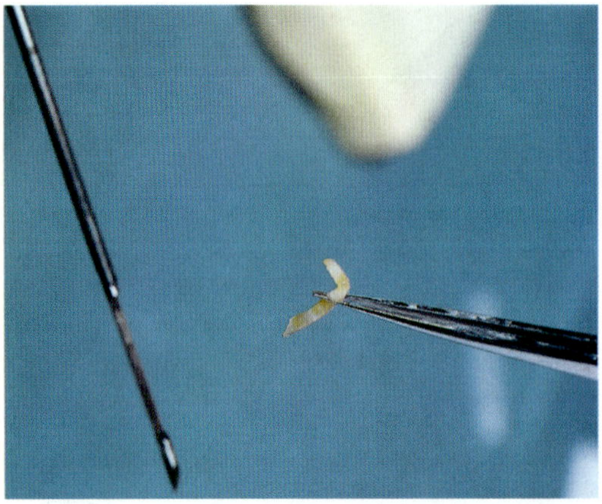

Fig. 15.6 The needle has been withdrawn from the trocar, and the tissue sample is retrieved from the 18-mm-long notch in the needle shaft.

lesions (Liberman et al. 1994). When these conditions are met, an almost 100 % accuracy rate is achieved even with very small lesions; this equals or surpasses the accuracy rate of open biopsies in patients with circumscribed, sonographically visible breast lesions (Parker et al. 1994). Although the automated core devices are used by most examiners, the recent introduction of a new device, the Mammotome (Biopsys Medical, Irvine, California) used in conjunction with stereotactic devices or ultrasound has gained widespread attention (Parker and Burbank 1996). The Mammotome overcomes several of the inherent drawbacks of automated core devices, which include the need for multiple needle insertions to acquire multiple samples, the need for pinpoint accuracy in targeting, the need to "fire" the device to acquire tissue – which at times may be scant – and lastly great difficulty in obtaining tissue with microcalcification (Parker and Burbank 1996). The Mammotome works on a different principle than automated biopsy guns. Instead of a Tru-Cut style of needle, which collects tissue in a notch and must be withdrawn after each pass, the Mammotome uses a vacuum chamber that helps pull tissue into the probe and transport it back, so that it does not have to be withdrawn each time. The Mammotome acquires larger amounts of tissue during each acquisition, and a given lesion can be canvassed much more quickly and completely, since the device remains within the breast while the tissue is being sampled (Parker et al. 1995a, 1995b, Parker and Burbank 1996). Parker et al. (1995) also found the Mammotome useful especially for stereotactic biopsy of microcalcifications. In their experience, successful, effortless, and speedy acquisition from most calcifications in a given cluster can be achieved – an important factor for ensuring a successful and accurate diagnosis.

In summary, although some investigators have successfully used FNAB for percutaneous breast biopsies, most clinicians, radiologists, and pathologists prefer histological specimens. Therefore, in most communities stereotactic or ultrasound-guided core breast biopsies have become a common and accepted alternative to surgical excisional biopsies. The introduction and increasing use of the Mammotome and successful percutaneous biopsy of microcalcification via this route should further decrease the need for open surgical biopsies.

Ultrasound-Guided Preoperative Localization

In patients with nonpalpable breast masses, preoperative localization of the clinically occult lesion is required. Even small mammographic densities can usually be visualized with modern, high-resolution ultrasound probes. Microcalcifications, on the other hand, can rarely be visualized with ultrasound. Approximately half of all nonpalpable lesions, usually detected by mammography, can be located in the ultrasound image (Potterton et al. 1994). Because of its simplicity, we prefer ultrasound localization even for lesions that are visible both mammographically and sonographically.

Once the lesion has been identified in the ultrasound image, various localization methods can be used. The simplest is to mark the location of the lesion on the skin, but this method does not indicate the depth

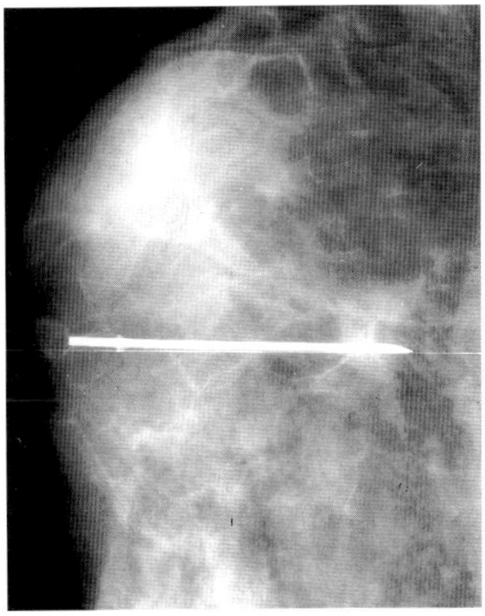

Fig. 15.7 Mammographic check of ultrasound-guided needle placement. A localization wire can now be introduced through the needle.

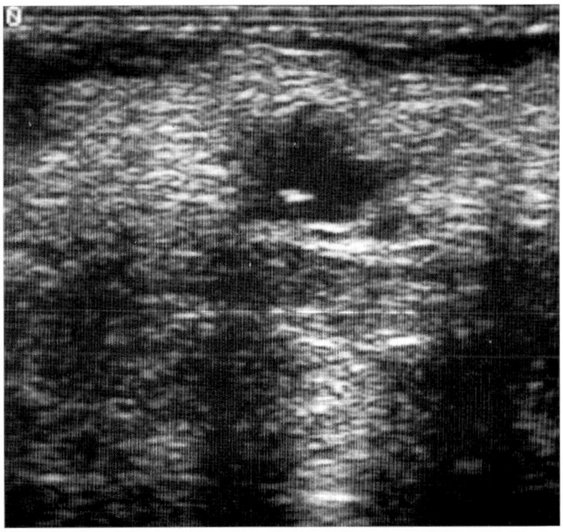

Fig. 15.8 Visualization of the needle tip at the center of an 18-mm hypoechoic invasive ductal carcinoma.

of the lesion. Needle localization solves this problem by transfixing the lesion and defining its depth (Fig. 15.7). Localization is most accurate when the needle is inserted parallel to the transducer face, as this provides a complete image of the needle path. Ultrasound can demonstrate the needle up to an angle of about 30°, allowing the needle tip to be placed in lesions only a few millimeters in diameter. One drawback of this method is that, as with mammographic needle guides, the path of the needle does not match the direct, anteroposterior approach taken by the surgeon. This requires a perpendicular insertion alongside the transducer. In this case only the needle tip is visible in the ultrasound image (Fig. 15.8), and usually the needle cannot be identified unless the echogenic tip is in motion. Schwartz et al. (1988) suggested that the surgeon should perform the breast ultrasound examination in the operating room, just before an anticipated biopsy. If the lesion cannot be easily localized after the incision is made, the authors recommend "gowning" the transducer and placing it in the open wound to help find the lesion. The drawback of this technique is that it sacrifices the spatial correlation between the sonographic and mammographic findings. To preserve this correlation, we obtain biplane mammograms after every ultrasound-guided localization to document the needle position. This enables the surgeon to select a suitable approach and to locate the lesion even if the needle has not been perfectly positioned.

If the needle itself is used for localization, there is a danger that it may become dislodged during patient transport or preoperative preparations. Also, a needle placed deeply in the breast may penetrate even more deeply if handled improperly, causing a pneumothorax or other injury. For many years, dye injection methods were widely used for the preoperative localization of clinically occult lesions. Dye solutions are easy to handle and produce a stained track that guides the surgeon to the targeted tissue. Dyes tend to spread and diffuse, however, and localization may become imprecise if too much time elapses between the dye injection and the surgery. Thus, the use of dye solutions requires a level of timing and organization that may not be available in emergency situations. As a result, wire localization has become the most common method for the preoperative localization of breast lesions.

The advantage of this technique is that the localizing wire provides the surgeon

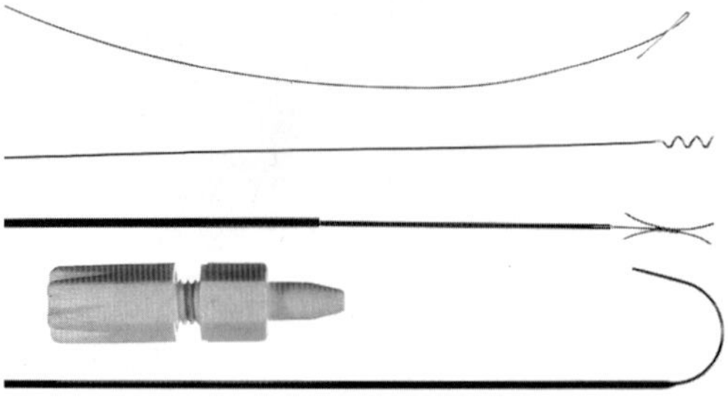

Fig. 15.9 Different types of localizing wires. From top to bottom: homemade Kopans-type hookwire; spiral-ended wire (Twistmarker, BIP); Ready-X localization needle; and Homer Mammalok wire with guide cannula.

with a relatively stable guide to the breast lesion. Various types of localizing wire are in use (Fig. 15.9), and it is difficult for any single wire to meet all requirements, some of which are mutually exclusive.

A localizing wire should be:

- Resistant to accidental withdrawal
- Resistant to forward displacement (hookwires)
- Resistant to transection by scissors or scalpel
- Resistant to tip breakage when traction is exerted on the wire
- Rigid enough to be palpable during surgery
- Flexible, to reduce patient discomfort

To avoid dislodgment during patient transfers and preoperative preparations, the tip of the wire should be securely anchored in the breast tissue, regardless of whether the surrounding tissue is fatty or fibrous. Also, the needle should not migrate more deeply during movements of the breast. This is a particular danger with curved-end wires that may engage and penetrate muscle (Davis et al. 1988). A localization wire should be resistant to inadvertent cutting by a pair of scissors or a scalpel. Transection of a very thin wire may occur during surgery without it being noticed (Homer 1983), and it may be difficult or impossible to find the small pieces of wire in the wound. A hookwire should not break off at the tip when the surgeon pulls on it to aid in the dissection (Bronstein et al. 1988). A rigid wire will make it easier for the surgeon to locate the tip intraoperatively, particularly if the surgeon is not dissecting along the wire itself. The wire can be made more rigid by threading a cannula over the wire just before surgery (Kwasnik et al. 1987). Alternatively, the guide cannula can be left indwelling in the breast if there is a brief interval between localization and surgery (Homer 1988). We prefer a hookwire attached to a flexible cable (Urrutia et al. 1988). This hook engages very securely in breast tissues of varying texture (Czarnecki et al. 1992). The projecting end of the wire is secured to the breast with sterile tape to prevent deeper migration. When localization is done the day before surgery, we ask our patients to wear a brassiere at night to prevent wire migration due to excessive breast movement.

In all biopsies of nonpalpable breast lesions, a specimen radiograph should be obtained to confirm that the lesion has been removed. If the lesion was properly localized, it may be possible to alert the surgeon to an incomplete resection or insufficient margins and recommend a selective reexcision. Even with a lesion that appeared only as a sonographic abnormality, a specimen radiograph is worthwhile, for when the specimen is freed from overlying tissues it will often show typical structures that confirm removal of the lesion. This is particularly helpful if the histological result does not conform to the expected diagnosis and there is doubt as to whether the lesion has actually been removed. A follow-up radiograph is usually rewarding in lesions that contain microcalcifications. In the absence of microcalcifications, both sonography and mammography are of limited value due to postoperative changes or scar formation.

16 Three-Dimensional Sonography of Breast Masses

Three-dimensional (3D) sonography is a new method of processing and analyzing a selected tissue volume in all spatial dimensions. While it cannot replace conventional sonography, it can complement it in selected areas. Three-dimensional ultrasound is still in its early stages, however, and while it has become feasible as a routine study, the technology is not available at all institutions.

The technical details of 3D ultrasound are beyond the scope of this book. Reference can be made to textbooks in which the technical principles of 3D ultrasound imaging are described in detail (Sohn and Bastert 1994, Sohn and Holzgreve 1995).

Advantages of 3D Sonography for Evaluating Breast Masses

The advantages of 3D sonography are as follows:

- It conveys a spatial, three-dimensional impression of the tumor and its relation to surrounding structures (e.g., the chest wall).
- The surface characteristics of the tumor (smooth or ill-defined) can be evaluated (Fig. 16.**1**).
- Series of sectional images can be generated at millimeter intervals, permitting a detailed survey of the internal structures of the tumor.
- Sectional images can be reconstructed in planes that are not accessible to conventional breast ultrasound (Fig. 16.**2**).

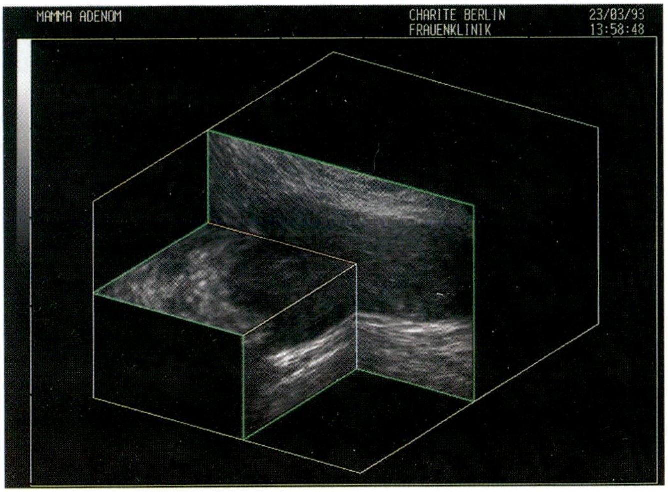

Fig. 16.**1** Three-dimensional breast ultrasound (Combison 530 with 10-MHz mechanical transducer, Kretztechnik), showing a 3D view of a fibroadenoma. The smooth surface of the tumor and its homogeneous internal structures are clearly appreciated.

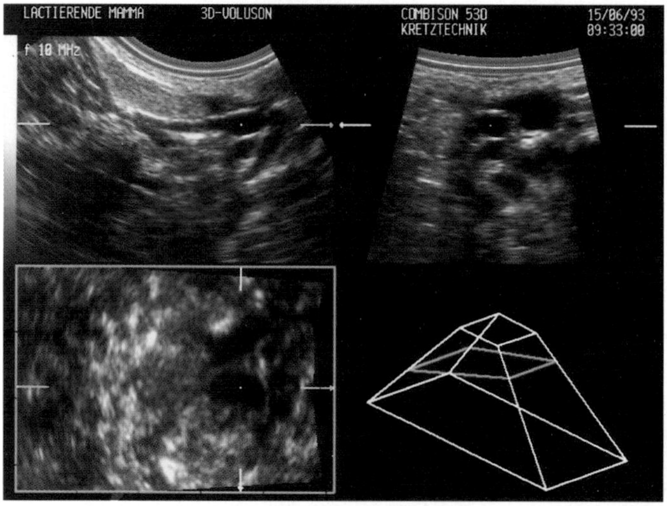

Fig. 16.2 Three-dimensional breast ultrasound. The display shows sectional images from various planes in a lactating breast. The dilated, anechoic ducts are visualized in longitudinal and transverse section.

- Tumor volumes can be objectively calculated (in two-dimensional ultrasound, the determination of tumor size depends on the image planes selected by the examiner).
- Standardization of the breast ultrasound examination may be feasible. For example, all of the glandular breast tissue can be imaged by holding the transducer perpendicular to the areola and selecting a large scan angle.
- The image data can be stored for later review by an experienced examiner.
- 3D images document a greater amount of information (allowing for more objective serial observations).
- The examination time is shortened for the patient. Image data are acquired from the region of interest, the patient is dismissed, and image planes can be selected arbitrarily for detailed scrutiny and dimensional measurements at a later time. (The examiner need not spend time defining the lesion on various sectional planes while the patient is present.)
- The same transducer can be used for conventional two-dimensional breast ultrasound.

Three-dimensional ultrasound increases the accuracy of breast tumor diagnosis (Sohn et al. 1992c) and greatly shortens the examination time for the patient.

The criteria for differentiating between benign and malignant lesions are the same as in two-dimensional ultrasound, and are easier to recognize in the freely selectable planes of the 3D image.

It is likely that, in the future, 3D ultrasound will have a key application in the precise calculation of tumor volumes in the follow-up of neoadjuvant chemotherapy and in monitoring the response to therapy with recurrent cancer. Software problems in 3D volumetrics still need to be resolved, however, in order to achieve accurate delineation of the tumor from surrounding tissues.

Figures 16.**1**–16.**8** illustrate some three-dimensional views of breast carcinomas.

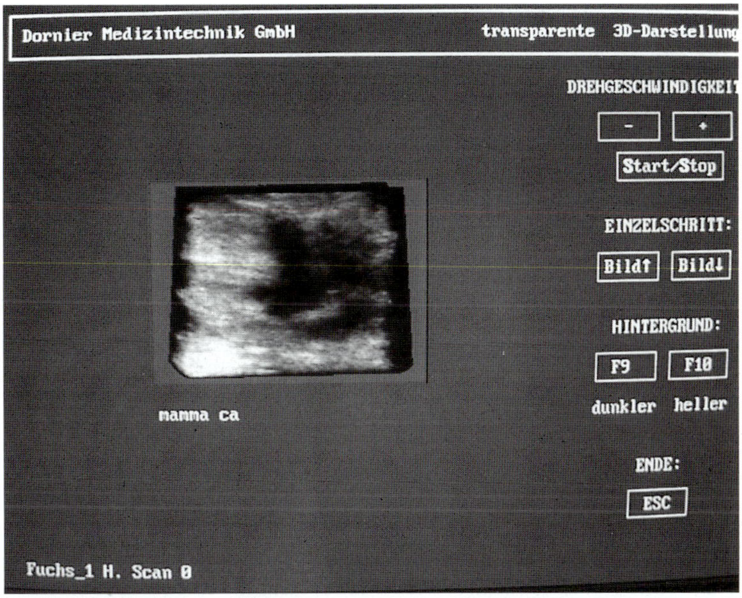

Fig. 16.**3** Three-dimensional view of a breast carcinoma.

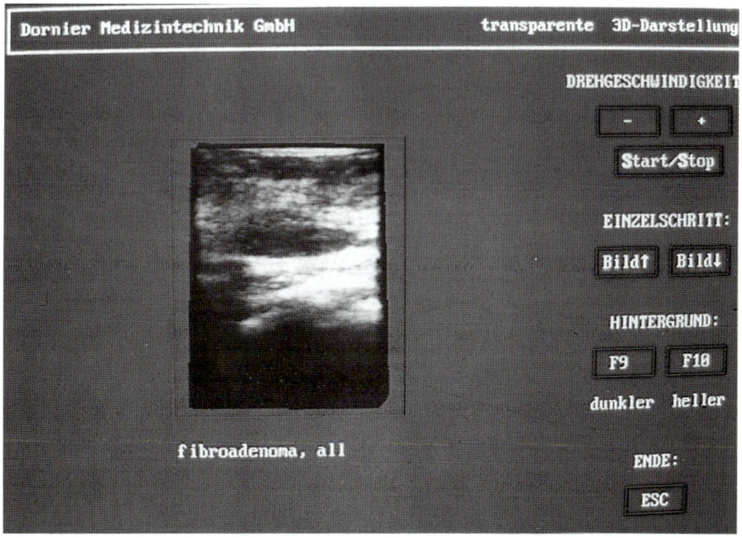

Fig. 16.**4** Three-dimensional view of a fibroadenoma of the breast.

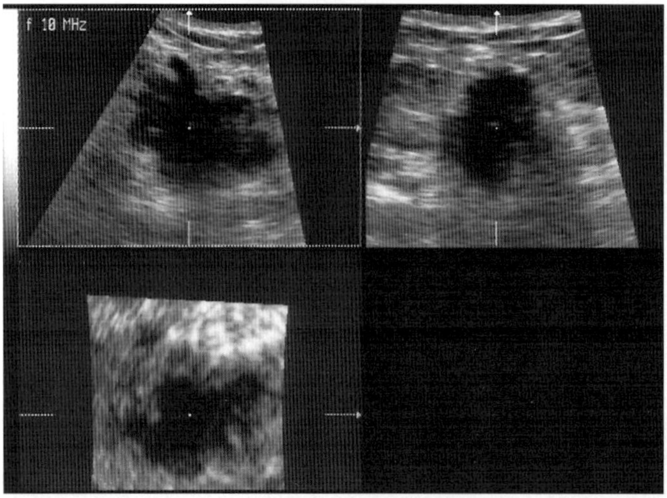

Fig. 16.**5** Three-dimensional sectional image analysis of a breast carcinoma.

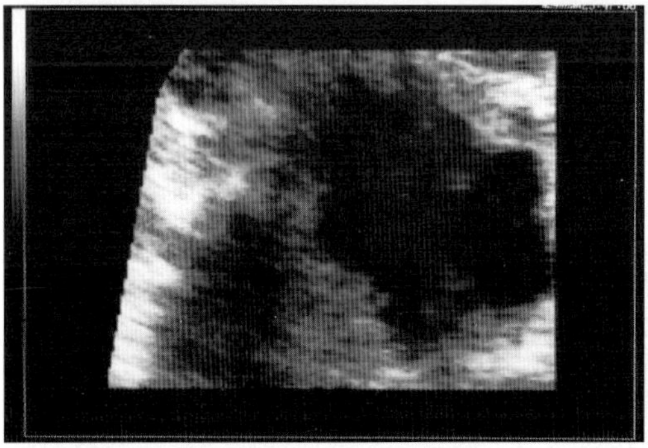

Fig. 16.**6** Three-dimensional transparent view of a breast carcinoma.

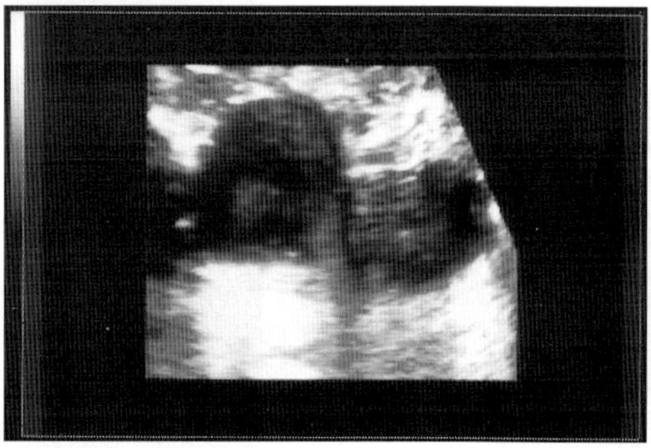

Fig. 16.**7** Three-dimensional view of a multifocal carcinoma.

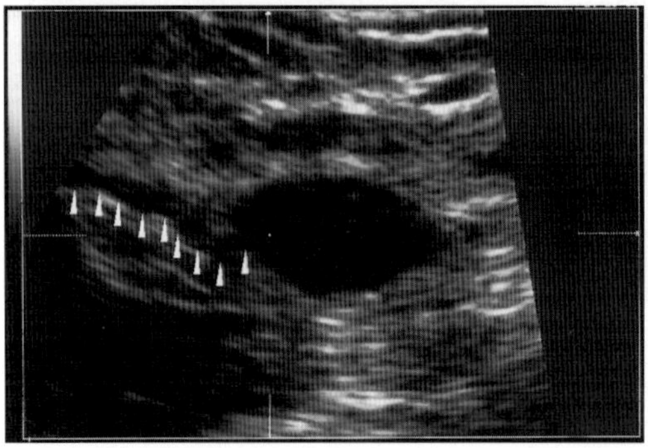

Fig. 16.**8** Three-dimensional view of a cyst communicating with a lactiferous duct.

17 Sonographic Evaluation of Breast Implants

C.I. Caskey and U.M. Hamper

Introduction

In April of 1992, the United States Food and Drug Administration (FDA) restricted the use of silicone gel-filled breast implants due to continued reports of adverse effects and unanswered questions concerning implant safety (Kessler 1992). These included questions regarding the true incidence of implant rupture, the unknown relationship between silicone and immune-related disorders, and the unknown relationship of breast cancer and implant use.

While the life expectancies of all silicone breast prostheses are unknown, scientific reports suggest that implant shells slowly degrade in vivo (deCamera et al. 1991). Consequently, manufacturers have routinely recommended removal of a ruptured prosthesis. In addition, the consistency of the gel becomes less viscous when intermixed with body fluids, making it more difficult to remove the implant. The identification of rupture as early as possible is important to facilitate safe operative removal, minimizing the length, extent, and cost of surgery.

Early and accurate diagnosis of failed implants poses a new challenge for radiologists. Comparative studies of imaging techniques (ultrasound, magnetic resonance imaging, computed tomography, and mammography) have demonstrated superior sensitivities and specificities for MRI and CT in the detection of implant rupture than for ultrasound or mammography (Berg et al. 1993, Everson et al. 1994, Gorczyca et al. 1994). However, the sensitivity and specificity of ultrasound for the detection of rupture improves with both the experience and the degree of involvement of the radiologist.

Technique and Normal Implant Appearance

An ultrasound examination of the breast to evaluate complications of implant use starts with taking the patient‘s implant history, including date of implantation, type of implant, additional surgery or complications, history of rupture, reason for placement, and symptoms.

The breast tissue and associated prostheses are best evaluated by the use of high frequency linear hand-held transducers. Scanning parameters should be adjusted to allow the ultrasound beam to penetrate the posterior wall of the implant and chest wall. This will usually be achieved with a 5-MHz or 7-MHz transducer.

The medial aspect of the breast is scanned with the patient in the supine position with her ipsilateral arm raised behind her head. In order to image the lateral aspect of the breast better, the patient is turned obliquely toward her contralateral side so that the lateral breast rests more flatly against the chest wall.

Scanning is performed in a sagittal radial fashion with documentation of representative areas in a "clock-face" manner. The use of compound imaging is particularly useful, as it allows an excellent overview of the breast implant (Fig. 17.**1**). Images of the axilla in the transverse and sagittal planes are also obtained for detection of adenopathy or free silicone. After the standard views are obtained, additional images are taken as needed to further elucidate a finding.

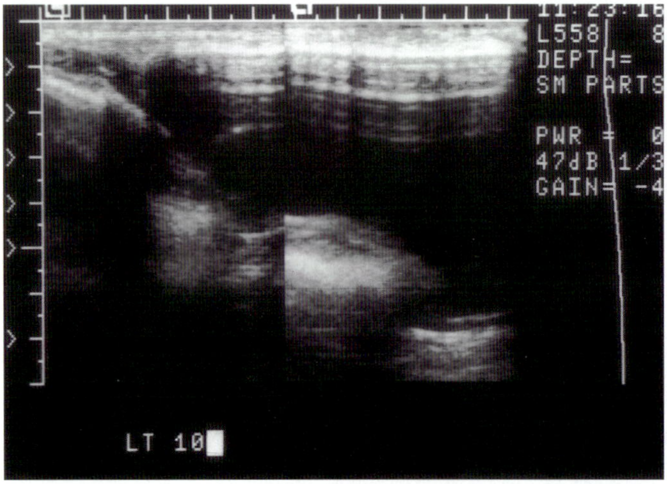

Fig. 17.**1** Ultrasound image of a normal single-lumen silicone gel-filled breast implant that had been in place for six years in a 38-year-old woman. Note the reverberation artifacts in the near field and the anechoic center.

The normal sonographic appearance of a breast implant is a triangular-shaped anechoic structure with a reverberation band anteriorly in the near field (Fig. 17.**1**). This "normal" appearance can vary depending on the exact structure of the implant. Anterior to the implant is an echogenic line of variable thickness, which represents the elastomer shell and the fibrous capsule.

A final impression is formed after all information is processed. The significance of minimal findings must be interpreted with respect to the global appearance. At our institution, results are reported as probabilities of rupture: normal, low probability of rupture, indeterminate for rupture, moderate probability of rupture, and high probability of rupture.

Implant Types

The first silicone breast implant was the Cronin implant introduced by Dow Corning in the 1960s. Since that time, multiple variations and changes have been made to the structure and the contents of the breast implant. It is essential to acquire a working knowledge of the more common implant types in order to be able to interpret the ultrasound examination accurately.

The most common implant type is the single-lumen silicone gel-filled implant. This prosthesis consists of a silicone elastomer shell filled with silicone gel. The elastomer shell may be smooth or textured. A textured shell is roughened by the creation of tiny finger-like projections in the shell. Texturing was introduced to decrease the incidence of breast hardening and capsular contractures.

Another prosthesis type is the polyurethane-covered single-lumen implant. It consists of a thin layer of polyurethane foam adherent to a single lumen silicone gel-filled implant. Marketed under various trade names (Natural-Y, Même, and Replicon), this implant was also manufactured to address the issue of capsular contractures. Unfortunately, the polyurethane rapidly breaks down after implantation, producing a known carcinogen, 2,4-toluenediamine, as a byproduct. This compound has been documented in trace amounts in the urine of women bearing these implants (Chan et al. 1991).

Two types of double-lumen implant are occasionally seen. The bilumen implant consists of a small outer lumen of saline surrounding a larger inner lumen of silicone gel. The expander or Becker implant is the reverse, consisting of an outer lumen of silicone gel and an inner expandable lumen of saline. This implant was designed to aid in breast reconstruction after mastectomy by allowing the saline lumen to gradually expand. While the sonographic appearance of the bilumen implant is indistinguishable from that of the single lumen, since the outer lumen is rarely detected with ultrasound, the normal appearance of the expander implant is more complicated and can mimic a ruptured implant.

The saline implant is the only implant that currently has FDA approval. This prosthesis consists of a silicone elastomer shell filled with saline.

Sonographic Signs of Implant Rupture

Breast implant ruptures can be classified as intracapsular (silicone contained by the fibrous capsule) or extracapsular (silicone migration outside the fibrous capsule). Most implant ruptures are contained ruptures, with no spread of silicone beyond the fibrous capsule. In one series of 22 proven implant ruptures, 95 % were intracapsular (Caskey et al. 1994).

Disorderly echoes present in what should be an anechoic structure are suggestive of implant rupture. Probably the most useful sign of implant rupture is echogenic lines of varying lengths, often seen coursing within the reverberation artifact or the interior of the implant, or both (Fig. 17.**2**). These lines represent portions of the ruptured elastomer shell that retract from the fibrous capsule and sink into the silicone gel. DeBruhl et al. (1993) described these lines as having a "stepladder" appearance (Fig. 17.**3a**). In addition, it has been shown that these lines correspond to the internal membranes described by Gorczyca et al. (1992, 1994) as a sign of implant rupture on MRI, or the "linguine sign" (Fig. 17.**3b**) .

The second most useful sign of implant rupture is the accumulation of low-level homogeneous echoes in the silicone gel within the interior of the implant (Fig. 17.**4**). These echoes are similar to the sonographic appearance of blood, i.e., endometrioma. These were seen in 54 % of the implant ruptures in our series (Caskey et al. 1994). The etiology of this echo pattern is unknown. One possibility is that large rents in the elastomer shell facilitate influx of body fluids, which then mix with the hydrophobic silicone gel. Then proteins or organic salts, or both, may mix with the silicone gel and cause a change in the echo texture.

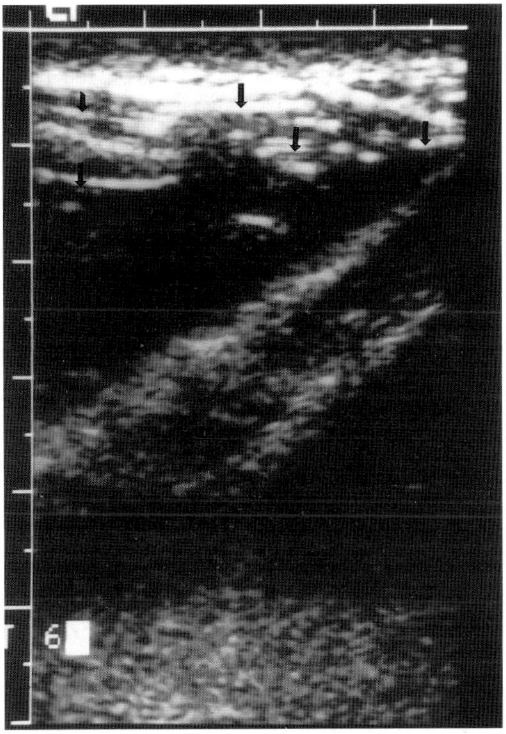

Fig. 17.**2** Ultrasound image of a single-lumen silicone implant in a 43-year-old woman who had had implants placed for augmentation 14 years previously. Note the echogenic lines (arrows) in the anterior reverberation band. Implant rupture was confirmed at surgery.

When present, the sonographic appearance of extruded silicone is the most specific sign for implant rupture. This is a unique sonographic pattern, which has been described as an echogenic area associated with a distal echogenic noise analogous in appearance to that of a snowstorm (Harris et al. 1993, Rosculet et al. 1992) (Fig. 17.**5**) In some cases this distal echogenic noise is nearly absent, and the echogenic area that corresponds to the free silicone blocks the transmission of sound. Another appearance

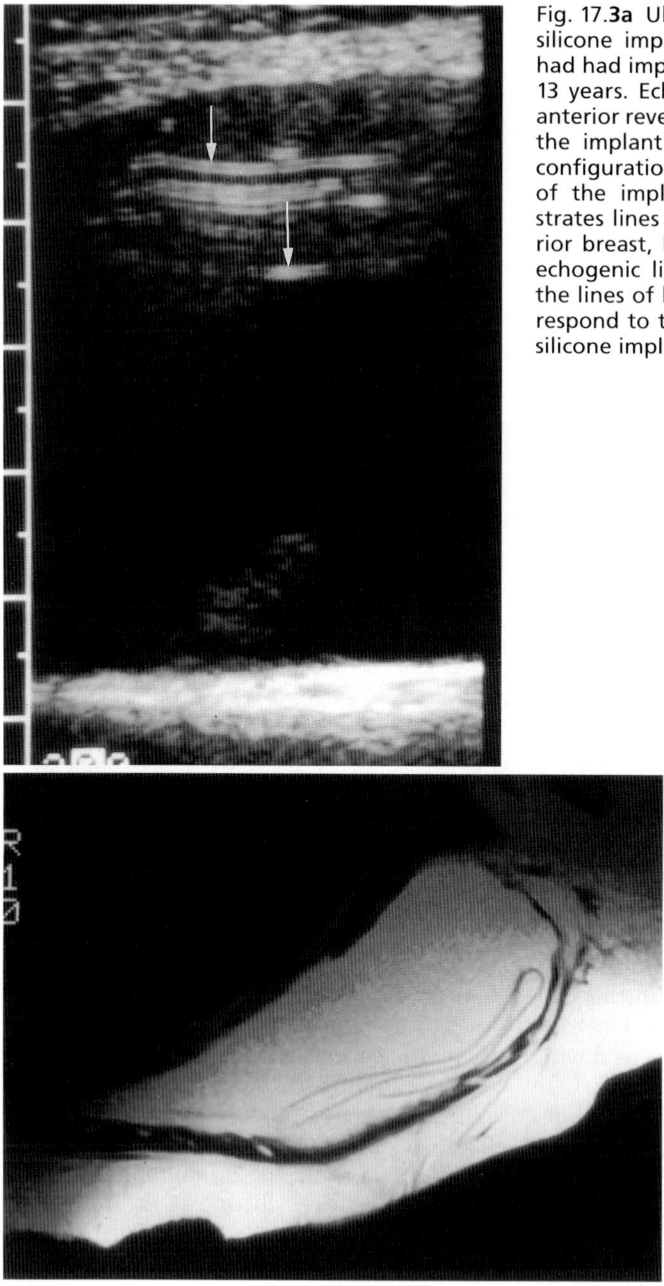

a

b

Fig. 17.3a Ultrasound image of a single-lumen silicone implant in a 60-year-old woman who had had implants in place for augmentation for 13 years. Echogenic lines are seen in both the anterior reverberation band and in the center of the implant (arrows), forming a "stepladder" configuration. **b** The magnetic resonance image of the implant in the same woman demonstrates lines of low signal intensity in the anterior breast, known as the "linguine" sign. The echogenic lines on the ultrasound image and the lines of low signal intensity on the MRI correspond to the ruptured elastomer shell of the silicone implant.

of free silicone is hypoechoic or anechoic collections that are similar to cysts but are strongly associated with this noise (Fig. 17.**6**). At present, there are two hypotheses concerning the way in which this phenomenon is produced. The first hypothesis suggests that the noise is due to reverberations within and between tiny droplets of silicone in the breast parenchyma (Harris et al. 1993). The second hypothesis proposes instead that the noise is due to phase aberration (Rubin et al. 1994). The intersection

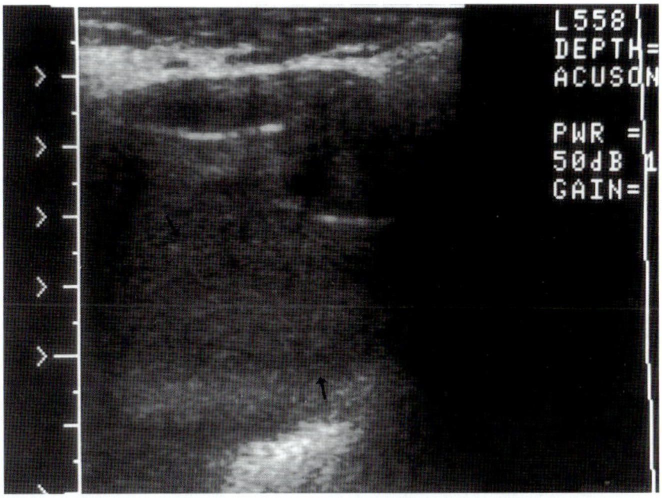

Fig. 17.**4** Ultrasound image of a single-lumen silicone implant in a 42-year-old woman who had had implants in place for 15 years. Note the diffuse low-level echoes (arrows) filling the implant – another finding associated with ruptured silicone implants.

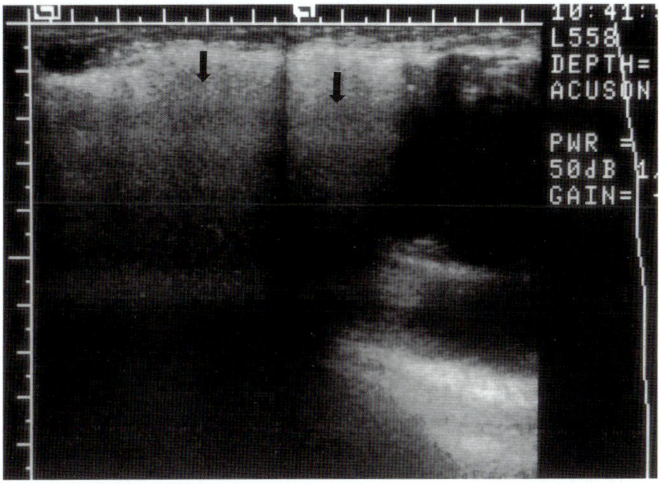

Fig. 17.**5** Ultrasound image, after mammographic compression, of a single-lumen silicone implant in a 37-year-old woman who had had implants placed 12 years previously. Note the area of bright echoes (arrows) obscuring the detail of the implant. This appearance, which is indicative of free silicone, has been compared to a "snowstorm."

of these tiny globules and the ultrasound beam produces changes in phase along the wavefront, creating incoherence in the sound beam, with random speckle noise.

Bulges in the contour of the implant are common but are an unreliable sign of implant rupture (Caskey et al. 1994). Nevertheless, large bulges have been the most striking finding in several proven cases of implant rupture and therefore should not be ignored.

All of the sonographic signs discussed above have sonographic mimics that add to the challenge of interpretation. For example, prominent echogenic fat collections can have a similar appearance to echogenic collections of free silicone (Fig. 17.**7**). On the other hand, the silicone snowstorm may be real but may represent residual material from a prior implant rupture and not from a rupture of the implant in question (Fig. 17.**8**). Invaginations or folds of the implant elastomer shell may be confused with the echogenic lines that represent the ruptured elastomer shell (Fig. 17.**9**). The sonographic appearance of a brightly echogenic line separating the outer silicone lumen and the inner saline lumen of a Becker expander

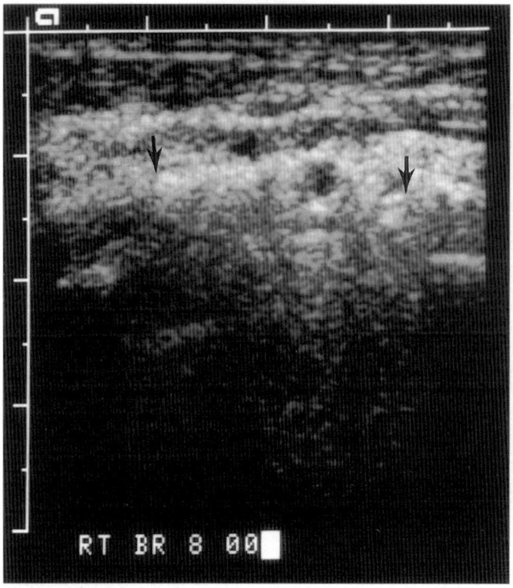

Fig. 17.**6** Ultrasound image of the breast of a 51-year-old woman with a history including a ruptured silicone breast implant. Extruded silicone was demonstrated at surgery. Note the areas of echogenic noise or "snowstorm" (arrows) associated with anechoic areas representing free silicone.

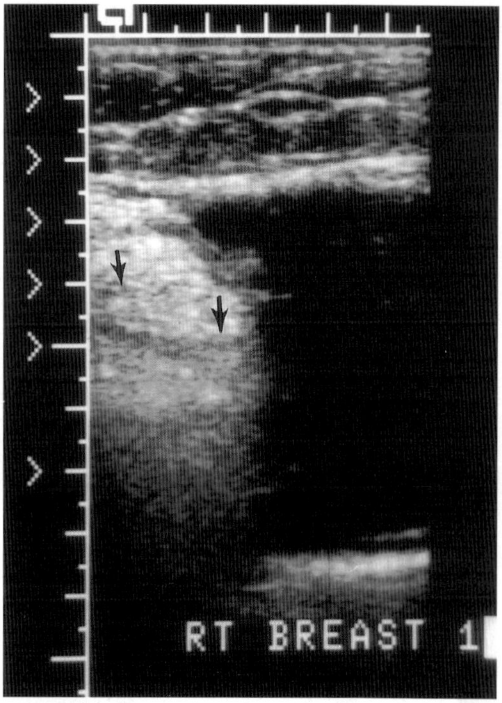

Fig. 17.**7** Ultrasound image of the breast of a 47-year-old woman who had had a single-lumen silicone implant in place for 12 years. Note the prominent echogenic fatty tissue (arrows) adjacent to the implant and partially obscuring the implant edge, which mimics free silicone.

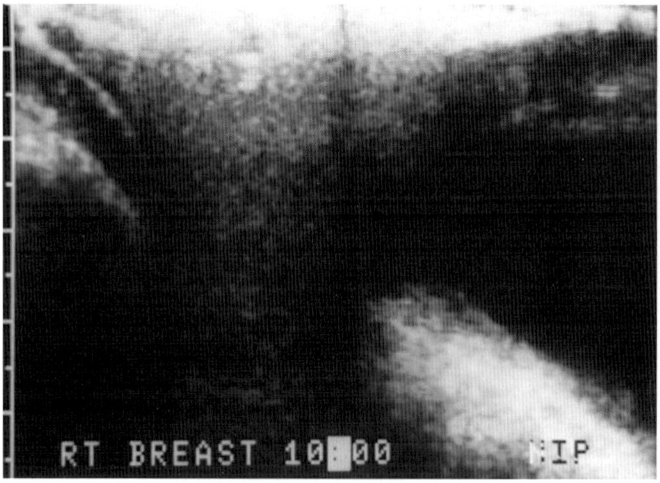

Fig. 17.**8** Ultrasound image of the breast of a 33-year-old woman with a history of a ruptured silicone implant. Note the echogenic noise obscuring the detail of the saline implant, which replaced a ruptured silicone implant.

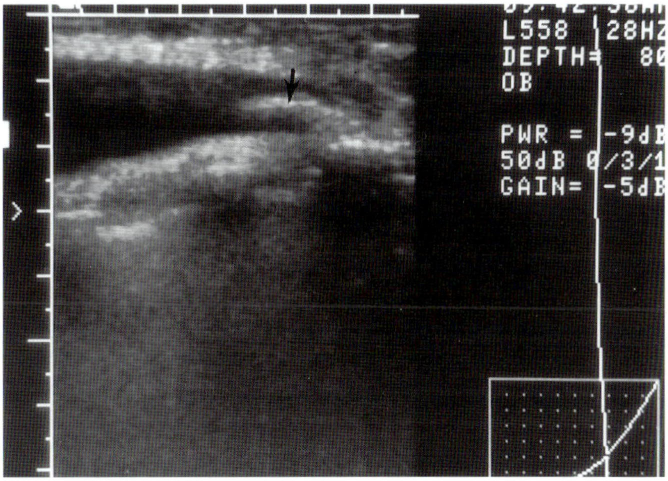

Fig. 17.**9** Ultrasound image of a polyurethane-covered breast implant that had been in place for two years in a 38-year-old woman. The prominent echogenic line (arrow) represents a fold of the polyurethane-covered elastomer shell, which can mimic a rupture.

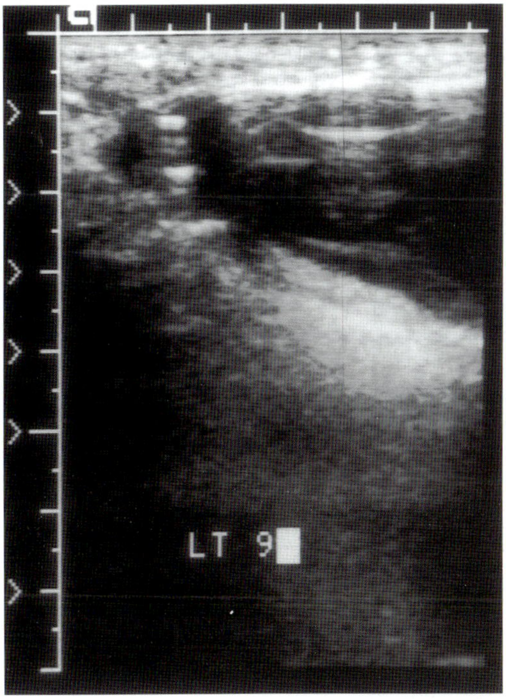

Fig. 17.**10** Ultrasound image of an expander implant (silicone outer lumen, saline inner lumen) placed in a 51-year-old woman for reconstruction. Note the echogenic lines representing the shell of the two lumens of this intact implant, which can mimic the findings of implant rupture.

implant is almost identical to the sonographic appearance of the ruptured elastomer shell of a single-lumen implant (Fig. 17.**10**) This again is evidence of the need to take an appropriate clinical history. Low-level homogeneous echoes have to be distinguished from overgain, reverberation, and scanning artifacts. Surgical practices such as the injection of saline directly into the silicone gel at or near the time of surgery in order to increase the volume of an implant to its desired size create striking internal echoes that may be misinterpreted as implant rupture (Fig. 17.**11**)

Other Complications of Implant Use: Ultrasound Findings

Although implant rupture with silicone extravasation is the most familiar complication of implant use, other implant-related disorders also exist and can be detected sonographically.

Peri-implant fluid collections are seen in specific clinical situations. For example, fluid collections adjacent to polyurethane-covered silicone gel implants are quite common (48 % in the series by Caskey et al. 1994, Berg et al. 1993) (Fig. 17.**12**). Fragmentation of polyurethane in vivo creates a

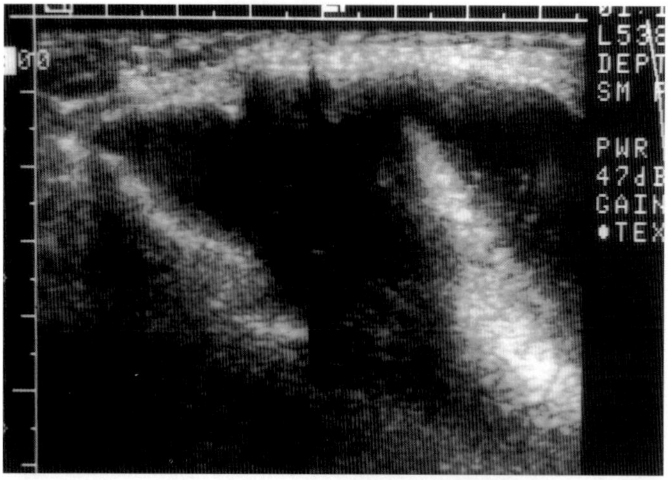

Fig. 17.**11** Ultrasound image of a silicone implant that had been in place for 10 years in a 41-year-old woman. Echoes are present in the lumen of the implant. Saline was injected into the silicone gel at initial implantation surgery to increase the volume of the prosthesis. This implant was intact at surgery.

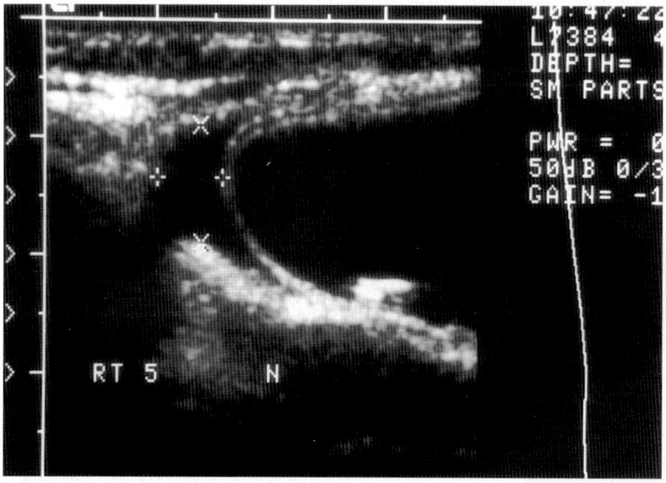

Fig. 17.**12** Ultrasound image of a polyurethane-covered implant that had been in place for three years for augmentation in a 48-year-old woman. An anechoic collection consistent with fluid is noted adjacent to the implant. This is a common finding in patients with polyurethane-covered implants.

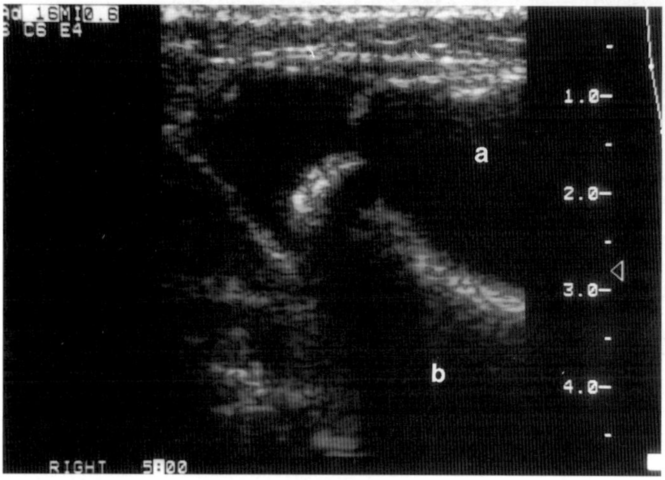

Fig. 17.**13** Ultrasound image of two stacked polyurethane-covered implants placed for reconstruction in a 57-year-old woman (a = anterior implant, b = posterior implant). Note the peri-implant fluid collection as well as the echogenic flap. This flap was observed to undulate on compression by the transducer, consistent with polyurethane fragmentation. At explantation, the polyurethane was found to be extensively fragmented.

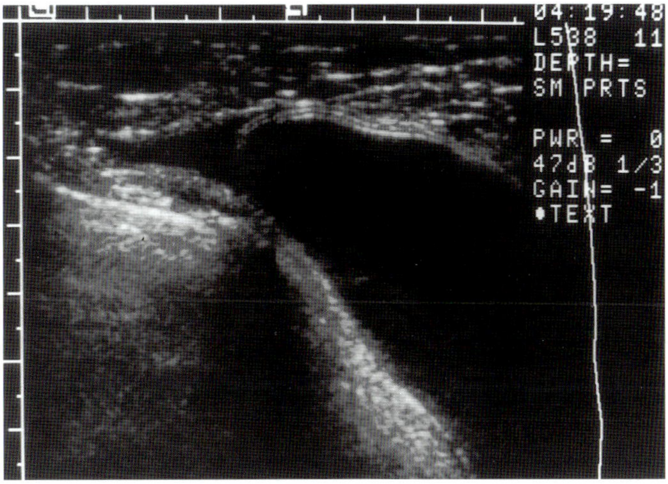

Fig. 17.**14** Ultrasound image of a saline implant in a 54-year-old woman. Note the fluid adjacent to the implant (arrow).

foreign-body reaction with chronic inflammation (Berrino et al. 1986), which is manifested sonographically as fluid collections. These collections may be anechoic and consistent with simple serous fluid or complex, with echoes representing debris of polyurethane fragmentation (Fig. 17.**13**). Peri-implant fluid accumulations are frequently associated with saline implants long after the immediate postoperative period (over 18 months) (Fig. 17.**14**). The etiology of these collections is not known, but it has been postulated that they may represent chronic inflammation induced by the textured implant surface. Other clinical settings associated with fluid collections include infections, malignant effusions, or ruptured saline or expander (saline component) implants. MRI easily detects small peri-implant collections; however, fragmentation of polyurethane has not been detected with MRI.

Summary

It has proved difficult to establish imaging criteria for breast implant rupture due to the wide variety of implant types, implant construction, and gel constituents. It has also been difficult to categorize and substantiate findings due to the litigious atmosphere that surrounds the investigation of these devices in the United States. Nevertheless, the interest in this area of medical imaging is continuing to grow as more and more radiologists are being asked to investigate the integrity of breast implants and the complications of their use.

18 Documentation in Breast Ultrasound

U. Siekmann and U.M. Hamper

Introduction

Since the criteria for a comprehensive breast ultrasound report are basically the same as the parameters required for an ultrasound report in general, it will be helpful to review some basic principles of the documentation of sonographic findings.

The ultrasound report provides a major clinical basis for diagnostic and therapeutic decision-making. It consists of verbal, written, and pictorial information, the pictorial documentation serving to illustrate and clarify the verbal descriptions. The desirable individual components of a complete written ultrasound report are summarized in Table 18.**1**.

The form of the documentation is crucial in terms of accessing the information and checking the validity and quality of the ultrasound services. This explains why computer-based data processing systems will assume growing importance in the hospital and office settings.

As diagnostic examinations become more frequent and complex, there is an inevitable proliferation of documentation sheets and diagnostic images, creating major logistical problems in terms of maintaining a well-organized filing system, keeping accurate records, and providing access in cases where records must be located and reviewed on or off-site.

There are various reasons why an organized and efficient approach to documentation is needed. Some are purely economical and based on cost containment; others are more legal in nature, relating to issues of competence and quality control. As growing numbers of third-party information requests are received in prenatal diagnosis (missed fetal anomalies) and other fields (Rauskolb 1994), it is easy to predict that the next few years will bring new standards of quality control and quality assurance in ultrasound services, including more stringent demands on documentation. This trend seems inevitable when we look at the broad field of obstetrics, where computer-based documentation systems have been established for some years. With the burgeoning costs of health care, there is an increasing reluctance to accept the almost exponential rise in expenditures that has occurred in the ultrasound sector. Besides facing limited reimbursements for examinations, physicians who use ultrasound are being challenged to demonstrate their competence as sonographers or sonologists and to raise their documentation standards. The latter requirement includes both an authorized form of written documentation and proof of technically acceptable image documentation that maintains a stable and high quality over an extended period of time. Using poorly exposed Polaroid photos or video printer images on paper of inferior quality to document ultrasound images will become a phenomenon of the past. Physicians who use ultrasound should make certain that their documentation meets the same quality standards that they would apply in selecting the ultrasound equipment itself. Proper image documentation on hard copy film, videotapes, or electronic media, for example, are part of an ultrasound accreditation requirement. In the United States, voluntary accreditation of ultrasound laboratories by the American Institute of Ultrasound in Medicine (AIUM) and the American College of Radiology (ACR) was initiated in 1995 in response to

Table 18.1 Possible format for systematic documentation of ultrasound findings

- Institution or facility where the examination is performed
  - Address, phone number, fax number, contact person
- Patient identification data
  - Last name, first name, date of birth, address
  - Identification number (for internal departmental use)
- Referring physician/referring facility or department
- Examiner
- Equipment specifications
  - Type, transducer, technique (Doppler)
- Indication for the examination
  - Presenting problem, special inquiry
- Documentation of findings, image documentation
  - Examination conditions
  - Scan planes
  - Delineation
  - Location, size, shape, echo pattern, isolated changes, organ-specific abnormalities
  - Other apparent abnormalities
- Serial examinations
  - Isolated focal lesions (size, contours, etc.)
  - Doppler flow changes
- Final assessment, comments
- Diagnosis
- Further recommendations, follow-ups, clinical procedure
- Additional documentation
  - Correlation between ultrasound findings and pathological diagnosis

general concerns among imaging specialists regarding the quality of ultrasound practiced. The purpose of these accreditation programs is to assure proper training, proper expertise, and proper understanding of the technology among the users of diagnostic ultrasound.

Computer-Based Documentation Systems

Text Data

The following considerations apply to the computer-based acquisition and processing of text data:

- Data acquisition and documentation must be complete. A consistent data entry format will provide a kind of checklist to help the examiner conduct a complete and systematic examination, without omitting mandatory measurements or evaluations. This option is particularly important for less experienced examiners and trainees.
- The findings should be entered in the correct form, and they should be easy to read and to print out. Any obvious peculiarities, such as atypical findings, should be specially marked so they can be quickly recognized.
- Besides simply documenting the data, an up-to-date computer system should include software that can evaluate the stored data from both a clinical and scientific standpoint, and is flexible in terms of the types of information that may be sought. Simple documentation software that lacks options for evaluation and statistical analysis would be only half a solu-

tion in terms of meeting prospective quality-control and quality-assurance demands.

- Equipment manufacturers should provide standard interfaces that allow direct data transfer between the ultrasound scanner and desktop computer. In turn, the documentation software should be configured in such a way that it writes the transferred data to the proper input lines, making it unnecessary to enter this information manually via the keyboard. This option saves a great deal of time and eliminates errors of data entry.
- The data transfer capability should include transfer of the corresponding image document. This follows the general recommendation that all measurable parameters be stored in the form of an image document. As far as hardware is concerned, a high-quality video grabber card should be used for image documentation, and complete image files should be stored on high-capacity removable media (e.g., magneto-optical disks).
- To avoid double entries in the clinical practice of data processing, it would be desirable to have the ultrasound documentation system incorporated into an interdepartmental system. For example, this system would allow patient identification data to be shared between the ultrasound documentation system and other systems in the facility (obstetric documentation system, computer-based surgical documentation, oncological data processing system). Intelligent coordination at the departmental level is the key to realizing the advantages of these various subsystems as components of an integrated solution, such as a picture archival and communication system (PACS), which can offer reliable and fast access to medical information.

The willingness of the user to master computer data entry increases as the user becomes more aware of how computerization shortens the documentation time and simplifies the writing of routine documents (physician letters, reports for inpatient and outpatient records).

- Databases (e.g., patient identification data, lists of referring physicians) should be available for all systems in order to avoid double entries. This requirement conforms to the above statement that ultrasound documentation and PACS capabilities should not be viewed in isolation but as an integral part of a coordinated departmental and interdepartmental system. The central clinical importance of ultrasound in all areas of our specialty underscores the importance of integrating it into a comprehensive documentation system. Initial results with a clinical information and management system (CIM) in Switzerland have been very promising (Baer et al. 1993). In the United States, evaluations of a sonographic PACS in clinical practice have shown promising results (Krampla et al. 1994, Patel et al. 1996).

Image Data

The adage that "a picture is worth a thousand words" is particularly true in ultrasound documentation. Requirements for extensive image documentation each year quickly demonstrate the need for adequate storage of the acquired information. This is an area in which state-of-the-art technical capabilities can and should be applied to benefit the user. Decreasing hardware costs should allow the upgrading of image documentation technology and archival solutions. Optical disks can provide years of degradation-free storage with immediate access to the stored images. If desired, the image data can be transferred to hard-copy media such as overhead transparencies, 35-mm slides (with annotations), or paper publications. Likewise, we currently have the technology to transmit image documents between institutions via high-speed data highways. These links allow for rapid online information exchange between hospitals or ultrasound departments, benefiting staff and patients by potentially eliminating the need for time-consuming and cost-intensive consultation visits.

Despite all the technical innovations in image documentation, it should be emphasized that even the most intelligent software usually cannot turn a primarily deficient image (due to faulty equipment settings, underexposure or overexposure, etc.) into a high-quality image through data manipulation. The primary signal must be identifiable as such and stored in its primary form, and any secondary manipulations must clearly identify the person performing the manipulation, when it was done, and what image parameters were modified. Edited images should be stored and administered in a separate file; the primary image itself should not be altered and must be preserved in the original format for legal reasons. If the image processing software did not offer this security option, the door would be open to tampering, with potentially severe legal consequences.

If the concept of image documentation on removable media is taken somewhat further, other applications become evident. For example, image and text files could be systematically combined to create a kind of electronic textbook with digitized images. The text and images could also be linked to documentation software, providing the user with online access to reference images that may be helpful in making a correct diagnosis. Online consultation systems could also be developed. At present, the technical possibilities of intelligent image processing software seem virtually limitless. The users of this software will ultimately determine the technical options that will be needed and those that will find clinical application.

Criteria for Reporting Breast Ultrasound Findings

In contrast to the established reporting schemes used in obstetric ultrasound, there are currently no uniform evaluation criteria, approved by professional societies, that are reflected in a generally valid protocol for the reporting of breast ultrasound findings. It is anticipated that in the future a systematic approach to breast ultrasound reporting similar to the American College of Radiology Breast Imaging Reporting and Data System (BI-RADS) will be established. Until this occurs, we can, however, list some basic guidelines that can help systematize and standardize the contents of the breast ultrasound report, and are desirable features to be included in a report:

- Lengthy, descriptive text entries should be avoided, as they create difficulties in subsequent computer handling and evaluation of the findings.
- The specific biophysical acoustic properties of the breast tissues should be taken into account in the interpretation of images.
- Specific criteria should be applied to the evaluation of focal sonographic lesions.
- Both the sonographic diagnosis and later clinical diagnosis (e.g., histology, cytology) should be included in the case documentation, as this provides a basis for checking the accuracy of the ultrasound diagnosis.
- Ultrasound-guided invasive procedures (e.g., cyst aspirations) should be documented.
- Finally, the documentation should include sonographic findings of the axilla as well as Doppler ultrasound findings, if these studies were performed.

Summary

The development and progress in electronic data processing systems has not bypassed the medical community. As routine documentation tasks grow more complex, physicians will experience almost daily the inadequacies of traditional documentation methods. With diagnostic ultrasound established at every modern hospital, large amounts of data are generated that require computer-assisted documentation and evaluation. Such a system must ensure the documentation of all services while providing options for quality assessment and quality assurance. Data access, integrity, and security must be established and guaranteed. It should be standard practice in the future to store all relevant data and the corresponding reference images in digitized form on appropriate storage media. The internal database structure should be compatible with other systems, such as surgical and oncological documentation, and should allow seamless interfacing between different picture filing and communications systems when needed.

A user-friendly, computer-based ultrasound documentation system should include a clear user interface with symbols for the most commonly used functions, pull-down menus, and mouse control. A Windows-type graphic user interface is recommended, as it already contains many useful resources such as printer drivers, simple word processors, network functions, etc. Windows users can choose from a variety of software titles for statistical data analysis, graphic displays, and many other applications. The system should have a networking capability that allows multiple ultrasound workplaces to be interconnected within the facility.

When electronic data processing is used for documentation and evaluation, parameters can be recorded in a standardized fashion that allows for internal quality control (with all individuals in a department using the same documentation scheme), as well as external quality control based on a comparison with data from other institutions. It is in the interests of all physicians who use ultrasound to set the very highest standards for their documentation and to make use of the undisputed advantages of state-of-the-art electronic data processing.

References

Adler DD, Carson PL, Rubin JM, Quinn-Reid D. Doppler ultrasound color flow imaging in the study of breast cancer: preliminary findings. Ultrasound Med Biol 1990; 16: 553–9.

Adler DD, Hyde DL, Ikeda DM. Quantitative monographic parameters as a means of distinguishing breast cancers from benign solid breast masses. J Ultrasound Med 1991; 10: 505–8.

Algire GB, Chalkley HW, Legallalis RY, Park HD. Vascular reactions of normal and malignant tissue in vivo. J Natl Cancer Inst 1945; 6: 46–73.

Andersson I, Aspergen K, Janzon L. Mammographic screening and mortality from breast cancer: the Malmö mammographic screening trial. Br Med J 1988; 207: 943–8.

Anton HW, Junkermann H, Wolf G, Teubner J. Lokalisation nicht-palpabler Läsionen in der Mammographie zur präoperativen Markierung und Gewebeentnahme. Radiologe 1993; 33: 271–6.

Audretsch W. Ultraschalldiagnostik bei Mammaprothesen nach operativer Behandlung von Mammatumoren oder Augmentationsplastik. Geburtshilfe Frauenheilkd 1975; 35: 853–8.

Audretsch W, Rezai M, Kolotas C, Zamboglou N, Schnabel T, Bojar H. Tumor-specific immediate reconstruction (TSR) in breast cancer patients. Sixth Annual Meeting, AWO/EUSOMA Workshop. Düsseldorf, 1995: 1–9.

Azavedo E, Svane G. Radiologic aspects of breast cancers detected through a breast cancer screening program. Eur J Radiol 1991; 3: 88–90.

Bader W, Otto WR, Böhmer S, Degenhardt E, Schneider J. Texturanalyse: Ein neues Verfahren zur Beurteilung mammasonographischer Herdbefunde. Bildgeb Imaging 1994; 61 (Suppl 2): 31.

Baer R, Brandao R, Langenegger D. Bewertung medizinischer Software. 2 vols. Zürich: BSG Unternehmensberatung und Institut für Informatik der Universität Zürich, 1993.

Baldt M von, Bankier A, Mallek R, Youssefzadeh G, Freilinger G, Wolf G. Langzeitveränderungen nach Implantaten von Mammasilikonprothesen. Röfo Fortschr Geb Röntgenstr Neuen Bildgeb Verfahr 1994; 160: 441–7.

Balu-Maestro C, Bruneton JN, Geoffray A, Chauvel C, Rogopoulos A, Bittman O. Ultrasonographic posttreatment follow-up of breast cancer patients. J Ultrasound Med 1991; 10: 1–7.

Bamber JC, Sambrook M, Minasian H, Hill CR. Doppler study of blood flow in breast cancer. In: Jellins J, Kobayashi T, editors. Ultrasonic examination of the breast. New York: Wiley, 1983: 371–8.

Barth V, Prechtel K. Atlas der Brustdrüse und ihre Erkrankungen. Stuttgart: Enke, 1990.

Bassett LW, Kimme-Smith C. Breast sonography: technique, equipment and normal anatomy. Semin Ultrasound CT MR 1989;10: 82–9.

Bassett LW, Ysrael M, Gold RH, Ysrael C. Usefulness of mammography and sonography in women less than 35 years of age. Radiology 1991; 180: 831–5.

Bässler R. Mamma. In: Remmele W, editor. Pathologie, vol. 3. Berlin: Springer, 1984: 305–91.

Bauer M, Schulz-Wendtland R, Kommoss F, Meisenbacher H. Hochgeschwindigkeitsstanze: Eine neue Methode zor histologischen Abklärung unklarer Mammaläsionen (n = 115) [abstract]. Abstractband zur 12. Wissenschaftlichen Tagung der Deutschen Gesellschaft für Senologie. Cologne, 1992.

Bell DS, Bamber JC, Eckersley RJ. Segmentation and analysis of colour Doppler images of breast tumour vasculature. Bildgeb Imaging 1993; 60 (Suppl 2): 51.

Berg WA, Caskey CI, Hamper UM, Kuhlman JE, Anderson ND, Chang BW, et al. Diagnosing breast implant rupture with magnetic resonance imaging, ultrasound, and mammography. RadioGraphics 1993; 13: 1323.

Berrino P, Galli A, Rainero ML. Long-lasting complications with the use of polyurethane-covered breast implants. Br J Plast Surg 1986; 39: 549.

Birdwell RL, Ikeda DM, Jeffrey SS, Jeffrey RB Jr. Preliminary experience with power Doppler imaging of solid breast masses. AJR Am J Roentgenol 1997; 169: 703–7.

Blohmer JU. Mammasonographie—Normale Anatomie. In: Sohn C, Holzgreve W, editors. Ultraschall in Gynäkologie und Geburtshilfe. Stuttgart: Thieme, 1995: 671–718.

Blohmer JU, Guski H. Sonographische Kriterien zur Differentialdiagnose von Mammatumoren. In: Sohn C, Holzgreve W, editors. Ultraschall in Gynäkologie und Geburtshilfe. Stuttgart: Thieme, 1995: 671–718.

Blohmer JU, Lau HU. Erste Erfahrungen mit der Farb-Doppler-Sonographie der Mamma. Gesellschaft für Geburtshilfe und Gynäkologie in Berlin [conference report]. Geburtshilfe Frauenheilkd 1993; 53: 730.

Blohmer JU, Chaoui R, Bollmann R, Lau HU. Die gepulste und farbkodierte Doppler-Mammasonographie: Stellenwert in der Differentialdiagnose von Mammatumoren [abstract]. Abstractband zur 13. Wissenschaftlichen Tagung der Deutschen Gesellschaft für Senologie. Berlin, 1993a.

Blohmer JU, Bollmann R, Chaoui R, Lau HU. Die Beurteilung der Dignität von Mammatumoren mit dem Ultraschall [abstract]. Ultraschall Klin Prax 1993b; 8: 150.

Blohmer JU, Bollmann R, Chaoui R, Lau HU. The assessment of breast vascularity using pulsed wave and colour Doppler sonography. Bildgeb Imaging 1993c; 60 (Suppl 2): 46.

Blohmer JU, Janda J, Guski H, Lau HU. Fibromatose der Mamma. Eine Falldarstellung und Literaturübersicht. Zentralbl Gynäkol 1994a; 116: 52–5.

Blohmer JU, Bollmann R, Chaoui R, Kürten A, Lau HU. Die Mastitis nonpuerperalis in der Realtime- und Farbdoppler-Sonographie. Geburtshilfe Frauenheilkd 1994b; 54: 161–6.

Blohmer JU, Bollmann R, Paepke S, Lau HU. Referenzwerte in der farbkodierten, gepulsten Dopplersonographie der Mamma. Bildgeb Imaging 1994c; 61 (Suppl 2): 30.

Blohmer JU, Bollmann R, Schmalisch A, Chaoui R, Lau HU. Die Differentialdiagnose von Mammatumoren durch den Vergleich der Durchblutung des Tumors mit der kontralateralen Brust mittels farbkodierter, gepulster Dopplersonographie. Geburtshilfe Frauenheilkd 1995a; 55: 1–6.

Blohmer JU, Schmalisch G, Hruby B, Chaoui R, Paepke S, Bollmann R. Sonographische Kriterien in der Differentialdiagnose von Herdbefunden der Mamma. Ultraschall 1995b; 16: 525.

Bostwick J III. Plastic and reconstructive breast surgery. St. Louis, MO: Quality Medical Publishing, 1990: 529–53.

Bouck N. Understanding tumor angiogenesis. Contemp Oncol 1994: 24–9.

Brenner H, Wiebelt H, Ziegler H. Die Entwicklung der Inzidenz und Prognose des Mammakarzinoms bei jungen Frauen vor dem Hintergrund von Veränderungen des Risikofaktorenprofils. Geburtshilfe Frauenheilkd 1990; 50: 683–8.

Britton PD, Coulden RA. The use of Doppler ultrasound in the diagnosis of breast cancer. Clin Radiol 1990; 42: 399–401.

Bronstein AD, Kilcoyne RE, Moe RE. Complications of needle localization. Arch Surg 1988; 123: 775–9.

Burg JP. Maximum entropy spectral analysis. 37th Annual International Meeting, Society of Exploration Geophysicists. Oklahoma City, Oklahoma: Society of Exploration Geophysicists, 1967.

Burns PN, Halliwell M, Wells PN, Webb AJ. Ultrasonic Doppler studies of the breast. Ultrasound Med Biol 1982; 8: 127–43.

Burns PN, Virjee JM, Gowland M, et al. The origin of Doppler shift signals from breast tumors. In: Jellins J, Kobayashi T. Ultrasonics examinations of the breast. New York: Wiley, 1983: 379–84.

Caskey CI, Berg WA, Anderson N, Sheth S, Chang BW, Hamper UM. Breast implant rupture: diagnosis by ultrasonography. Radiology 1994; 190: 819.

Cazzialanza E, Magnani P, Segalini A, Canepari M. New uses of mammary ultrasonography. Aesthet Plast Surg 1994; 18: 189–93.

Chan SC, Birdsell DC, Gradeen, CY. Detection of toluenediamines in the urine of a patient with polyurethane-covered breast implants. Clin Chem 1991; 37: 756.

Ciatto S, Roselli Del Turco M, Bravetti P. Nonpalpable breast lesions: stereotaxic fine-needle aspsiration cytology. Radiology 1989; 173: 57–9.

Ciatto S, Bravetti P, Cecchini S, Grazzini G, Iossa A, Cariaggi P, et al. The role of fine needle aspiration cytology in the differential diagnosis of suspected breast cancer local recurrences. Tamori 1990; 76: 225–6.

Ciatto S, Catania S, Bravetti P, Bonardi R, Carriagi P, Pacifico E. Fine-needle cytology of the breast: a controlled study of aspiration versus nonaspiration. Diagn Cytopathol 1991; 7: 125–7.

Cole-Beuglet C, Goldberg BB, Kurtz AB, Patchepdy AS, Shaber GS, Rubin CS. Clinical experience with a prototype real time dedicated breast scanner. AJR Am J Roentgenol 1982; 139: 903–11.

Cole-Beuglet C, Soriano RT, Kurtz AB, Goldberg BB. Fibroadenoma of the breast: sonomammography correlated with pathology in 122 patients. AJR Am J Roentgenol 1983; 140: 319–75.

Cosgrove D. Doppler competes for breast evaluation role. Diagn Imaging 1992; 8: 40–1.

Cosgrove DO, Bamber JC, Davey JB, Mac Kinna JA, Sinnett HD. Color Doppler signals from breast tumors: work in progress. Radiology 1990; 176: 175–80.

Czarnecki DJ, Berridge DL, Splittgerber GE, Goell WS. Comparison of the anchoring strengths of the Kopans and Hawkins II needle-hook-wire systems. Radiology 1992; 183: 573–4.

Davis PS, Wechsler RJ, Feig SA, March DE. Migration of breast biopsy localisation wire. AJR Am J Roentgenol 1988; 150: 787–8.

DeBruhl ND, Gorczyca DP, Ahn CY, Shaw WW, Bassett LW. Sonographic evaluation of silicone breast implants. Radiology 1993; 189: 95.

deCamera DL, Sheridan JM, Kammer BA. Rupture and aging of silicone breast implants. Paper presented at 1991 meeting of the American Society of Plastic and Reconstructive Surgeons.

Delorme S. Dopplersonographie des Mammakarzinoms. Radiologe 1993; 33: 287–91.

Delorme S, Anton HW, Knopp MV, Betsch B, Trost U, Junkermann I, et al. Vaskularisation des Mammacarcinoms: quantitative und morphologische Beurteilung mittels farbcodierter Sonographie [abstract]. Ultraschall Klin Prax 1991; 6: 219.

Dock W. Duplex sonography of mammary tumors: a prospective study of 75 patients. J Ultrasound Med 1993; 2: 79–82.

Dongen JA van, Fentiman IS, Harris JR, Holland R, Peterse JL, Salvadori B, et al. In-situ breast cancer: the EORTC consensus meeting. Lancet 1989; ii: 25–7.

Dow Corning Corporation. Package insert for Silicone Gel Mammary Implant. Midland, Michigan: Dow Corning/Wright, January 1991: 8.

Dowlatshaki K, Gent HJ, Schmidt R, Jokich PM, Bibbo M, Sprenger E. Nonpalpable breast tumors: diagnosis with stereotaxic localization and fine needle aspiration. Radiology 1989; 170: 427–33.

Duda VE, Rode G, Schlief R.Echocontrast agent enhanced color flow imaging of the breast. Ultrasound Obstet Gynecol 1993; 3: 191–4.

Dussik KT. Über die Möglichkeit hochfrequente mechanische Schwingungen als diagnostisches Hilfsmittel zu verwerten. Z Ges Neurol Psychiatr 1942; 174: 152–68. Cited after Eckel K, editor. Die Entdeckung des ersten bildgebenden Verfahrens der Ultraschalldiagnostik durch K.-Th. Dussik vor 50 Jahren. Ein historischer Rückblick 1942–1992. Ultraschall Klin Prax 1992; 7: 299–305.

Ernst R, Weber A, Liebe, Friemann J. Wert der Sonographie in der präoperativen Diagnostik des multizentrischen multifokalen Mammakarzinoms. In: Hansmann M, editor. Ultraschalldiagnostik 86. Berlin: Springer, 1986.

Ernst R, Weber A, Bauer KH, Friemann J, Zumtobel V. Perioperative Ultraschalluntersuchung der Brustdrüse beim Mammakarzinom. Zentralbl Chir 1990; 115: 963–75.

Everson LI, Parantainen H, Detlie T, Stillman AE, Olson PN, Landis G, et al. Diagnosis of breast implant rupture: imaging findings and relative efficacies of imaging techniques. AJR Am J Roentgenol 1994; 163: 57.

Feldmann HU, Schindler JE. Die "Wechseljahre" der Frau: Der Niedergang der Ovarien vollzieht sich häufig über mehr als ein Jahrzehnt. Gyne 1995; 3: 1–5.

Finlay ME, Liston JE, Lunt LG, Young JR. Assessment of the role of ultrasound in the differentiation of radial scars and stellate carcinomas of the breast. Clin Radiol 1994; 49: 52–5.

Finsterer H, Prechtel K. Mammazytologie. Möglichkeiten und Grenzen. Beitr Onkol 1990; 38: 93–105.

Fleischer AC, Jones HW III. Early detection of ovarian carcinoma with transvaginal sonography. New York: Raven Press, 1993.

Folkman J. Tumor angiogenesis: therapeutic implications. N Engl J Med 1971; 285: 1182.

Folkman J. How is blood vessel growth regulated in normal and neoplastic tissue? Cancer Res 1986; 46: 467–73.

Folkman J. The role of angiogenesis in tumor growth. Semin Cancer Biol 1992; 3: 65–71.

Folkman J, Klagsbrun M. Angiogenic factors. Science 1987; 235: 442–7.

Fornage BD. Ultrasound of the breast. Ultrasound Quart 1993; 11: 1–39.

Fornage BD, Morel M, Toubas O. Accuracy of sonography in the size of determination of breast carcinoma. Radiology 1987; 165: 36.

Fornage BD, Lorigan JG, Andry E. Fibroadenoma of the breast: sonographic appearance. Radiology 1989; 172: 671–5.

Fornage BD, Sneige N, Faroux MJ, Andry E. Sonographic appearance and ultrasound-guided fine-needle aspiration biopsy of breast carcinomas smaller than 1 cm^3. J Ultrasound Med 1990; 10: 559–68.

Fornage BD, Coan JD, David SL. Ultrasound-guided needle biopsy of the breast and other interventional procedures. Radiol Clin North Am 1992; 30: 167–85.

Fornage BD, Sneige N, Singletary SE. Masses in breasts with implants: diagnosis with US-guided fine-needle aspiration biopsy. Radiology 1994a; 191: 339–42.

Fornage BD, Ross MI, Singletary SE, Paulus DD. Localization of impalpable breast masses: value of sonography in the operating room and scanning of excised specimens. AJR Am J Roentgenol 1994b; 163: 569–73.

Forouhi P, Walsh JS, Anderson TJ, Chetty U. Ultrasonography as a method of measuring breast tumour size and monitoring response to primary systemic treatment. Br J Surg 1994; 81: 223–5.

Fournier D von, Anton HW, Junkermann H, Bastert G, van Kaick G. Brustkrebsscreening. Radiologe 1993; 33: 227–35.

Frischbier HJ. Beitrag zur kontroversen Einschätzung des Mammographie-Screenings bei asymptomatischen Frauen zwischen dem 40. und 50. Lebensjahr. Geburtshilfe Frauenheilkd 1994; 54: 1–11.

Gerlach B, Holzgreve W. Mammasonographie: Erfahrungen, Entwicklungen und Ergebnisse im Stufe-III-Zentrum der UFK Münster (1987–1992). Ikon 1993; 3: 1–24.

Gorczyca DP, Sinha S, Ahn CY, DeBruhl ND, Hates MK, Gausche VR, et al. Silicone breast implants in vivo: MR imaging. Radiology 1992; 185: 407.

Gorczyca DP, DeBruhl ND, Ahn CY, Hoyt A, Sayre JW, Nudell P, et al. Silicone breast implant ruptures in an animal model: comparison of mammography, MR imaging, US and CT. Radiology 1994; 190: 227.

Hachiya J, Seki T, Okada M, Nitatori T, Korenaga T, Furuya Y. MR imaging of the breast with Gd-DTPA enhancement: comparison with mammography and ultrasonography. Radiat Med 1991; 9: 232–40.

Hackelöer BJ, Duda V, Lauth G. Ultraschall-Mammographie. Berlin: Springer, 1986.

Hardy JR, Powles TJ, Judson I, Heron C, Williams M, Cherryman G, et al. How many tests are required in the diagnosis of palpable breast abnormalities? Clin Oncol 1990; 2: 148–52.

Harlow CL, Schackmuth EM, Bregman RS, Zeligman BE, Coffin CT. Sonographic detection of hematomas and fluid after imaging guided core breast biopsy. J Ultrasound Med 1994; 13: 877–82.

Harper P. Ultrasound mammography. Baltimore: University Park Press, 1985.

Harris KM, Gannott MA, Shestak K, Losken HW, Tobon H. Silicone implant rupture: detection with US. Radiology 1993; 187:761.

Harter LP, Curtis JS, Ponto G, Craig PH. Malignant seeding of the needle track during stereotaxic core needle breast biopsy. Radiology 1992; 185: 713–4.

Hayes R, Michel M, Nunnerley HB. Acute inflammation of the breast: the role of breast ultrasound in diagnosis and management. Clin Radiol 1991; 44: 253–6.

Heilenkötter U, Jagella P. Farbdopplersonographie exstirpationsbedürftiger Mammatumoren – Darstellung einer Untersuchungsmethode. Geburtshilfe Frauenheilkd 1993; 53: 247–52.

Hergan K, Amann T, Oser W. Sonoanatomie der Axilla. Ultraschall Med 1991; 12: 236–43.

Hermanek P, Scheibe O, Spiessl B, Wagner G. UICC: TNM-Klassifikation maligner Turnoren, 2. Revision. Berlin: Springer, 1992.

Heywang SH, Wolf A, Pruss E, Hilberta T, Eiermann W, Permanetter W. MRI of the breast: use and limitations. Radiology 1989; 171: 95–103.

Heywang-Köbrunner SH. Nonmammographic breast imaging techniques. Curr Opin Radiol 1992; 4: 146–54.

Holland R, Hendricks JHCL, Nravunac M. Mammographically occult breast cancer: a pathologic and radiologic study. Cancer 1983; 52: 1810–9.

Holland R, Veling SHJ, Mravunac M, Hendriks JHCL. Histologic multifocality of Tis, T1–2 breast carcinomas: implications for clinical trials of breast-conserving surgery. Cancer 1985; 56: 979–90.

Homer MJ. Transection of the localization hooked wire during breast biopsy. AJR Am J Roentgenol 1983; 141: 929–30.

Homer MJ. Localization of nonpalpable breast lesions with the curved-end, retractable wire: leaving the needle in vivo. AJR Am J Roentgenol 1988; 151: 919–20.

Horak ER, Leek R, Klenk N, et al. Angiogenesis, assessed by platelet/endothelial cell adhesion molecule antibodies, as indicator of node metastasis and survival in breast cancer. Lancet 1992; 340: 1120.

Huber S, Delorme S, Knopp MV, Junkermann H, Zuna I, von Fournier D, van Kaick G. Computer-assisted quantitative assessment of color Doppler sonography in the evaluation of breast tumors. Bildgeb Imaging 1993; 60 (Suppl 2): 18.

Ishii M. Ultrasonographic diagnosis of breast disease: a review of diagnostic criteria of sonomammography on real-time scanner [in Japanese]. Nippon Igaku Hoshasen Gakkai Zasshi 1993; 53: 1141–59.

Jackson VP. The role of US in breast imaging. Radiology 1990; 177: 305–11.

Jackson VP. The current role of US in breast imaging. Radiol Clin North Am 1995; 33: 1161–70.

Jackson VP, Kelly-Fry E, Rothschild PA, Holden RW, Clarke SA. Automated breast onography using a 7.5 MHz PVDR transducer: preliminary clinical evaluation. Radiology 1986; 159: 679–84.

Jackson VP, Reynolds HE, Hawes DR. Sonography of the breast. Seminars Ultrasound CT MR 1996; 17: 460–75.

Jellins J. Combining imaging and vascularity assessment of breast lasions. Ultrasound Med Biol 1988; 14: 121–30.

Jellins J, Kossoff G, Reeve TS, Barraclough BH. Ultrasonic grey scale visualization of breast disease. Ultrasound Med Biol 1975; 1: 393–404.

Jonat W. Aktuelle Aspekte in der Diagnostik des Mammakarzinoms. Stuttgart: Enke, 1989.

Junkerman H, Anton HW, Krapfl E, Harcos A, von Fournier D. Abklärung von Mammaläsionen durch Stanz-, Drill- und Feinnadelbiopsie. Radiologe 1993; 33: 267–70.

Kaiser WA, Diedrich K, Reiser M, Krebs D. Moderne Diagnostik der Mamma. Geburtshilfe Frauenheilkd 1993; 53: 1–14.

Kaplan SS, Racenstein MJ, Wong WS, Hansen GC, McCombs MM, Bassett LW. US-guided core biopsy of the breast with a coaxial system. Radiology 1995; 194: 573–5.

Karstrup S, Solving J, Nolsoe CP, Nilsson P, Khattar S, Loren I, et al. Acute puerperal breast abscesses: US-guided drainage. Radiology 1993; 188: 807–9.

Kassenärztliche Bundesvereinigung: Qualifikationsvoraussetzungen gemäss § 135 Abs. 2 SGB V zur Durchführung von Untersuchungen in der Ultraschalldiagnostik (Ultraschall-Vereinbarung). Dtsch Arztebl 1993; 90B: 390–403.

Kaufmann M, von Minckwitz G, Finn HP, Schmid H, Goerttler K, Gastert G. Combination of grading and new biological factors (S-phase fraction and epidermal growth factor receptor) can predict relapse and survival in patients with node-negative primary breast cancer. Onkologie 1994; 17: 166–72.

Kedar RP, Cosgrove DO, Smith IE, Mansi JL, Bamber JC. Breast carcinoma: measurement of tumor response to primary medical therapy with color Doppler flow imaging. Radiology 1994; 190: 825–30.

Kelly-Frey E. Influences on the development of ultrasound pulse-echo breast instrumentation in the United States. In: Harper, P, editor. Ultrasound mammography. Baltimore: University Park Press, 1985.

Kessler DA. The basis of the FDA's decision on breast implants. N Engl J Med 1992; 326: 1713.

Kindermann G, Genz T. Treatment of primary breast cancer. In: Burghardt E, editor. Surgical gynecologic oncology. Stuttgart: Thieme, 1993.

Kindermann G, Willgeroth E. Detection of breast cancer. In: Burghardt E, editor. Surgical gynecologic oncology. Stuttgart: Thieme, 1993.

Konishi YK. Clinical application of color Doppler imaging to the diagnosis of breast disease. Toshiba Med Rev 1992; 42: 12–27.

Kopans D, Meyer J, Sadowsky N. Breast imaging. N Engl J Med 1984; 310: 960–6.

Kopans DB, Meyer JE, Linfors KK. Whole-breast US imaging: four-year follow-up. Radiology 1985; 157: 505–7.

Krampla W, Mosser H, Hruby W. Integration of ultrasound in a fully digital radiology department. Invest Radiol 1994; 29: 733–76.

Kratchowil A, Kaiser P. Die Darstellung der Erkrankungen der weiblichen Brust im Ultraschallschnittbildverfahren. In: Bock J, Ossoing K, editors. Ultrasono Graphia Medica, Vol. 111. Vienna: Verlag der Wiener Medizinischen Akademie, 1969.

Kremkau EW. Instrumentation. Diagn Imaging 1993; 2: 11–6.

Kubek KA, Chan L, Frazier TG. Color Doppler flow as an indicator of nodal metastasis in solid breast masses. J Ultrasound Med 1996; 15: 835–41.

Kurjak A, Salihagic A, Kupesic-Urek S. Clinical value of assessment of gynaecological tumour angiogenesis by transvaginal colour Doppler. Ann Med 1992; 24: 97–102.

Kwasnik EM, Sadowsky NL, Vollmann RW. An improved system for surgical excision of needle-localized nonpalpable breast lesions. Am J Surg 1987; 154: 476–67.

Löfgren M, Andersson I, Bondeson L, Lindholm K. X-ray guided fine-needle aspiration for the cytologic diagnosis of nonpalpable breast lesions. Cancer 1988; 61: 1032–7.

Lee SK, Lee T, Lee KR, Su UG, Liu RJ. Evaluation of breast tumors with color Doppler imaging: a comparison with image-directed Doppler ultrasound. J Clin Ultrasound 1995; 23: 367–73.

Leonard C, Harlow CL, Coffin C, Drose J, Norton L, Kinzie J. Use of ultrasound to guide radiation boost planning following lumpectomy for carcinoma of the breast. Int J Radiat Oncol Biol Phys 1993; 27: 1193–7.

Leucht W. Teaching atlas of breast ultrasound. Stuttgart: Thieme, 1992.

Liberman L, Giess CS, Dershaw DD, Louie DC, Deutch BM. Non-Hodgkin lymphoma of the breast: imaging characteristics and correlation with histopathologic findings. Radiology 1994a; 192: 157–60.

Liberman L, Dershaw DD, Rosen RP, Abramson AF, Deutsch BM, Hann LE. Stereotaxic 14-gauge breast biopsy: how many core biopsy specimens are needed? Radiology 1994b; 192: 793–5.

Liston JC, Malata CM, Varma S, Scott M, Sharpe DT. The role of ultrasound imaging in the diagnosis of breast implant rupture: a prospective study. Br J Plast Surg 1994; 47: 477–82.

Ljung BM. Fine-needle aspiration of the breast. In: Wied GL, Keebler CM, Koss LG, Patten SE, Rosenthal DL, editors. Compendium on diagnostic cytology. Chicago: Tutorials of Cytology, 1992.

Madjar H, Schillinger H. Einführung in die Doppleranalyse zur Mammadiagnostik. In: Hansmann M, editor. Ultraschalldiagnostik. Berlin: Springer, 1986.

Madjar H, Jellins J, Schillinger H, Hillemanns HG. Differenzierung von Mammakarzinomen durch CW-Doppler-Ultraschall. Ultraschall Med 1986; 7: 183–4.

Madjar H, Giese E, Schillinger H. Durchblutungsmessungen an Mammatumoren. Vergleich mit Prognosefaktoren. Arch Gynecol Obstet 1989a; 245: 697.

Madjar H, Sauerbrei W, Schillinger H. Aktueller Stand der Dopplertechniken. In: Gebhardt J, et al., editors. Ultraschalldiagnostik 89. Berlin: Springer, 1989b.

Madjar H, Sauerbrei W, Münch S, Prömpeler H, Schillinger H. Methodenanalyse zur Doppleruntersuchung der weiblichen Brust. Ultraschall 1989c; 10: 196–201.

Madjar H, Münch S, Sauerbrei W, et al. Differenzierte Mammadiagnostik durch CW-Doppler-Ultraschall. Radiologe 1990a; 30: 193.

Madjar H, Sauerbrei W, Münch S, Prömpeler H, Schillinger H. Methodenanalyse zur Doppleruntersuchung der weiblichen Brust. Ultraschall Med 1990b; 4: 196–201.

Madjar H, Prömpeler H, Wilhelm CH. Doppler zur Diagnostik und Therapie von Brusterkrankungen [abstract]. Ultraschall Klin Prax 1991a; 6: 220.

Madjar H, Sauerbrei W, Münch S, Schillinger H. Continuous-wave and pulsed Doppler studies of the breast: clinical results and effect of transducer frequency. Ultrasound Med Biol 1991b; 17: 31–9.

Madjar H, Sauerbrei W, Rachowska A, Pfleiderer A. Vergleich von hochauflösender Sonographie und Mammographie. Ultraschall Klin Prax 1991c; 6: 290–7.

Madjar H, Prömpeler H, Kornmoss E, Göppinger A. Ergänzt der Farbdoppler die Mammadiagnostik? Radiologe 1992a; 32: 568–75.

Madjar H, Vetter M, Prömpeler HJ, Wieacker R, Schillinger H. Untersuchungen zur normalen Vaskularisation der weiblichen Brust durch Doppler-Ultraschall. Ultraschall Med 1992b; 13: 171–7.

Madjar H, Ladner HA, Sauerbrei W, Oberstein A, Prömpeler H, A. Pfleiderer: Preoperative staging of breast cancer by palpation, mammography and high-resolution ultrasound. Ultrasound Obstet Gynecol 1993a; 3: 185–90.

Madjar H, Prömpeler H, Schürmann R, Göppinger A, Breckwoldt M, Pfleiderer A. Verbesserung der Durchblutungsdiagoostik von Brusttumoren durch Echokontrastmittel. Geburtshilfe Frauenheilkd 1993b; 53: 866–9.

Madjar H, Vetter M, Prömpeler H, Breckwoldt M, Pfleiderer A. Doppler measurement of breast vascularity in women under pharmacologic treatment of benign breast disease. J Reprod Med 1993c; 38: 935–40.

Madjar H, Makowiec U, Mundinger A, Du-Bois A, Kommoss E, Schillinger H. Einsatz der hochauflösenden Sonographie zur Brustkrebsvorsorge. Ultraschall Med 1994a; 15: 20–3.

Madjar H, Prömpeler H, Wolfahrt R, Bauknecht T, Pfleiderer A. Farbdopplerflussdaten von Mammatumoren. Ultraschall Med 1994b; 15: 69–76.

Marquet KL, Funk A, Fendel H, Handt S. Der echodichte Randsaum und hyperreflexive Ausläufer: Sensible Kriterien maligner Prozesse in der Mammasonographie. Geburtshilfe Frauenheilkd 1993; 53: 20–3.

Matsuo S, Eto T, Soejima H, Ohara O, Hidaka O, Miyazaki J, Tsunoda T, Kanematsu T. A case of intracystic carcinoma of the breast: the importance of measuring carcinoembryonic antigen in aspirated cystic fluid. Breast Cancer Res Treat 1993; 28: 41–4.

Mendelson EB. Breast imaging. Diagn Imaging 1993; 3: 53–5.

Mendelson EB. Breast ultrasound 1994. In: Leopold GR, editor. 1994 AIUM syllabus for categorical course on women's imaging. Rockville, MD: American Institute of Ultrasound in Medicine, 1994: 83–8.

Michelow BJ, Hartrampf CR Jr, Bennett GK. TRAM flap safety optimized with intraoperative Doppler. Plast Reconstr Surg 1990; 86: 143–6.

Minasian H, Bamber JC. A preliminary assessment of an ultrasonic Doppler method for the study of blood flow in human breast cancer. Ultrasound Med Biol 1982; 8: 357–64.

Moriggl B, Steinlechner M. Ultrasonoanatomy for evaluation of the local lymphatic groups of the mamma. Surg Radiol Anat 1994; 16: 77–85.

Mosny DS, Nitz U. Behandlungsfehler in der Brustchirurgie aus forensischer Sicht. Gynäkologe 1994; 27: 249–55.

Nishimura S, Matsusue S, Koizumi S, Kashihara S. Architectural distortion of subcutaneous fascial layer in breast tumors: ultrasonographic evaluation. Ultrasound Med Biol 1992; 18: 815–20.

Nyirjesy I, Billingsley ES. Management of breast problems in gynecologic office practice using sonography and fine-needle aspiration. Obstet Gynecol 1992; 79: 699–702.

Pahnke VG, Kitschke HJ, Bernauer M, Koll R. Mastitis nonpuerperalis—eine Erkrankung mit zunehmender klinischer Relevanz? Geburtshilfe Frauenheilkd 1985; 45: 29–35.

Pamilo M, Soiva M, Lavast EM. Real-time ultrasound, axillary mammography, and clinical examination in the detection of axillary lymph node metastasis in breast cancer patients. J Ultrasound Med 1989; 8: 115–20.

Parker SH. Percutaneous large core breast biopsy. Cancer 1994; 74 (Suppl 1): 256–62.

Parker SH, Burbank F. A practical approach to minimally invasive breast biopsy. Radiology 1996; 200: 11–20.

Parker SH, Lovin JD, Jogbe WI, Burke BJ, Hopper KD, Yakes WF. Nonpalpable breast lesions: stereotactic automated large-core biopsies. Radiology 1991; 180: 403–7.

Parker SH, Jobe WE, Dennis MA, Stavros AT, Johnson KK, Yakes WE, et al. US-guided automated large-core breast biopsy. Radiology 1993; 187: 507–11.

Parker SH, Burbank F, Jackman RJ, Aucreman CJ, Cardenosa G, Cink TM, et al. Percutaneous large-core breast biopsy: a multi-institutional study. Radiology 1994; 193: 359–64.

Parker SH, Stavros AT, Dennis MA. Needle biopsy techniques. Radiol Clin North Am 1995a; 33: 1171–86.

Parker SH, Dennis MA, Stavros AT. Critical pathways in percutaneous breast intervention. Radiographics 1995b; 15: 946–50.

Patel MD, Callen PW, Mar YB, Filly RA, Goldenstein RB, Feldstein VA. Evaluation of a sonographic PACS in clinical practice: analysis of technical and analytical time savings. J Ultrasound Med 1996; 15: 755–62.

Peters-Engl C, Medl M, Leodolter S. The use of colour-coded and spectral Doppler ultrasound in the differentiation of benign and malignant breast lesion. Br J Cancer 1995; 71: 137–9.

Plate KH. Angiogenese und Anti-Angiogenese. Dtsch Ärztebl 1993; 90A: 2987–95.

Pohlmann R, Richter R, Parow E. Über die Ausbreitung und Absorption des Ultraschalls im menschlichen Gewebe und seine therapeutische Wirkung am Ischias und Plexusneuralgie. Dtsch Klin Wochenschr 1939; 7: 251–4.

Potterton AJ, Peakman DJ, Young JR. Ultrasound demonstration of small breast cancers detected by mammographic screening. Clin Radiol 1994; 49: 808–13.

Röder HU, Schäfer L, Schmidt B, Walter E. Übereinstimmung von mammographischer und pathologisch-anatomischer Tumorausdehnung beim Mammakarzinom. Röfo Fortschr Geb Röntgenstr Neuen Bildgeb Verfahr 1991; 154: 321–5.

Radmann D, Heinrich J. Sonographische Diagnostik des Mammakarzinoms. Gynäkol Prax 1993; 17: 675–84.

Rauskolb R. Ultraschalluntersuchungen im Rahmen der Pränataldiagnostik aus forensischer Sicht. Gynäkologe 1994; 27: 191–6.

Raza S, Baum JK. Solid breast lesions: evaluation of Power Dopper US. Radiology 1997; 203: 164–8.

Richter K. Technique for detecting and evaluating breast lesions. J Ultrasound Med 1994; 13: 797–802.

Rosculet KA, Ikeda DM, Forrest ME, Oneal RM, Rubin JM, Jeffries DO, et al. Ruptured gel-filled silicone breast implants: sonographic findings in 19 cases. AJR Am J Roentgenol 1992; 159: 711.

Rosen PP, Fracchia AA, Urban JA, Schottenfeld D, Robbins GE. Residual mammary carcinoma following simulated partial mastectomy. Cancer 1975; 35: 739–47.

Rubin JM, Helvie MA, Adler RS. US appearance of ruptured silicone breast implants [letter]. Radiology 1994a; 190: 583.

Rubin, JM, Cude RO, Carson PL, Bree RL, Adler RS. Power Doppler US: a potentially useful alternative to mean frequency-based color Doppler US. Radiology 1994b; 190: 853–6.

Salomon A. Beiträge zur Pathologie und Klinik der Mammakarzinome. Arch Klin Chir 1913; 103: 573–8.

Scatarige JC, Hamper UM, Sheth S, Allen HA III. Parasternal sonography of the internal mammary vessels: technique, normal anatomy and adenopathy. Radiology 1989; 172: 453–7.

Schepps B, Scola FH, Frates RE. Benign circumscribed breast masses: mammographic and sonographic appearance. Obstet Gynecol Clin North Am 1994; 21: 519–37.

Schild R, Fendel H. Die dopplersonographische Differenzierung von benignen und malignen Mammatumoren. Geburtshilfe Frauenheilkd 1991; 51: 696–702.

Schild R, Schroers B, Funk A, Buro K. Dopplersonographische Untersuchungen von Mammatumoren in CW-Technik. Zentralbl Gynäkol 1993; 115: 483–7.

Schön G, Strasser K, Dünser M, Buchberger W, Margreiter R. Riesiges Cystosarcoma phylloides. Mammographische und sonographische Befunde eines aussergewöhnlichen Falles. Akt Radiol 1994; 4: 41–3.

Schwartz GE, Goldberg BB, Rifkin MD, D'Orazio SE. Ultrasonography: an alternative to x-ray-guided needle localization of nonpalpable breast masses. Surgery 1988; 104: 870–3.

Shapiro S, Strax PH, Venet L. Periodic breast cancer screening in reducing mortality from breast cancer. JAMA J Am Med Assoc 1971; 215: 1777–85.

Sickles EA, Filly RA, Callen PW. Breast cancer detection with sonography and mammography: comparison using state-of-the-art equipment. AJR Am J Roentgenol 1983; 140: 843–5.

Sickles EA, Fily RA, Callan PW. Benign breast lesions: ultrasound detection and diagnosis. Radiology 1984; 151: 467–86.

Silverstein MJ, Poller DN, Waisman JR, Colburn WJ, Barth A, Gierson ED, et al. Prognostic classification of breast ductal carcinoma in situ. Lancet 1995; 345: 1154–7.

Sohn C, Bastert G. Die dreidimensionale Ultraschalldiagnostik. Berlin: Springer, 1994.

Sohn C, Holzgreve W. Ultraschall in Gynäkologie und Geburtshilfe. Stuttgart: Thieme, 1995.

Sohn C, Meyberg G. Erste Erfahrungen mit einer neuen Farbtechnik: Die Ultraschall-Angiographie. Zentralbl Gynäkol 1995; 117: 90–6.

Sohn C, Stolz W. Dopplersonographische Durchblutungsmessung von Brusttumoren [abstract]. Ultraschall Klin Prax 1991; 6: 219.

Sohn C, Grotepass J, Schneider W, Sohn G, Funk A, Jensch P, et al. Dreidimensionale Darstellung in der Ultraschalldiagnostik. Erste Ergebnisse. Dtsch Med Wochenschr 1988; 113: 1743–7.

Sohn C, Grischke EM, Wallwiener D, Kaufmann M, von Fournier D, Bastert G. Die sonographische Durchblutungsdiagnostik gut- und bösartiger Brusttumoren. Geburtshilfe Frauenheilkd 1992a; 52: 397–403.

Sohn C, Stolz W, Grischke EM, Wallwiener D, Bastert G, von Fournier D. Die dopplersonographische Untersuchung von Mammatumoren mit Hilfe der Farbdopplersonographie, der Duplexsonographie und des CW-Doppler. Zentrabl Gynäkol 1992b; 114: 249–53.

Sohn C, Stolz W, Kaufmann M, Bastert G. Die dreidimensionale Ultraschalldarstellung benigner und maligner Brusttumoren–erste klinische Erfahrungen. Geburtshilfe Frauenheilkd 1992c; 52: 520–5.

Sohn C, Grischke EM, Schild R. Dopplersonographie in der Gynäkologie--Durchblutungsdiagnostik von Tumoren. In: Sohn C, Stolz W, Bastert G, editors. Dopplersonographie in der Gynäkologie und Geburtshilfe. Stuttgart: Thieme, 1993a.

Sohn C, Grischke EM, Stolz W, Bastert G. Untersuchungen zum Zusammenhang zwischen dem Grad der Durchblutung und dem biologischen Verhalten von Mammatumoren. Ultraschall Klin Prax 1993b; 8: 11–4.

Soo MS, Willigford ME, Walsh R, Bentley RC, Kornguth PJ. Papillary carcinoma of the breast: imaging findings. Am J Roentgenol 1995; 164: 321–6.

Stavros AT, Dennis MA. The ultrasound of breast pathology. In: Parker SH, Jobe WE, editors. Percutaneous breast biopsy. New York: Raven Press, 1993: 111–27.

Stavros AT, Thickman D, Rapp CL, Dennis MA, Parker SH, Sisney GA. Solid breast nodules: use of sonography to distinguish between benign and malignant lesions. Radiology 1995; 196: 123–34.

Stomper PC, Davis SP, Sonnenfeld MR, Meyer JE, Greenes RA, Eberlein TJ. Efficacy of specimen radiography of clinically occult non-calcified breast lesions. AJR Am J Roentgenol 1988; 151: 43–7.

Svane G, Potchen EJ, Sierra A, Azavedo E. Screening mammography: breast cancer diagnosis in asymptomatic women. St. Louis: Mosby, 1993.

Teboul M. A new concept in breast investigation: echo-histological acinoductal analysis or analytic echography. Biomed Pharmacother 1988; 42: 289–96.

Teubner J, Müller A, van Kaick G. Echomorphologie der Brustdrüse. Vergleichende sonographische, radiologische, anatomische und histologische Untersuchungen von Mammapräparaten. Radiologe 1983; 23: 97–107.

Teubner J, van Kaick G, Junkermann H. 5-MHz Realtime-Sonographie der Brustdrüse. Teil 1: Gerätetechnische Untersuchungen. Radiologe 1985a; 25: 449–56.

Teubner J, van Kaick G, Junkermann H, Pickenhan L, Wesch H, Eggert-Kruse W, et al. 5-MHz Realtime-Sonographie der Brustdrüse. Teil 2: Untersuchungstechnik und diagnostische Wertigkeit. Radiologe 1985b; 25: 457–67.

Teubner J, Bohrer M, van Kaick G, Georgi M. Echomorphologie des Marnmakarzinoms. Radiologe 1993; 33: 277–86.

Tulusan AH. Pathology. In: Burghardt E, editor. Surgical gynecologic oncology. Stuttgart: Thieme, 1993.

Tulusan AH, Reitzenstein M, Ronay G, Schmidt C, Adam R, Lang N: Pathologic-anatomical aspects of breast cancer, with therapeutic considerations. In: Bohmert HH, Leis HP, Jackson IT, editors. Breast cancer: conservative and reconstructive surgery. Stuttgart: Thieme, 1989: 35–8.

Urrutia EJ, Hawkins MC, Steinbach BG, Meacham MA, Bland KI, Copeland EM, et al. Retractable-barb needle for breast lesion localization: use in 60 cases. Radiology 1988; 169: 845–7.

Venta LA, Dudiak CM, Salomon CG, Flisak ME. Sonographic evaluation of the breast. Radiographics 1994; 14: 29–50.

Walsh JS, Dixon JM, Chetty U, Patterson D. Colour Doppler studies of axillary node metastases in breast carcinoma. Clin Radiol 1994; 49: 189–91.

Weidner N, Semple JP, Welch WR, Folkman E. Tumor angiogenesis and metastasis: correlation in invasive breast carcinoma. N Engl J Med 1991; 324: 1–8.

Wild JJ, Reid JM. Further pilot echographic studies on the histologic structure of turnours of the living intact breast. Am J Pathol 1952; 28: 839–54.

Woolt B. On estimating the relation between blood group and disease. Ann Hum Genet 1955; 19: 251–3.

Index

Note: page numbers in *italics* refer to figures and tables

D

E

N

O

P

Q

R

S

T